Second Edition

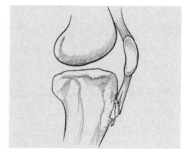

Primary
Orthopedic
Care

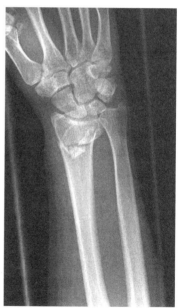

Christy L. Crowther, RN, MS, CRNP
Chesapeake Orthopaedic and Sports Medicine Center
Glen Burnie, Maryland
Clinical Instructor, Department of Family Medicine
University of Maryland School of Medicine
Baltimore, Maryland

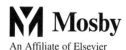 Mosby
An Affiliate of Elsevier

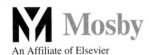

An Affiliate of Elsevier

11830 Westline Industrial Drive
St. Louis, Missouri 63146

PRIMARY ORTHOPEDIC CARE, 2nd edition   0-323-02365-7
Copyright © 2004, Mosby, Inc. All rights reserved.

No part of this publication may be reproduced or transmitted in any form or by any means, electronic or mechanical, including photocopying, recording, or any information storage and retrieval system, without permission in writing from the publisher. Permissions may be sought directly from Elsevier's Health Sciences Rights Department in Philadelphia, PA, USA: phone: (+1) 215 238 7869, fax: (+1) 215 238 2239, e-mail: healthpermissions@elsevier.com. You may also complete your request on-line via the Elsevier Science homepage (http://www.elsevier.com), by selecting 'Customer Support' and then 'Obtaining Permissions'.

Previous edition copyrighted 1999
International Standard Book Number 0-323-02365-7

Executive Publisher: Barbara Nelson Cullen
Acquisitions Editor: Sandra Clark Brown
Developmental Editor: Adrienne Simon
Publishing Services Manager: Deborah Vogel
Project Manager: Mary Drone

Printed in the United States
Last digit is the print number: 9   8   7   6   5   4   3   2   1

In memory of K.B.C.

Primary

Orthopedic

Care

Contributor

Ray Pensy, MD
Chief Resident, Orthopedic Surgery
University of Maryland Department of Orthopedics
Baltimore, Maryland

Chapter 4: *Wrist and Hand*

Reviewers

Judith L. Barron, BS, MS
Registered Nurse- Nurse Inspector
Long Beach Unified School District
Long Beach, California

Jean E. Lee, MSN, FNP-BC, ANP-C
Primary Care Nurse Practitioner
Department of Veteran Affairs
Kansas City, Missouri

Dorothy B. Liddel, MSN, RN, ONC
Retired Associate Professor
Columbia Union College
Takoma Park, Maryland

Musculoskeletal complaints continue to comprise a large percentage of visits to primary care providers. A basic knowledge and understanding of relevant anatomy, commonly encountered conditions, and appropriate initial treatment are important to provide quality patient care. Hopefully this edition has clarified and expanded the earlier text.

The intent of this book is to be a basic, user-friendly clinical resource for primary care nurse practitioners, physicians, and physician assistants. If a greater depth of anatomy, pathology, and treatment is required, the reader should put this book down and read something else. There are many excellent (and more expensive) works on the market that provide definitive treatment and care for orthopedic problems.

I would like to express my thanks to Ray Pensy, M.D., for his expertise and outstanding contribution to revising and updating Chapter 4. His work, contributed during his immensely busy schedule, is a wonderful addition to this book.

Adrienne Simon, my developmental editor at Mosby, has been a constant source of patience and encouragement, both of which I greatly appreciate. Thanks again to the third-year family practice residents at The University of Maryland School of Medicine who unfailingly encourage me to try and stay current. Most of all, I hope that you, the reader, find this book helpful in your daily practice.

Christy L. Crowther, RN, MS, CRNP

Contents

CHAPTER 3

CHAPTER 4

CHAPTER 5

CHAPTER 6

CHAPTER 7

Chapter 1

Cervical Spine

ANATOMY

Bony Structures

The cervical spine consists of seven vertebrae, which comprise a "firm but flexible" shaft. Stability of the neck is sacrificed for mobility. Anatomy is frequently divided into the "upper" cervical spine, consisting of the first and second cervical vertebrae (C1-C2), and the "lower" cervical spine, which is made up of the third through seventh vertebrae (C3-C7).

Compared with the vertebrae of the thoracic and lumbar spine, the cervical vertebrae bear the least amount of weight and are relatively smaller and thinner. The lateral diameter of the cervical vertebrae is greater across than its anteroposterior (AP) diameter. The first and second vertebrae form a unique articulation. C1, also known as the *atlas*, is a bony ring from which two lateral masses extend and articulate with the two occipital condyles of the skull. C2, also known as the axis, provides a weight-bearing surface on which C1 rotates. The axis has a distinctive, vertically projecting process called the *odontoid*. The primary function of the odontoid process is to protect against horizontal displacement of C1. When palpating down from the posterior occiput, the first palpable posterior spinous process is C2, since C1 has only a rudimentary process (Figures 1-1 through 1-4).

Approximately one-half of the rotation of the neck occurs at C1 and C2. This unique articulation also allows for approximately 25% of normal cervical extension but

very little flexion. Range of motion (ROM) at this articulation is limited by the suboccipital muscles. Rotation of the cervical spine greater than 45 to 50 degrees can impede blood flow in the vertebral arteries and lead to vertigo, nausea, tinnitus, or, in at-risk patients, even stroke.

Each vertebra bears the weight of those above it (Figure 1-5). Most of the weight is borne by the vertebral body. Each vertebra articulates with the inferior and superior facet joints of the adjoining vertebrae, but the facet joints themselves support very little weight. These facet articulations are classified as *synovial joints*; as such, they have a synovial capsule around them. The primary movement of the facet joint is gliding. Relative laxity of the synovial joint capsule allows for both flexion and extension. The greatest amount of flexion and extension in the cervical spine occurs at C5 and C6; as a result, this is the most common location of degenerative changes in the cervical spine. The adjacent vertebrae, C4-C5 and C6-C7, allow considerable flexion and extension but to a lesser degree than C5-C6. At C7, mobility markedly decreases as the cervical spine meets with the much more inflexible thoracic spine.

The vertebral foramina in the cervical spine are fairly large to allow passage of the spinal cord. Anteriorly the foramina are surrounded by the vertebral body; anterolaterally the pedicles encompass the spinal opening. Just lateral to the anterior portion of the vertebral body are the transverse processes. Each process contains an opening through which the vertebral arteries and nerves pass

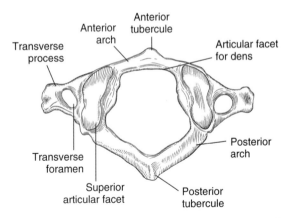

Figure 1-1   The superior view of C1, also known as the atlas. The articular facets meet with the occipital condyles of the skull. Note the articular facet for the dens.

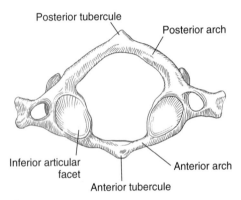

Figure 1-2   The inferior portion of C1 articulates with the superior facets of C2.

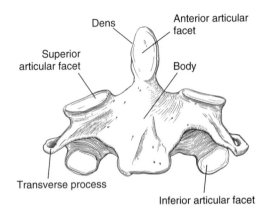

Figure 1-3   C2, or the Axis. The odontoid process (or peg) is situated on the anterior portion of the bone.

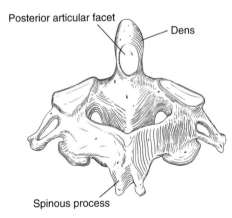

Figure 1-4   The first posterior spinous process of the cervical spine is at C2.

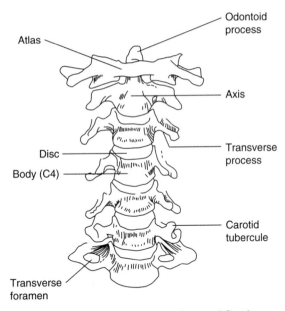

Figure 1-5   The seven cervical vertebrae and five intervertebral cervical disks.

(Figure 1-6). The pedicles connect with similar notches on adjacent vertebrae at the articular facets. From the facets, extending medially and posteriorly, are the laminae. The laminae fuse posteriorly to form the posterior spinous process. The spinous processes in the cervical spine are relatively short until the level of C7 (Figures 1-7 and 1-8). The posterior spinous process of C7 is

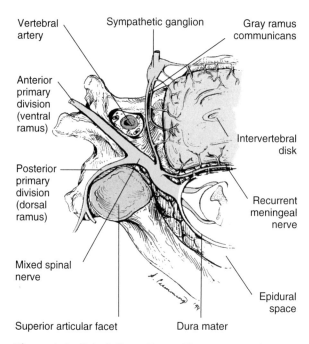

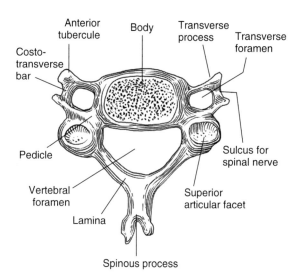

Figure 1-6   Spinal Nerve Roots. The roots contain separate sensory (posterior) and motor (anterior) branches after they exit the spinal ganglia. (From Cramer GD, Darby SA: *Basic and clinical anatomy of the spine, spinal cord, and ANS*, ed 1, St Louis, 1995, Mosby.)

quite long and usually palpated easily at the base of the posterior neck.

The seventh cervical vertebra is a transitional bone that connects the cervical and thoracic vertebrae. Functionally, it is more of a thoracic than a cervical vertebra. It is not unusual for C7 to lack a transverse foramen on one or both sides. Alternately, the transverse process may also abnormally develop into a cervical rib at either C6 or C7. These ribs may be bilateral or unilateral.

Cervical Nerves and Neurologic Function

Eight cervical nerves exit the spinal canal at the level above the corresponding vertebra. For example, the sixth cervical nerve exits at the C5-C6 foramina. Once exited from the spinal cord, the cervical nerves are termed *nerve roots*. Unlike the remainder of the spinal nerve roots, the upper cervical roots run almost horizontally out of the spinal column rather than obliquely.

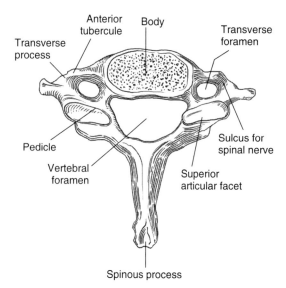

Figures 1-7 and 1-8 Differences in size of the spinous processes of the cervical spine vertebrae. **Figure 1-7,** Superior view of C4 vertebral body; **Figure 1-8,** Superior view of C7 vertebral body.

At C5-7 the spinal nerves run obliquely, this time in an inferiorly directed fashion.[8] The motor (anterior) and sensory (posterior) branches of each nerve root remain separate until they fuse in the spinal ganglion. Nerve root pain is commonly associated with three sites along the nerves: (1) nerve fibers of the dural sheath surrounding the nerve root, (2) irritation of the sensory root, or (3) irritation of sensory fibers of the motor root. In addition to the motor and sensory components, the fifth, sixth, and seventh cervical nerves are associated with specific reflexes.

Evaluation of the neurologic function of the cervical nerves is more easily accomplished through physical examination. Clinical assessment of C1-C4 is difficult and generally not indicated in a primary care setting; consequently, the first four cervical nerves are not included.

The fifth cervical nerve exits the spinal cord at the C4-C5 foramen. It divides into the suprascapular and axillary nerves, which innervate the supraspinatus and deltoid muscles, thus allowing abduction of the shoulder. The musculocutaneous nerve that branches off from the C5 and C6 nerves controls elbow flexion. The biceps tendon reflex is primarily a function of C5, although C6 also provides some innervation. Sensation of C5 encompasses the lateral deltoid and arm from the shoulder to the elbow.

C6 provides sensation to the lateral forearm, thumb, index finger, and one half of the long finger. Extension of the wrist is attributable to the integrity of both C6 and C7; ulnar deviation of the wrist during active wrist extension may indicate a lesion at C6. Testing the brachioradialis reflex at the wrist is the best reflex to evaluate C6 integrity.

Although sensation to the long finger is a function of C7, the digit may also be supplied by C6 and C8; therefore sensation of C7 cannot be fully evaluated by clinical examination. Triceps strength during elbow extension, the triceps reflex, wrist flexion, and finger extension strength are all functions of C7. The radial nerve is a branch of C7. If C7 is nonfunctional, radial deviation of the hand will occur during wrist extension. Sensation to the medial forearm and the ring and little fingers is supplied by C8. The median and ulnar nerves are branches of C8; the ulnar branch is easily evaluated by testing sensation on the ulnar aspect of the little finger. Flexion of the fingers at the metacarpophalangeal (MCP) joint and extension of the thumb rely on integrity of C8. There is no specific reflex associated with C8 testing. Table 1-1 summarizes cervical nerve root evaluation.

Musculature and Soft-Tissue Structures

More than a dozen muscles stabilize and provide movement of the neck; as a result, muscular problems of the neck are not uncommon. Overuse, trauma, and disease processes affecting structures adjacent to the neck muscles can also be sources of muscular pain. The main mass of neck extensor muscles is in the atlanto-occipital area (Figure 1-9).

TABLE 1-1	**Cervical Nerve Root Evaluation**		
Nerve Root	**Sensation**	**Muscle Action**	**Reflex**
C4	Upper shoulder and chest	Shoulder elevation	None
C5	Lateral arm from shoulder to elbow	Shoulder abduction	Biceps
		Elbow flexion	
	Lateral deltoid	Biceps contraction	
C6	Lateral forearm	Wrist extension	Partial biceps
	Thumb	Partial biceps contraction (elbow flexion)	Brachiocadialis
	Index finger		
	Half of long finger		
C7	Long finger—variable	Elbow extension	Triceps
		Wrist flexion	
		Finger flexion	
C8	Ring, little fingers	Finger flexion at metacarpophalangeal joints	None
	Distal half of forearm (ulnar aspect)	Thumb extension	

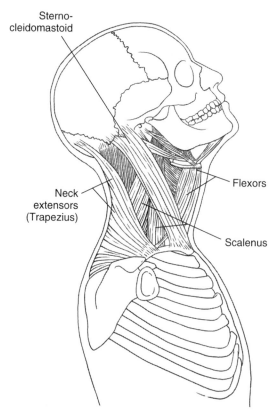

Figure 1-9 Primary extensor and flexor muscles of the neck. The scalene muscles aid in flexion, the sternocleidomastoid muscle assists in rotation, and the trapezius muscles help in extension of the neck.

Most of the neck flexors overlie C4. Muscular problems of the neck frequently involve the sternocleidomastoid and trapezius. The sternocleidomastoid muscle, which originates at the sternoclavicular area and inserts into the mastoid process of the temporal bone, flexes the head on the chest and assists in rotating the head toward the contracting muscle. The trapezius muscles are located posteriorly and originate at the occiput and posterior spines of C7 to the 12th thoracic vertebra (T12), inserting into the scapular spine and acromion process of the scapula. Movement of the shoulder girdle is a primary function of the trapezius muscles. Cervical strain often affects the trapezius muscles and causes stiffness or painful movement of the neck.

Although muscles provide support and some stability to the neck, the craniocervical ligaments are the predominant stabilizers of the cervical spine (Figure 1-10). Supporting ligaments of the cervical spine are both internal and external craniocervical structures. The internal craniocervical ligaments are located on the posterior aspect of the vertebral bodies, within the vertebral canal, and near the articular facets of the lateral masses. These ligaments aid in restricting excessive movement of the cervical spine. The external craniocervical ligaments provide additional stability for movement of the cranium and the atlas and axis vertebrae. The ligaments supporting the neck are broad and dense. In fact, stability of C1 and C2 is almost entirely a function of ligamentous support.

Between each vertebral body of the lower cervical spine is a fibrocartilaginous tissue complex that forms the intervertebral disk. The disks act as shock absorbers, connecting adjacent vertebrae and allowing for movement of the neck.[9] There is no disk between the occiput and C1 or between C1 and C2; therefore the five cervical disks begin at C2-C3.

The intervertebral disks are made up of an outer layer of tough fibrous tissue called the annulus fibrosus and a soft, pulpy center called the nucleus pulposus. The disks are thicker anteriorly than posteriorly, which contributes to the normal lordotic curve of the cervical spine.

EXAMINATION OF THE CERVICAL SPINE

Neurologic Examination

An examination of the cervical spine consists in large part of evaluating the cervical nerves as already noted. Each cervical nerve tested (usually C5 through C7) is evaluated for its motor, sensory, and reflex components. Figure 1-11 illustrates the approximate dermatomal distribution of the cervical and thoracic nerve roots. Reflexes should be graded as to their briskness. A fairly standard grading system is outlined in Table 1-2.

The motor component of C5 is tested by having the patient flex the elbow to 90 degrees and then abduct the arm against resistance. Having the patient actively flex and extend the elbow against resistance will also provide

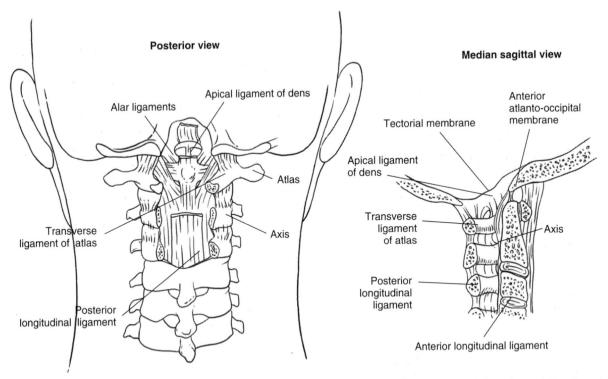

Figure 1-10   Ligamentous stabilization of the cervical spine. The alar and transverse ligaments of the atlas stabilize C1 and C2. The anterior and posterior longitudinal ligaments prevent vertebral subluxation, but these can be damaged with extremes of extension and flexion.

an evaluation of C5. Biceps flexion is predominately a function of C5, although there is also a small component of C6 innervation. Testing sensation over the lateral deltoid muscle provides an indication of the integrity of the C5 nerve root and its axillary nerve branch. The biceps reflex is tested to assess C5 function; again, C6 plays a small part in this reflex.

Isolated muscle testing of C6 cannot be clinically evaluated since C5 plays a role in biceps testing and C7 is partially responsible for wrist extension. Wrist extension is tested by stabilizing the patient's forearm with the examiner's hand while the patient extends the wrist against the examiner's other hand. The sensory branch of C6 is intact if the patient can discern light touch to the lateral forearm, thumb, and index finger. A brisk brachioradialis reflex, which is tested at the wrist, indicates an intact C6 nerve.

Elbow extension, wrist flexion, and finger extension at the MCP joints are muscle movements innervated by C7. Sensation to the middle finger is supplied by C7, but it may also be a function of C6 and C8. The triceps reflex is a function of the C7 portion of the radial nerve.

Motor integrity of C8 allows finger flexion at the MCP and distal interphalangeal joints. Flexion of the fingers against resistance is accomplished by having the patient make a loose fist and then interlock his or her fingers with those of the examiner. The examiner then attempts to pull the patient's fingers out of the flexed position. The nerve is intact if the patient's fingers remain flexed against resistance. Normal sensation to the ring and little fingers indicates integrity of C8. There is no reflex purely associated with C8.

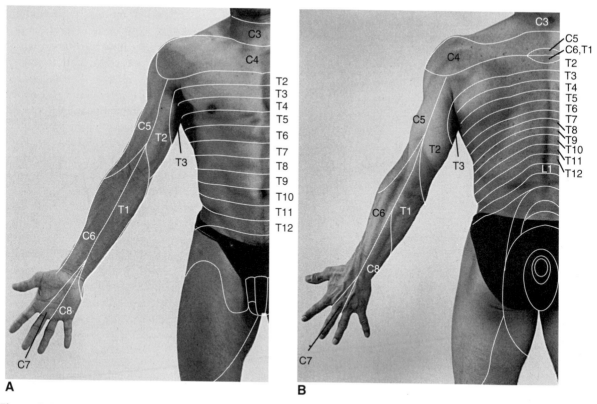

Figure 1-11 Approximate location of the cervical and thoracic nerve root dermatomes, showing anterior **(A)** and posterior **(B)** distributions. Exact dermatomal regions vary by individual. (From Reider B: *The orthopaedic physical examination*, Philadelphia, 1999, WB Saunders, p 322.)

Musculoskeletal Examination

A thorough examination includes noting active and passive neck movement, as well as resisted isometric movements. Differentiation between a true pathologic condition and psychogenic or nonorganic neck pain can be difficult when evaluating the cervical spine.

Active ROM is evaluated first. When assessing active movements, the examiner should note the patient's willingness to perform the movement, as well as any limitation of motion. The normal movements of the cervical spine are forward flexion, extension (or backward flexion), rotation to both sides, and lateral flexion to both sides. Table 1-3 shows the normal amount of active movement in each plane.

If active movement is limited, the examiner should ask the patient to lie in a supine position and then gently passively move the patient's neck. Resisted isometric movements consist of the patient maintaining the endpoint of each movement while the examiner attempts

TABLE 1-2	Standard Grading Scale for Spinal Reflexes

Grade	Reflex Tone
0	Absent
1	Diminished
2	Average
3	Exaggerated
4	Clonus

TABLE 1-3	Normal Range of Motion in the Cervical Spine

Movement	Degrees	Evaluation
Flexion	80-90	*Cervical flexion*
Extension	70	*Cervical extension*
Rotation	70-90 right and left	*Cervical rotation*
Lateral flexion	20-45 right and left	*Cervical lateral bending*

(From Hartley, A: *Practical joint assessment, upper quadrant: a sports medicine manual*, ed 2, St Louis, 1995, Mosby.)

to move the neck. Resisted movements should not be attempted if there is obvious muscle atrophy or weakness. Muscle strength should be recorded. A standard system for grading muscle strength is noted in Table 1-4.

A physical examination can reveal clues to nonorganic causes of neck pain. Frequently pain will not follow any dermatomal distribution. A pain drawing is a simple way for the patient to localize various sensations. Figures 1-12 and 1-13 illustrate both a normal pattern for cervical nerve root pain (see Figure 1-12) and nonorganic pain (see Figure 1-13).

Patients complaining of neck pain often experience weakness in an upper extremity. When testing individual hand grip strength in the patient with neck pain, the examiner should repeat, testing both hand grips simultaneously, if the symptomatic arm has a weak grip. A patient who magnifies his or her symptoms will have either bilaterally weak or bilaterally strong hand grips, since the brain is not usually quick enough to transmit differing messages to each hand.

PATHOLOGIC CONDITIONS AND TREATMENT

Cervical Strain

Cervical strain, whether acute or chronic, is one of the most common neck complaints seen in primary care orthopedics. Acute cervical strain refers to damage and inflammation to the soft tissues of the neck, caused either by overuse or overstretching of tensed muscles. The trauma preceding onset of symptoms is frequently a fall or motor vehicle accident; it may also be preceded by heavy

TABLE 1-4	Muscle Strength Testing	
Muscle Tone	**Grade**	**Movement**
Normal	5	FROM against maximal resistance
Good	4	FROM against moderate resistance
Fair +	3	FROM against gravity with minimal resistance
Fair	3	FROM against gravity only
Poor	2	FROM with gravity eliminated
Trace	1	+ Muscle contraction; no joint motion
Zero	0	No palpable muscle contraction

Normal strength is usually given a grade of 5. *FROM*, Full range of motion.

PAIN DRAWING

Name: _____   Date: _____

A Pain Drawing is a way to accurately describe and "map out" all of your symptoms. Please take time to understand the symbols and draw them in the areas where you feel symptoms.

N N N N N	Dull Aching	X X X X X X X	Burning	= = = = =	Numbness
/// /// /// /// ///	Stabbing	• • • • • • • • • •	Pins & Needles	S S S S S S	Muscular Cramp

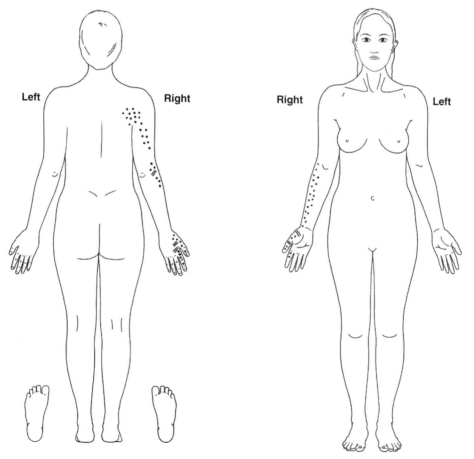

Figure 1-12 A pain drawing illustrating a normal dermatomal pattern of pain, such as that caused by a herniated cervical disk. The practitioner may substitute any symbols for those given.

PAIN DRAWING

Name: _____   Date: _____

A Pain Drawing is a way to accurately describe and "map out" all of your symptoms. Please take time to understand the symbols and draw them in the areas where you feel symptoms.

$N\,N\,N$ $N\,N$	Dull Aching	$X\,X\,X\,X$ $X\,X\,X$	Burning	$=\,=\,=$ $=\,=$	Numbness
$/\!/\!/$ $/\!/\!/$ $/\!/\!/$ $/\!/\!/$ $/\!/\!/$	Stabbing	$\cdot\;\cdot\;\cdot\;\cdot$ $\cdot\;\cdot\;\cdot\;\cdot$	Pins & Needles	$S\,S\,S$ $S\,S\,S$	Muscular Cramp

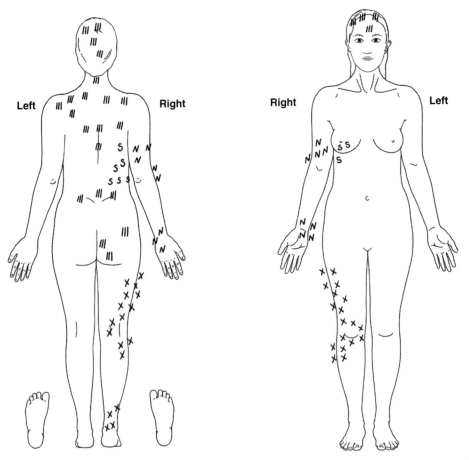

Figure 1-13 An example of a pain drawing that follows no known dermatomal pattern. Note the presence of pain symbols outside the body; this is not uncommon.

lifting or overhead work. Chronic cervical strain can occur in patients who spend long hours at computer terminals or engage in other activities that cause prolonged flexion or extension of the neck. The severity of cervical strain varies from a mild discomfort to a more serious injury that involves ligamentous damage. When cervical ligaments are affected, the injury becomes a cervical sprain.

History

Typically symptoms do not develop until a few hours after the injury and may not appear for 24 to 48 hours. It is important that the examiner ask about activity of the preceding few days, because some patients do not make the connection between activity and delayed onset of symptoms.

Patients typically relate a history of increasing posterior neck stiffness and pain associated with difficulty moving the neck in a normal fashion. One side of the neck may be more tender than the other. Pain frequently radiates to the occiput and across both shoulders and into the deltoid muscles; tingling of the fingers may also occur. Occipital headaches are not uncommon. Lateral flexion of the neck toward the affected side tends to increase pain. If muscle spasm is present, lateral flexion away from the affected side may reduce pain.

Physical Examination

Patients typically guard neck movements, moving slowly and cautiously. Since there is usually no point tenderness to palpation of the posterior processes, the examiner should consider a possible fracture if tenderness exists. Diffuse tenderness in the posterior neck and across the trapezius muscles is common. Muscle spasm may be palpable. Pain tends to increase with lateral flexion, but there is no limit in ROM. Axial compression (Spurling's maneuver) does not increase pain with a cervical strain, but generally pain will increase with cervical nerve root disease[31] (Figures 1-14 and 1-15).

Diagnosis

Diagnosis is based on history and examination. There are no specific x-ray findings on AP and lateral views, although lateral x-ray films of the cervical spine may show flattening of the normal lordotic curve. Flattening of the curve may indicate muscle spasm. If there is con-

cern about ligamentous laxity, flexion and extension films should be obtained.

Treatment

Treatment is primarily symptomatic. Moist heat for 10 to 15 minutes at a time twice a day helps relieve muscle spasm. Nonsteroidal antiinflammatory drugs (NSAIDs) are beneficial in reducing pain and inflammation. The use of muscle relaxants is not generally indicated. Home stretching exercises can help reduce spasm and pain, but some patients will respond better with a formal physical therapy program. Symptoms usually resolve within 2 to 3 weeks.

Whiplash

Whiplash is a term used to describe an acceleration-deceleration type of injury that results from extreme hyperextension followed by forced forward flexion, causing injury to the neck muscles and supporting structures (Figure 1-16). The true pathology also involves shear, tension, and rotational forces on the spine. Severity of injury ranges from cervical strain to conditions as serious as tearing the anterior portion of a cervical disk. Preexisting spinal alignment may contribute to the severity of an acute injury.[18] The most common mechanism of whiplash injury is a motor vehicle accident in which the patient is hit from behind.

In the case of an auto accident, it is important that the examiner note how and where the neck injury occurred, as well as whether the patient was restrained and where she or he was sitting. If only a lap belt was in use, strain on the neck can actually be increased, since the seat belt restrains the patient's trunk but not the neck. The use of headrests may reduce shear forces on the neck.[29] In accidents of 15 mph or less, the passenger in the right front seat is more at risk for whiplash than the driver; in accidents above 20 mph, the driver is more likely to sustain whiplash.

History

The cervical spine is the most common location for spinal cord injuries, since the cervical area has the greatest movement of the spinal column.[7] Flexion-extension injuries in combination with a rotatory component of neck movement are often associated with damage more serious than a flexion-extension injury alone. Flexion-extension-rotation injuries can occur in contact sports

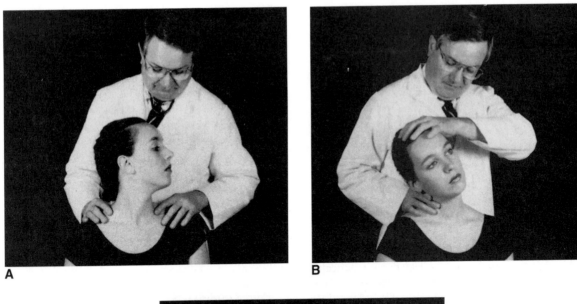

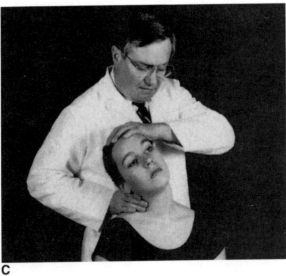

Figure 1-14 Spurling's Maneuver or Test. A, While seated comfortably and with an erect posture, the patient actively rotates the head from side to side. Localization of pain is noted. **B,** The patient's head is laterally flexed toward the side of complaint. Gradually the examiner applies progressive downward pressure to the head and neck. Reproduction of symptoms or collapse sign at this point constitutes a positive test. The balance of the test should not be completed. **C,** From the laterally flexed position, the neck is extended as far as the patient can tolerate. The examiner applies progressive downward pressure. Reproduction of radicular symptoms suggests nerve root compression. Localized spinal pain suggests facet involvement. (From Evans RC: *Illustrated orthopedic physical assessment,* ed 2, St Louis, 2001, Mosby.)

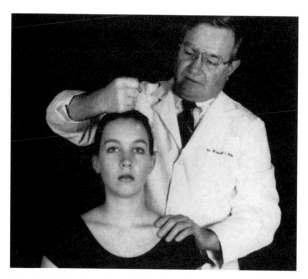

Figure 1-15   Spurling's Maneuver or Test. A vertical blow is delivered to the uppermost portion of the cranium. The examiner may wish to interpose a hand between the concussing hand and the patient's skull. The head and neck are first in a neutral position for this procedure and then positioned into lateral flexion and extension for a repeated procedure. The test will stimulate any nerve root irritation or other pain-sensitive structures related to disk disease and cervical spondylosis. Use of this modification should not be a surprise to the patient. (From Evans RC: *Illustrated orthopedic physical assessment,* ed 2, St Louis, 2001, Mosby.)

(e.g., football) or in motor vehicle accidents where the patient's vehicle is struck obliquely from behind. In the case of a motor vehicle accident, the examiner should note the amount of damage to the patient's vehicle. Secondary gain—particularly monetary compensation—is often a factor in the patient's symptoms and recovery.[5,11,28] There is some evidence that patients involved in litigation have more pain and a longer recovery period from neck injuries.

Pain and decreased ROM are the predominant symptoms of whiplash. Pain usually begins soon after the injury but may not occur for a few days. The pain pattern is similar to that of cervical strain; however, unlike cervical strain, pain radiates down the arms more often in whiplash. This radiating pain does not necessarily indicate nerve root involvement. Dysphagia, headache, and blurred vision are not uncommon.

Physical Examination

Range of motion is limited and uncomfortable. Swelling of the anterior neck is indicative of severe whiplash, and the patient may have objective neurologic signs such as decreased reflexes at C5-C6. The presence of Horner's syndrome is evidence of significant injury, and these patients should be referred to a neurologist.

Tenderness occurs in the occipital area and along the trapezius muscles, where spasm may be palpable. The

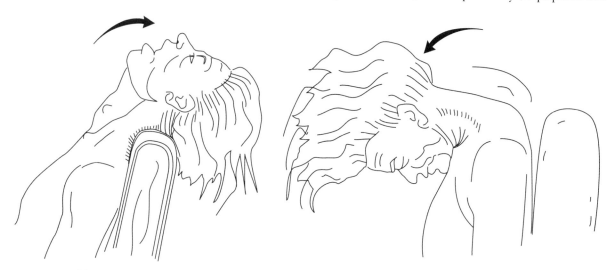

Figure 1-16   Hyperextension followed by forced flexion of the cervical spine, causing whiplash.

examiner should palpate the posterior spinous processes for any point tenderness. Pain and tenderness that is well localized over a bony prominence may indicate a fracture; these patients should be referred to an orthopedic surgeon. Patients with bilateral tingling of the upper extremities or other bilateral neurologic complaints should have the cervical spine immobilized and then be urgently referred to an emergency department, orthopedic surgeon, or neurosurgeon.

Diagnosis

History and examination are the critical factors in making a correct diagnosis. Findings on AP and lateral cervical spine films are not necessarily diagnostic in themselves, but they are useful for assessing preexisting degenerative changes of the spine, which may raise the practitioner's awareness of associated symptoms.

An x-ray study should begin with a lateral view, since the height of both disk spaces and vertebral alignment are easily seen. A flattening, or even a reversal of the normal lordotic curve of the cervical spine, is best seen in the lateral view and is generally indicative of muscle spasm. An AP view is best for showing fractures of the articular masses or vertebral bodies. Rotational abnormalities are also easily discernible on an AP view. Flexion and extension films will exaggerate any ligamentous instability, making it easier to see. Some ligamentous injuries should not be evaluated on flexion and extension x-ray films; they may cause subluxation of one or more vertebrae when the neck is maximally flexed or extended. A subluxation of more than 3 mm on the lateral view is a sign of cervical instability; these patients should be referred to an orthopedic surgeon. Patients who complain of neck instability may have more serious injury. If serious ligamentous injury is suggested, the patient should have the neck immobilized and be referred to an emergency department or a specialist as soon as possible. If ligamentous instability is suggested, it is appropriate to call for emergency medical services to immobilize the patient's neck before transporting.

Treatment

Initial treatment of cervical strain or mild whiplash without evidence of neurologic deficit consists primarily of NSAIDs and rest. A soft cervical collar may be worn only for the first 24 to 48 hours to reduce stress on the neck muscles. It is important to understand that a soft collar will not significantly restrict movement of the cervical spine. Ice packs to the areas of pain and tenderness may be applied for 10 to 15 minutes every hour for the first 1 to 2 days after injury since cold reduces tissue inflammation. After 48 to 72 hours, the use of moist heat and gentle ROM exercises may decrease muscle spasm and pain. If the patient has a severe pain, mild oral narcotics such as acetaminophen with codeine or hydrocodone may reduce pain, especially at night. Some patients benefit from a course of physical therapy. Spinal manipulation is sometimes recommended, but it is not without risks, including a potential for neurologic damage.[14,24] Most patients will recover fully within a few months.

Fractures

Fractures to the cervical spine are usually the result of significant trauma. Direct blows to the head, diving accidents, falls, and motor vehicle accidents are common causes of bone injury. Most patients who sustain a cervical fracture have been or will be evaluated in an emergency department or by a specialist. Occasionally, however, a patient who was inebriated at the time of injury may sober up later and notice neck pain. These patients generally do not recall any injury, but obvious bruising or other skin trauma may suggest an injury more serious than cervical strain.

The risk of permanent or life-threatening injuries associated with cervical spine fractures necessitates extreme caution in moving or examining any patient with a possible cervical fracture. Significant pain and nuchal rigidity are associated with fractures; pain is usually prominent and ROM is greatly decreased. Neurologic symptoms such as weakness, numbness, or tingling of the extremities are often present. If either history or examination leads to the suggestion of fracture, the patient should have the neck immobilized and be sent to an emergency department for radiologic and neurologic evaluation. Individuals over the age of 65 are more prone to having multilevel injures and neurologic deficit.[17]

DEGENERATIVE DISEASES

Degenerative Disk Disease and Spondylosis

In a normal, healthy adult, the intervertebral disks provide approximately one quarter of the length of the vertebral column. With increasing age, disk degeneration becomes more prevalent, but it is not always symptomatic. Cervical disk disease is generally a slow, progressive process, although acute pain may occur. As adults age, the water content of the nucleus pulposus diminishes, and the spongy material becomes more similar to the relatively more rigid annulus fibrosus. Microfissures occur in both the annulus fibrosus and nucleus pulposus. As the disk heights decrease, the ligaments around the spinal canal, particularly the ligamentum flavum, thicken. The intervertebral disk spaces become narrower, and osteophytes tend to form on the adjacent vertebral bodies. Osteophyte formation may cause narrowing of the spinal canal, or *spinal stenosis*. When the osteophytes irritate the spinal cord or the exiting nerve root, cervical radiculopathy results. This type of lesion is known as a *hard-disk* problem and is typically found in the older adult population. Overall, hard-disk problems are more common than soft-disk lesions.

Hard-disk disease, also known as *spondylosis*, is present in more than half of individuals over age 50.[9] Cervical spondylosis is the term used to describe degenerative changes throughout the spine, including disks, ligaments, and vertebral bodies. The pathophysiologic characteristic of cervical spondylosis is altered biomechanics of the spine's motion segment, resulting in accelerated degenerative changes. Spondylosis can cause neck pain alone (known as axial pain), upper extremity pain from cervical radiculopathy (when nerve roots are compressed), or cervical myelopathy (due to spinal cord compression).

Development of transverse osteoarthritic bars from the midline of the spinal canal posteriorly can be seen on radiographs (osteophytes may also be present laterally); these osteophytes then compress the cervical nerve roots. Spurring is frequently found in the facet joints.

Bony spurring of the vertebrae can affect the size and shape of the spinal canal, even to the extent of causing acquired spinal stenosis. Spinal stenosis is any narrowing of the spinal or nerve root canal or the intervertebral foramina. Depending on its location, spinal stenosis can be asymptomatic or cause neck stiffness, myelopathy, pain, or radiculopathy.[4] Typically affected individuals note gradual, progressive weakness and sensory changes of the extremities. Symptomatic spinal stenosis is best diagnosed based on history, plain x-rays, and MRI.

Symptoms of cervical spondylosis include pain and stiffness in the neck, shoulder, and upper extremities. Cervical radiculopathy causes arm pain; weakness and sensory changes may or may not be present. Symptoms of cervical myelopathy may present initially as a gait or balance problem.[10] Hyperreflexia may be present. Upper extremity sensory complaints tend to be in a global rather than dermatomal distribution.

Soft-disk herniation occurs when the soft nucleus pulposus extrudes through the surrounding annulus fibrosus. The usual inciting mechanism for such a herniation is trauma that causes a tear in the annulus fibrosus. Sudden onset of acute pain may indicate a disk herniation.

Disk lesions of either variety most often affect the C5-C6 and C6-C7 interspaces (Figure 1-17). When a nerve root is involved, numbness and tingling occur in

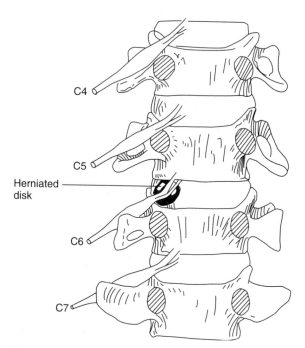

Figure 1-17   Illustration of a herniated cervical disk (C5-C6) causing pressure on the C6 nerve root.

one or both upper extremities. Clinical evaluation of the cervical nerves will help localize the disk lesion (Figure 1-18). For example, a C5-C6 disk herniation will cause a C6 nerve root irritation, and the patient will have numbness and tingling along the C6 nerve distribution and usually go with that thumb and index finger. Table 1-5 summarizes common findings associated with various levels of degenerative disk disease.

History

In addition to the neurologic signs associated with disk diseases, stiffness and neck or arm pain are predominant symptoms. Any movement that increases intradiskal pressure, such as coughing, sneezing, or Valsalva's maneuver, may exacerbate pain. Arm (radicular) symptoms may be worse than neck (axial) pain. Pain is usually eased by rest and is less severe on waking in the morning. In patients younger than 50 years of age, pain may shift from one side to the other. Elderly patients are more likely to develop a bilateral disk lesion and have pain in both arms. Referred pain in the scapular region that extends toward the shoulder(s) is not uncommon. Unlike osteoarthritis, patients with disk degeneration may have periodic pain-free episodes.

Physical Examination and Diagnosis

Examination may reveal decreased ROM and tenderness in the suprascapular area. Passive ROM may be more uncomfortable than active ROM; extension is usually more painful than flexion. Pain with rotation toward the painful side suggests disk protrusion. Cervical radiculopathy is clinically confirmed if pain and/or radicular symptoms worsen when axial loading (Spurling's maneuver or test, see Figures 1-13 through 1-16) is performed.[31] To perform this maneuver the patient laterally flexes the head toward the painful side. The practitioner then places his or her hands on the crown of the patient's head and presses downward. If this maneuver causes an increase in pain or other symptoms, a herniated disk is likely.

Flexion of the neck that causes an electric shock-type sensation is known as Lhermitte's sign and may indicate cord compression. Heel-to-toe walking, walking on tiptoe, and heel walking should also be assessed since balance difficulty or spasticity suggests cervical myelopathy. Myelopathy is an upper motor neuron disorder; as such, hyperreflexia or a positive Babinski's sign may be present.

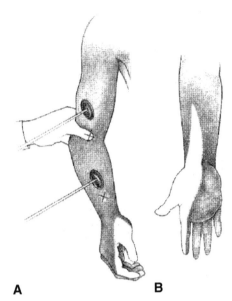

A   **B**

Figure 1-18 Area of abnormal sensation associated with herniated cervical disk causing impingement of the C6 nerve root. **A,** Decreased sensation of thumb and index finger. Biceps and brachioradialis reflexes are diminished. **B,** Decreased sensation is most easily assessed on the palmar surface of the hand. (From Olson WH: *Symptom-oriented neurology: handbook for primary care,* ed 7, St Louis, 1994, Mosby.)

Plain x-ray films (AP and lateral views) are helpful in evaluating disk space height. Narrowing of the intervertebral disk space raises the suggestion of disk disease. An x-ray film will reveal osteophytes on the vertebral bodies and posterior facet joints. Spurring (osteophytes), best seen on lateral films on either the anterior or posterior vertebral bodies, can also be evaluated. A computed tomography (CT) myelogram is sometimes used to evaluate the extent of spinal stenosis. Magnetic resonance imaging (MRI) provides the best images for evaluating the spinal cord, disks, and other soft tissue structures.

Treatment

In the absence of significant neurologic symptoms, such as muscle wasting, anesthesia of an extremity, or absence of a reflex, a course of conservative therapy is appropriate. Conservative therapy, consisting of NSAIDs, rest, and physical therapy may ease symptoms.[26] A soft cervical collar may decrease symptoms by reducing nerve root irritation. Once the acute pain subsides, simple, gentle ROM

TABLE 1-5		**Common Findings in Degenerative Cervical Disk Disease**			
Level of Disk Herniation	**Nerve Root**	**Pain**	**Numbness**	**Muscle Weakness**	**Reflex Change**
C4-C5	C5	Base of neck Shoulder Anterolateral aspect of arm	Deltoid Lateral arm	Deltoid Biceps Supraspinatus Infraspinatus	Decreased or absent biceps

C5-C6	C6	Neck
		Shoulder
		Medial border of scapula
		Occasionally, lateral aspect
		  of arm
			Thumb
			Index finger
			Half of middle finger
			Lateral forearm
				Biceps (mild)
				Wrist extension
					Decreased
					  brachioradialis

C6-C7	C7	Same as C6 nerve	Middle finger	Triceps Finger
				  extension
				Wrist flexion
					Decreased or
					  absent triceps

C7-T1	C8	Neck
		Medial border of scapula
		Anterior chest
		Medial aspect of upper
		  arm and forearm
			Little and ring fingers
			Distal forearm
			  (ulnar aspect)
				Finger flexion	None

exercises may relieve some associated neck muscle spasm (Figure 1-19). Some clinicians include the use of a soft cervical collar worn only at night to reduce intradiskal pressures and nerve root irritation.

If there is no decrease in symptoms after 4 to 6 weeks or if symptoms become worse at any time, the patient should be referred to an orthopedic surgeon or neurosurgeon. Surgical treatment of spondylosis has been shown to be of most benefit in patients with cervical radiculopathy.[9]

Osteoarthritis

History and Physical Examination

Osteoarthritis (OA), also known as degenerative joint disease, can affect any weight-bearing joint, including the intervertebral joints of the cervical spine. In the spine it is the associated degenerative disk disease rather than the bony changes in vertebrae that causes most of the clinical complaints.

Degenerative bony changes of the cervical spine are almost universally present in individuals over the age of 50 years. The most common region of the cervical spine to be affected is C5-C7, since this site is where most neck flex-

ion occurs, but OA can affect any of the cervical vertebrae. Severe OA of the facet joints can cause spinal stenosis.

Osteoarthritis of the atlanto-odontoid joint (occiput-C1) is commonly found in patients who complain of suboccipital headache.[33] The bony changes associated with OA at the uppermost cervical level are rarely visible on plain x-ray films because overlying bones obscure the atlanto-odontoid joint. If clear visualization of this area is necessary, CT is preferable to x-ray evaluation.

Diagnosis

Diagnosis of OA is based on history, examination, and radiographic findings. The patient is usually older than 50 years and has a history of neck pain and morning stiffness that diminishes with activity. However, the overall course is progressive in nature. If there are osteophytes impinging on the nerve roots or intervertebral disks, radicular symptoms may occur. Neck extension decreases neural foraminal size, causing nerve root irritation and increased pain.

Treatment

Treatment is mainly symptomatic, since there is no definite correlation between the severity of symptoms and

Exercises:
Stand under a hot shower for five to ten minutes and
perform the following exercises, twice daily if possible.

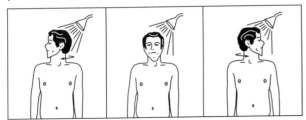

1. Stand erect. Turn head slowly as far as
   possible to the right. Return to normal
   center position and relax. Turn head
   slowly as far as possible to the left.
   Return to normal center position and
   relax.

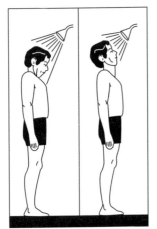

2. Stand erect. Try to touch your
   chin to your chest, slowly.
   Raise head backwards, looking
   up at ceiling, slowly.

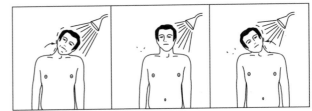

3. Stand erect. Try to touch left ear to the left shoulder.
   Return to normal center position and relax. Try to
   touch right ear to the right shoulder. Return to normal
   center position and relax.

Figure 1-19   Simple cervical range-of-motion exercises, performed in a hot shower, may reduce spasm and pain.

radiographic findings. Three primary goals of treatment
are to relieve pain, improve function, and prevent disability.[16] Acetaminophen, topical analgesics such as capsaicin cream, or NSAIDs may relieve pain. Moist heat
will improve blood flow and may reduce stiffness, as may
gentle ROM exercises. Patient education is directed at
providing realistic expectations of activity and the slow
progressive nature of the disease. If numbness, weakness, or tingling of the extremities are present or
develop, the patient should be referred to an orthopedic
surgeon or neurosurgeon.[1]

Rheumatoid Arthritis

Rheumatoid arthritis (RA) frequently affects the cervical spine; in fact, it has been identified as the second
most common site of RA after the hands and feet. Most
frequently, RA affects the upper spine (C1-C2), but it
also can cause erosive changes in the lower cervical spine
(C3-C7). RA can also cause disk space narrowing, osteoporosis, and diskitis.[12] The clinical course of RA is
highly variable; therefore the severity of cervical spine
involvement is also unpredictable. However, the severity

of systemic RA and cervical spine damage do correspond.[6,20] The inflammatory process of RA affects connective tissue throughout the body, including ligaments and the synovium of the joint capsules. The ligaments suffer microtears, disruption of collagen, and deposition of fibrin. Ligamentous instability and degradation, in conjunction with the erosive changes in the joints, lead to increased risk of subluxation of the vertebrae.

Subluxations of the cervical spine fall into one of three categories: anterior atlantoaxial subluxation (AAS), vertical subluxation (VS) of the odontoid, or subaxial subluxation (SS).[20] Severe subluxations can lead to paralysis or even death as a result of cord compression. The most common type of subluxation is AAS, which occurs when there is greater than 3 mm of space between the ring of C1 and the anterior portion of the odontoid. Vertical subluxation of the odontoid (C2) is associated with more advanced disease and occurs when the articulations of the occiput-C1 and C1-C2 are destroyed and C1 collapses down onto C2. The danger of VS is the migration of the odontoid process into the foramen magnum. Subaxial subluxations affect the lower cervical spine and are believed to be the result of a postinflammatory ankylosis, which stiffens the spine and reduces its mobility. In the lower cervical spine SS causes multiple-level subluxations, or a "staircase" deformity.

The diagnosis of any of these subluxations is made by a lateral x-ray film.[22] The subluxation may be magnified by flexion of the neck during the film, but AAS or VS deformities can be difficult for the nonspecialist to visualize, and these patients should be referred to a rheumatologist or an orthopedic surgeon who treats the cervical spine.

History

Most patients with RA of the cervical spine have a history of symptoms involving the wrists and hands or feet. Neck pain and stiffness is an unusual presenting symptom of RA. Generally neck ache and stiffness in a patient with RA indicate cervical spine involvement. Symptoms tend to remit and flare in accordance with other joint involvement. Suboccipital pain may be caused by anterior subluxation of C1 on C2.

Physical Examination

Early in the course of the RA, there are few specific physical findings other than decreased ROM and stiffness

with movement. Radicular pain may occur later. Pain radiating to the occiput is the most common symptom of AAS, but occipital headache is not diagnostic. The presence of AAS in rheumatoid arthritis tends to indicate a poorer prognosis.[21] Motor weakness should be carefully and thoroughly evaluated, since it may be an early sign of spinal cord compression.

Diagnosis

The presence of RA, combined with symptoms of neck ache, is suggestive of cervical involvement. An x-ray evaluation will help differentiate RA from OA, because osteophytes are not evident with RA and the vertebrae tend to appear osteopenic. A common site of RA involvement is C3-C4; this region is where subluxation is most common in the lower cervical spine. The C5-C6 area is involved more commonly in OA, and osteophytes are usually evident on the vertebrae.

If subluxation of the cervical spine is suggested or if neurologic symptoms appear, MRI is the diagnostic tool of choice. In addition to evaluating the extent of cord compression associated with subluxation, MRI can evaluate the extent of pannus formation, visualize the presence of extradural nodules that may also compress the cord, and reveal abnormalities that cannot be visualized on x-ray films.

Treatment

Generally treatment of RA is directed in conjunction with or dictated by a rheumatologist. Early in the disease, NSAIDs (including cyclooxygenase-2 [COX-2]–specific agents) are used to decrease the inflammatory response and subsequent neck pain. Early, more aggressive treatment of RA tends to have a better outcome. Most individuals with RA should be on disease-modifying antirheumatic drugs within 3 months of diagnosis.[3] The use of more potent agents should be left to the expertise of a rheumatologist. Radiographic evidence of instability (noted on flexion/extension views) is reason to refer the patient for surgical stabilization.[2]

Nonpharmacologic therapies include physical therapy, occupational therapy, and psychosocial counseling. Physical therapy can strengthen neck muscles and relieve some stiffness. Improving the performance of everyday activities through improving body mechanics or through the use of assistive devices is in the realm of occupational therapists. Referral to a psychologist or social worker may be necessary if neck involvement affects the patient's life to the extent that coping mechanisms and interpersonal relationships are compromised.

Infection

Infections of the cervical spine are less common than those of the lumbar spine. However, increasing incidence of human immunodeficiency viral infection and intravenous drug use are leading to increasing numbers of spinal infections. Postsurgical or other iatrogenic causes, such as invasive testing, trauma, and lymphatic seeding of extrapulmonary tuberculosis, can also cause cervical spine infection.[15,30]

Cervical spine infections include osteomyelitis, diskitis, epidural infections, and meningitis.[25] Atlantoaxial subluxation may occur as a result of bony and ligamentous destruction from the infection. Treatment depends on the cause and site of the infection. Successful treatment relies on using the correct antimicrobial agent for the infecting organism, appropriately removing any sequestered nidus, and maintaining adequate antibiotic levels. *Staphylococcus aureus* remains the most common infecting organism, but any pathogen, including viruses[15] and fungi, may cause infection. *Pseudomonas aeruginosa* is a common pathogen among intravenous drug abusers.

History

Patients will usually note localized pain and tenderness of a few months' duration. (Unfortunately, localized pain occurs later in the course of the disease.) Early in the course of infection, the pain may be diffuse and associated with shoulder pain or headache, thus making early diagnosis of infection difficult. Pain is worsened by activity yet not relieved by rest. Movements that jar the spine, such as walking down stairs or stepping off a curb, may increase pain. Diabetic patients, especially men over the age of 50 with a history of recent upper respiratory, sinus, urinary tract, or skin infection, may be predisposed to infection. Intravenous drug users with neck pain should be evaluated for infection.

Physical Examination

A physical examination will reveal localized tenderness and soft-tissue swelling. Muscle spasm may occur, and torticollis may be present.[13] Neurologic signs are usually absent early in the disease course, and this absence may result in a delayed diagnosis.[13] Myelopathy is a late finding of cervical spine infection.

Diagnosis

A diagnosis is based on the history, a clinical examination, the suggestion of disease, and the exclusion of other causes of neck pain. Typical systemic signs of infection, such as fever, chills, and anorexia, may not be present. Leukocytosis may be absent early, but a complete blood count with a differential should always be sent. The erythrocyte sedimentation rate (ESR) is almost always elevated, sometimes significantly so. Blood and urine cultures should also be sent to identify the causative pathogen.

Radionucleotide scanning used to be the "gold standard" for detecting cervical spine infections, but its lack of specificity in spite of great sensitivity has caused this method to be largely supplanted by MRI. Arthritis, fracture, and tumor will all cause positive findings on a bone scan, although a combination of technetium-99m– and gallium- or indium-111–labeled white blood cells will help differentiate infection from inflammatory causes.[27]

MRI is the preferred diagnostic tool for identifying cervical spine infections. This imaging technique is as sensitive as and more specific than a bone scan. One drawback of MRI is that end plates of the vertebrae are somewhat difficult to visualize; consequently, early erosive changes attributable to infection may not be visualized, and other changes within the bone may need to be differentiated from other processes, such as acute rheumatoid arthritis. Gadolinium-enhanced MRI reduces these problems and improves specificity for diagnosing infections.[27] The primary disadvantage to MRI is its cost; it is significantly more expensive than a bone scan.

A CT image, including high-resolution reformatted CT scanning, is useful for diagnosing osteomyelitis or disk space infections and spinal cord destruction.[13,27] A CT scan will visualize vertebral end-plate changes earlier than MRI.

Once the history, clinical findings, and imaging studies lead to a diagnosis of infection, the most important step is identifying the causative organism. Ideally a bone culture is obtained to identify the organism; in reality, this is not always practical or possible. Referral to an orthopedic surgeon or infectious disease specialist is appropriate at this point.

Treatment

Treatment of cervical spine infections is based on the location and type of infection and the causative organism. Surgical drainage of the epidural abscess or the removal of vertebral sequestrum and incision and drainage of infected material can be combined with antibiotic therapy. Any material obtained during surgery should be sent for culture and Gram's stain. Generally, treatment of spinal infections begins with a 4- to 6-week course of intravenous antibiotic therapy. Effectiveness of therapy is evaluated by improved clinical status and a decrease in ESR.

Torticollis

Torticollis, or wryneck, is a disorder of the cervical muscles or fascia that results in an abnormal rotation and tilting of the head. Most cases occur in infants or pediatric patients and resolve spontaneously.

In adults, torticollis is associated with a cervical fracture (especially of the dens), RA, tumors or neoplasms of the posterior cranial fossa or spinal cord, or trauma to the C1-C2 articulations; it may also be idiopathic in origin. A traumatic cause of torticollis is the most important consideration in adults since an undetected and untreated injury can have significant associated morbidity. Spasmodic torticollis, which is relatively rare, primarily occurs in adults with a history of emotional disturbances.

The pathologic abnormality of torticollis is attributable to a subluxation and fixation of the facet joints. The facet joints may become "locked" when they sublux, and anterior or posterior displacement of the cervical spine may also occur.

History

The patient may have a history of trauma, rheumatoid arthritis, or neoplasm, or there may be no known precipitating factor. Sometimes a stiff or painful neck may be the only complaint preceding the onset of symptoms.

Physical Examination and Diagnosis

A diagnosis is determined by a physical examination. Usually the head is tilted in one direction, and spasm of the neck muscles (particularly the sternocleidomastoid) causes rotation of the head toward the other side. By itself, the presence of torticollis is not necessarily a major concern; a careful evaluation of possible underlying causes is of primary importance so that treatment is directed appropriately.

An x-ray study may reveal bony malalignment or lesions. MRI best evaluates soft-tissue lesions or tumors.

Treatment

If no underlying abnormality is present, treatment is initially conservative. Bed rest, NSAIDs, gentle passive stretching, and a soft cervical collar may alleviate some symptoms. Muscle relaxants and benzodiazepines do not offer significant relief. If there is no improvement in 1 to 2 weeks, or there are any abnormal neurologic findings, the patient should be referred to an orthopedic surgeon or neurosurgeon.

DIFFERENTIAL DIAGNOSES—RED FLAGS

When evaluating a patient with any cervical spine abnormality, one of the most important determinations the practitioner can make is whether symptoms are primarily neurologic, muscular, or mechanical in origin. Disorders of primary neurologic dysfunction tend to be more serious than those of muscular origin. Examples of symptoms predominantly neurologic in origin include radicular symptoms, such as numbness, tingling, and decreased reflexes. Mechanical instability of the cervical spine may be attributable to trauma or changes associated with rheumatoid arthritis. A disorder of muscular origin is generally not as serious as a primary neurologic or mechanical abnormality. However, muscular symptoms are frequently the result of pathologic neurologic or mechanical processes. Certain findings, from either history or a clinical examination, are suggestive of serious pathologic conditions (see the Red Flags box on p. 24). Patients exhibiting these symptoms or signs can be appropriately referred to a neurologist or orthopedic surgeon for further evaluation and management.

EVALUATION MODALITIES

Imaging

Knowing what type of test to order and when to order it is often a function of clinical expertise. A basic knowledge of the scope and limitations of various diagnostic modalities is important to the proper evaluation and treatment of cervical spine disorders.

Plain X-Ray Films

The most commonly used diagnostic tool in evaluating the cervical spine is the plain x-ray film. An x-ray study is noninvasive, painless, and relatively inexpensive. No special preparation of the patient is required. Plain films are useful for determining the alignment of the spine, presence of fractures, lytic lesions of the bone, degenerative changes such as osteophytes, and disk space heights. AP and lateral projections are useful in evaluating disk space height and spinal alignment. Flexion and extension views should be obtained if there is a question of ligamentous instability. Oblique views will show foraminal narrowing. An open-mouth odontoid view is necessary to properly evaluate C1-C2.

Interpretation of x-ray films is based on a systematic evaluation of the bony structures and associated spaces. Developing a system of viewing films is as important as identifying abnormalities. The key to evaluating x-ray films is consistently using whatever system the practitioner has developed. The following steps may prove helpful:

1. General overview: Physically take a step or two back from the film. Note any gross asymmetry or deformity. Note the overall alignment, size, and shape of the bones, as well as their density.
2. Close inspection: Examine the continuity of individual vertebral bodies; note any breaks or irregularities (fractures or osteophytes) in the edges of the vertebrae. Note any change in the density of each vertebra.
3. Specific area: Compare the area of physical findings or symptoms with the corresponding area on the x-ray film. Note any alteration in disk space height, localized periosteal reaction (seen as fuzziness of the bony edge), or local lesions.
4. Associated structures: Search for increased soft-tissue density, which appears whiter, and

unusual calcifications. (In soft tissue, they may indicate resolving hematoma. Calcification of vertebral arteries may be the cause of vertigo or dizziness. The presence of air in the soft tissues may indicate deep infection.)

As noted earlier in this chapter, x-ray studies have several limitations. Joint structures, such as cartilage and synovium, are not visualized; soft tissue and surrounding spaces are difficult to evaluate. Early changes associated with infection or with nerve root or spinal cord impingement are not visible.

Computed Tomography

A CT image offers improved visualization of soft tissues, air-fluid levels in abscesses, and greater detail of bony structures. When combined with intravenous contrast material, CT is especially useful for evaluating lesions of muscle or the lymphatic system or for evaluating vascular structures. Spiral (or helical) CT generates three-dimensional images of various structures and is useful for reconstructing osseous structures to locate obscure fractures or to assess enlarged cervical lymph nodes accurately. The scan times are shorter in spiral CT than conventional CT, so the patient is exposed to less radiation.[19] Spiral CT is being increasingly used.

Limitations of CT include the interference and artifact caused by metallic objects (such as bullet fragments, metallic dental fillings, or surgical clips). Motion of the patient will result in poor quality films, although the faster scan times of spiral CT help overcome this problem. Little special preparation of the patient is required, but prostheses, including dentures, should be removed to decrease the incidence of artifact.

Magnetic Resonance Imaging

The scanning technique of choice for evaluating soft tissue is MRI. Patients are not exposed to ionizing radiation; and differentiation of muscle, fat, and fluid is best seen with MRI.

It is important to note a few basics of MRI. An MRI is based on the physical properties of various body tissues. Images are usually either T1-weighted or T2-weighted; these classifications, called spin sequences, are based on differences in the makeup of tissues. For example, water appears brighter than oil on

T2-weighted images. Inflammation, cervical disks, cerebrospinal fluid, and fluid-filled abscesses appear brighter than surrounding structures on T2-weighted images.[19] The brightness of the images is referred to as the signal; a low signal on T2-weighted images appears dark, and tissue with a high signal on T2-weighted images appears bright. The same is true of T1-weighted images. T1-weighted studies are used to maximize the contrast between intraspinal fat, which is bright, and disk material, nerve roots, and bone.

Just as three-dimensional CT is becoming more common, three-dimensional MRI is gaining greater popularity, particularly for evaluating degenerative disk disease.[23] The primary advantage of this modality is improved accuracy in assessing disk abnormalities. For evaluation of infection, tumor or postoperative soft tissue changes, adding gadolinium, a contrast material, improves MRI specificity.[26]

MRI is useful for evaluating disk disease, cysts, herniated disks, and differentiation of postoperative causes of pain (scar tissue versus recurrent disk herniation, neoplasms, tumors, and inflammatory conditions).[19] An MRI should not be used for patients with pacemakers, cerebral aneurysm clips, and metallic orthopedic implants, because of problems associated with alterations in the pacemaker settings and potential movement of metallic objects. Tattoos (including tattooed eyeliner) may contain metallic-based pigments, which will heat up with MRI and can cause a local burning sensation and inflammation.

Patients having MRI should remove all jewelry, makeup, and deodorant. They should also be instructed to call the radiology center in advance to obtain any special instructions before their examination. Patient motion, coil size, and magnet strength all affect MRI quality.[19] A final consideration in ordering an MRI is whether the patient is claustrophobic; open MRI is available, but the quality of the images may be inferior to the standard machine.

In summary, plain x-ray studies are the simplest, easiest, most inexpensive imaging technique for evaluating the cervical spine. A CT image is especially useful for more detailed evaluation of bone, particularly fractures or suspected fracture. An MRI is the preferred imaging choice for evaluating soft tissue, disk, and spinal cord abnormalities.

INDICATIONS FOR REFERRAL

See the following Red Flags Box for referral information.

Red Flags *for Cervical Spine Disorders*

Patients with these findings may need to be referred for more extensive work-up.

Sign/Symptom	Response
Gradually increasing intensity of pain that does not resolve or diminish	Suggests a serious lesion, such as spinal cord compression
Pain that expands into surrounding dermatomes	Indicative of an expanding lesion, such as tumor or metastases
Bilateral arm pain	Indicative of an involvement of both nerve roots, a finding that is unusual for disk problems (except over age 50)
Arm pain that persists longer than 6 months, unrelieved by rest; associated with weight loss	(Pain from herniated disk generally resolves in 6 months or less); indicative of neoplasm or metastases
Painful, limited range of motion	Indicative of a lesion of the upper cervical spine (C1-C2), ankylosing spondylitis, fracture or subluxation, or bone disease
Pain only with lateral flexion away from the painful side	Suggestive of lesion of lung apex (disk abnormality is usually painful in most planes of motion)
Pain and weakness with resisted neck movement	Indicative of a fracture of first rib, vertebral metastases, or retropharyngeal tendonitis (resisted movements are painful but not weak in disk disease)
Muscular weakness without pain	Indicative of an anterior nerve root lesion
Horner's syndrome (ptosis, miosis, and loss of sweating on ipsilateral side of face caused by injury to sympathetic nerves)	May be indicative of tumor or other lesion in the thorax or superior pulmonary sulcus; involves the cervical sympathetic ganglia at the base of the neck
Hoarseness	Suggestive of epidural or retropharyngeal abscess or of cervical muscle rupture, which may cause hematoma that impinges on laryngeal nerve

REFERENCES

1. Albert TJ, Murrell SE: Surgical management of cervical radiculopathy, *J Am Acad Orthop Surg* 7(6):368, 1999.
2. Alberstone CD, Benzel EC: Cervical spine complications in rheumatoid arthritis patients, *Postgrad Med* 107(1):199, 2000.
3. American College of Rheumatology: Guidelines for the management of rheumatoid arthritis (2002 update), *Arthritis Rheum* 46(2):328, 2002.
4. Best JT: Understanding spinal stenosis, *Orthopaedic Nurs* 21(3):48, 2002.
5. Cassidy JD and others: Effect of eliminating compensation for pain and suffering on the outcome of insurance

claims for whiplash injury, *N Engl J Med* 342:1179, 2000.

6. Casey ATH, Crockard HA: In the rheumatoid patient: surgery to the cervical spine, *Br J Rheumatol* 34:1078, 1995.

7. Chiles BW, Cooper PR: Acute spinal injury, *N Engl J Med* 334(8):514, 1996.

8. Ebraheim NA et al: Anatomic study of the cervicothoracic spinal nerves and their relation to the pedicles, *Am J Orthop* 29(10):770, 2000.

9. Emery SE: Cervical degenerative disk disorders. In Beatty JH, editor: *Orthopaedic knowledge update,* ed 6, Rosemont, Ill, 1999, American Academy of Orthopaedic Surgeons.

10. Emery SE: Cervical spondylotic myelopathy: diagnosis and treatment, *J Am Acad Orthopaedic Surgeons* 9(6):377, 2001.

11. Feffari R, Russell AS: Whiplash: heading for a higher ground, *Spine* 24:97, 1999.

12. Gornisiewicz M, Moreland LW: Rheumatoid arthritis. In Robbins L et al, editors: *Clinical care on the rheumatic diseases,* ed 2, Atlanta, 2001, American College of Rheumatology.

13. Ghanayem AJ, Zdeblick TA: Cervical spine infections, *Orthop Clin North Am* 27(1):53, 1996.

14. Kapral MR, Bondy SJ: Cervical manipulation and risk of stroke, *CMAJ* 165(7):907, 2001.

15. Kreitzer JM, Freedman GM, Kihtir S: Cervical radicular pain caused by herpes simplex virus-type 1 infection: a case report, *Mt Sinai J Med* 69(1-2):107, 2002.

16. Lozada CJ, Alman RD: Osteoarthritis. In Robbins L and others, editors: *Clinical care of the rheumatic diseases,* ed 2, Atlanta, 2001, American College of Rheumatology.

17. Lomoschitz FM et al: Cervical spine injuries in patients 65 years old and older: epidemiological analysis regarding the effects of age and injury mechanism on distribution, type, and stability of injuries, *Am J Radiol* 178(3):573, 2002.

18. Maiman DJ, Yoganandan N, Pinter FA: Preinjury cervical alignment affecting spinal trauma, *J Neurosurg* 97(suppl 1):57, 2002.

19. Murphy RB and others: Imaging of the cervical spine and its role in clinical decision making, *J South Orthop Assoc* 9(1):24, 2000.

20. Oda T and others: Natural course of cervical spine lesions in rheumatoid arthritis, *Spine* 20(10):1128, 1995.

21. Riise T, Jacobsen BK, Gran JT: High mortality in patients with rheumatoid arthritis and atlantoaxial subluxation, *J Rheumatol* 28(11):2425, 2001.

22. Roche CJ, Eyes BE, Whitehouse GH: The rheumatoid cervical spine: signs of instability on plain cervical radiographs, *Clin Radiol* 57(4):241, 2002.

23. Ross JS: Three-dimensional magnetic resonance techniques for evaluating the cervical spine, *Spine* 20(9):1099, 1995.

24. Rothwell DM, Bondy SJ, Williams JI: Chiropractic manipulations and stroke: a population-based case-control study, *Stroke* 34(5):1054, 2001.

25. Ruiz A and others: MR imaging of infections of the cervical spine, *Magn Reson Imaging Clin North Am* 8(3):561, 2000.

26. Slipman CW and others: Chronic neck pain: mapping out diagnosis and management, *J Musculoskeletal Med* 19(6):242, 2002.

27. Stabler A, Reiser MF: Imaging of spinal infection, *Radiol Clin North Am* 39(1):115, 2001.

28. Swartzman LC, Teasell RW, McDermid AJ: The effect of litigation status on adjustment to whiplash injury, *Spine* 21(1):53, 1996.

29. Tencer AF, Mirza S, Bensel K: Internal loads in the cervical spine during motor vehicle rear-end impacts: the effect of acceleration and head-to-head restraint proximity, *Spine* 27(1):34, 2002.

30. Tirri R, Vitiello R, DiMartino G: Pott's disease of the lower cervical spine in a diabetic patient, *Monaldi Arch Chest Dis* 55(3):205, 2000.

31. Tong HC, Haig AJ, Yamakawa K: The Spurling test and cervical radiculopathy, *Spine* 27(2):156, 2002.

32. Tseng SH and others: Ruptured cervical disc after spinal manipulation therapy: report of two cases, *Spine* 27(3):E80, 2002.

33. Zapletal J et al: Relationship between atlanto-odontoid osteoarthritis and idiopathic suboccipital neck pain, *Neuroradiology* 38:62, 1996.

Chapter 2

Shoulder

Descriptions ranging from "inherently unstable" to a "balance of form and function" have been used to describe the shoulder. Like the hip, the shoulder is a ball-and-socket joint, but it differs in a number of significant respects. First, whereas the hip is a weight-bearing joint, the shoulder is a suspension joint. Of all the joints in the body, the shoulder has the greatest mobility. Mobility, however, comes at the sacrifice of stability. The hip socket, the *acetabulum*, is deep and encompasses greater than 50% of the femoral head; the shoulder socket, the *glenoid*, is shallow and comes in contact with relatively little surface area of the head of the humerus, similar to the golf ball resting on a tee.[19] The lack of bony stability allows increased joint mobility; the muscles, tendons, and ligaments are the predominant stabilizers, rather than bone.

ANATOMY AND BONY STRUCTURES

The shoulder girdle is comprised of three bones (humerus, scapula, and clavicle) and four articulations. The articulations are named for their anatomic locations: coracoclavicular (CC), acromioclavicular (AC), glenohumeral (GH), and coracoacromial (CA). Only one, the GH, is considered a true synovial joint.

Of the osseous structures, the scapula is the most complex. It is a roughly triangular bone that is relatively flat and suspended between the second and seventh ribs by numerous back muscles. There are three primary palpable landmarks on the scapula: the spine, acromion, and coracoid processes. (Figure 2-1 illustrates the primary structures of the shoulder.) The spine is situated on the posterior aspect of the scapula and extends laterally and obliquely to the upper portion of the bone. The acromion process arises from the lateral portion of the scapular spine and is the most lateral projection of the scapula. Generally there are three basic shapes of the acromion. These are classified as type I, which is fairly straight; type II, which curves downward; and type III, which has a hooked or beaked end (Figure 2-2). A fourth type, in which the undersurface is convex, has also been identified.[34]

The acromion articulates with the lateral end of the clavicle, forming the AC joint. When injured, the AC ligament, which connects these two bones, is the structure referred to as a *separated shoulder*.

The glenoid fossa, or process, is a concave projection from the lateral portion of the scapula. In posteroanterior diameter it is the thickest portion of the scapula.[10] The glenoid has a fibrocartilaginous covering called the *labrum*. The cartilage is thicker near the outer edges than it is in the center; thus the area of contact between the humeral head and the glenoid is increased. The labrum also improves conformity of the glenoid and humerus by deepening the glenoid socket. The concave surface of the glenoid assists in maintaining the humeral head in the center of the glenoid fossa. Loss of glenoid concavity through loss of bone (from trauma or disease) or loss of cartilage (from degenerative disease) contributes to shoulder instability.[15]

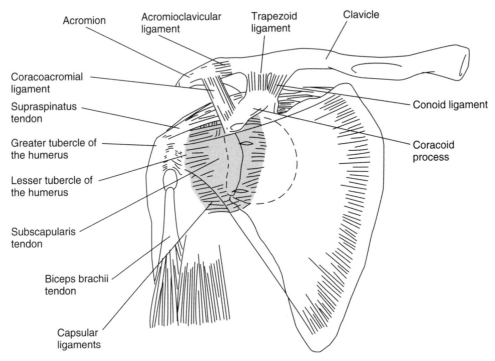

Figure 2-1   Primary structures of the shoulder joint (anterior view). (From Greenfield G, Stanish WD: Relieving shoulder pain without surgery, *Physician Sportsmedicine* 22:68, 1994.)

The GH articulation forms what is commonly called the *shoulder joint*. This joint links the humerus and the thorax. Stability of the joint and, in fact, of the entire shoulder depends on keeping the humeral head centered in the glenoid fossa,[14] which is accomplished through a complex interaction of muscles, ligaments, and tendons.

The clavicle originates at the sternum just above the first rib and extends nearly horizontally to the AC joint. In addition to the stability provided by the AC ligament, several muscles and the CC ligament help maintain the position of the clavicle.

Part of the third bone of the shoulder girdle, the humeral head, is the "ball" of the ball-and-socket joint. The primary humeral structures associated with the shoulder are the head, the anatomic neck, the greater and lesser tuberosities, and the surgical neck. The humeral head articulates with the glenoid fossa, forming the GH joint. Inferior to the humeral head is the anatomic neck, a narrowed section that separates the

head from the tuberosities. Each tuberosity provides attachment for the muscles of the rotator cuff. The supraspinatus, infraspinatus, and teres minor muscles attach at the greater tuberosity; the subscapularis attaches on the lesser tuberosity. The bicipital groove separates the two tuberosities; the long head of the biceps tendon lies in this groove. Just inferior to the tuberosities lies the surgical neck of the humerus; this is the most common area in which proximal humerus fractures occur.

SOFT-TISSUE STRUCTURES

Muscles

Although the shoulder girdle provides more than 40 attachments for muscles, fewer than 10 muscles are involved in most outpatient treatment. Four of the most important muscles are those of the rotator cuff: the

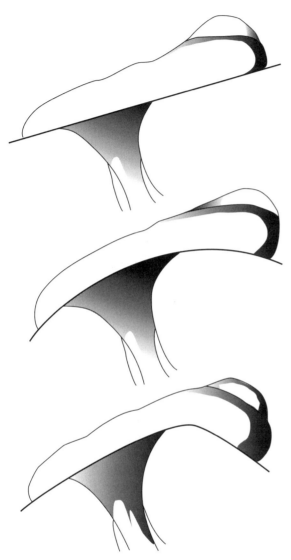

passes through the relatively small subacromial space that lies between the humeral head and the CA ligament. It is at this point that the muscle and its tendon are relatively avascular. The supraspinatus muscle stabilizes in the glenoid fossa, and, in combination with the deltoid, assists in shoulder abduction.[1] The subacromial bursa which is about the size of a 50-cent piece, lies between the supraspinatus tendon and deltoid muscle, beneath the acromion. The bursa extends back to the CA ligament. Lying transversely over the inferior portion of the scapula are the infraspinatus and teres minor muscles. The infraspinatus muscle is primarily responsible for lateral (external) rotation of the arm. Abduction and flexion of the arm are assisted by the teres minor. Located on the anterior surface of the scapula, the subscapularis is the predominant muscle involved in medial (internal) rotation of the arm.

As the muscles of the rotator cuff form their tendinous attachment to the humerus, they become a fibrous capsule complex, which firmly attaches distally to the anatomic neck of the humerus.[2] Overuse, overstretching, and trauma all render the tendons of the shoulder muscles susceptible to inflammation and injury. These maladies may range from bicipital tendonitis to impingement syndrome and rotator cuff tears.

A fifth muscle, the deltoid, overlies the SIT muscles at their insertions on the humeral tuberosities; it is clinically important to be able to differentiate deltoid abnormalities from those of the rotator cuff (Figure 2-3). The deltoid is the primary abductor of the humerus and initiates a great deal of other shoulder motion before various other elements of the rotator cuff are recruited.

Stabilization of the shoulder by the rotator cuff occurs through a system of mechanisms that prevent (1) superior translation of the humeral head, (2) anterior dislocation (the rotator cuff pulls the humeral head posteriorly during lateral raising of the arm), and (3) posterior dislocation during the same motion.[33] The net effect is to stabilize and centralize the humeral head in the glenoid fossa during movement. Each muscle assists with specific movements. The supraspinatus assists with abduction and forward flexion, the infraspinatus and teres minor externally rotate the humerus, and the subscapularis internally rotates the humerus.

Figure 2-2   Types of Acromion Processes. Type I *(top)* is flat; type II *(middle)* is curved; type III *(bottom)* is hooked. (From American Academy of Orthopaedic Surgeons: *Orthopaedic knowledge update 4*, Rosemont, Ill, 1993, AAOS.)

supraspinatus, infraspinatus, teres minor (SIT) muscles, and subscapularis. Maintaining the head of the humerus in the glenoid fossa is the primary function of the rotator cuff. The supraspinatus muscle lies over the superior portion of the scapula (above the scapular spine) and

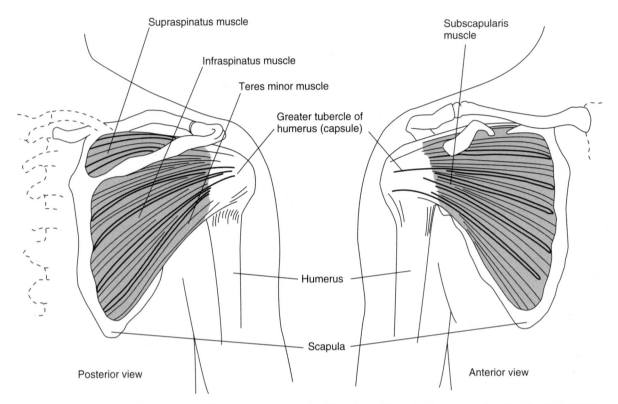

Figure 2-3   Muscles of the rotator cuff. (From Glockner SM: Shoulder pain: a diagnostic dilemma, *Am Fam Physician* 51:7, 1995.)

Ligaments

The ligaments of the shoulder are considered to be passive or static stabilizers in that they are lax during most of the shoulder's range of motion (ROM).[14,33] This arrangement allows great mobility but provides little stability. Ligaments, in concert with the muscles of the shoulder, work synergistically to maintain joint stability. The interplay of these stabilizers has been hypothesized to be a type of reflex arc.[13]

Neurovascular Structures

Several important nerves affect and transverse the shoulder. Those most vulnerable to direct injury are the brachial plexus with its associated nerve branches, the spinal accessory nerve, and the long thoracic nerve. The spinal accessory nerve, which lies fairly superficially, provides the only innervation to the trapez-

ius muscle. Most damage to the brachial plexus is caused by shoulder dislocation, which results in a traction type of injury. Dislocation causes traction on the nerve, resulting in brachial plexus injury. Direct trauma resulting in a scapular fracture may damage either the spinal accessory or the long thoracic nerve. Injury to any of the cervical nerves at or above the level of C6 will result in alteration of sensation or movement of the shoulder.

The subclavian artery and vein, the two main vascular structures of the upper extremity, are contained in the thoracic outlet. Trauma, particularly fractures of the clavicle, can injure these vessels. The axillary vein, which also lies anteriorly, is subject to injury because of its relatively unprotected, superficial position.

Multiple vessels supply the rotator cuff. This fact helps explain the spontaneous healing of some rotator cuff tears in younger patients. However, the relatively avascular insertion of the supraspinatus tendon on the humeral head may be a factor in the large number of rotator cuff tears occurring in this area.

GENERAL EXAMINATION

Before the examiner can localize a shoulder abnormality, he or she must have knowledge of normal shoulder movement. Once ROM is assessed, movement should be evaluated in terms of smoothness and strength.

Assessing Range of Motion

Various methods for describing shoulder ROM have been published. Regardless of which method is used, the primary purpose of ROM testing is twofold: (1) to assess how ROM affects the patient's daily activities; and (2) to assist the examiner in localizing the abnormality. Because the shoulder has the greatest mobility of any joint in the body, evaluating shoulder ROM can be confusing. Subtle reductions in various planes of motion can indicate abnormality.

The primary movements of the shoulder are forward flexion (or elevation), extension, abduction, adduction, and internal and external rotation. Shoulder motion frequently involves combinations of these movements. For example, tucking in the back of one's shirt combines extension with internal rotation. Figures 2-4 through 2-8 illustrate normal ROM for the shoulder.

A rapid method of assessing the shoulder is to evaluate flexion, abduction, adduction, and internal and external rotation. Initially the patient should perform all movements actively without any resistance. Forward flexion and abduction are normally 0 to 180 degrees; pain that occurs with either motion in the arc between 70 and 120 degrees suggests impingement or AC joint arthritis.

Abduction is tested by asking the patient to flex both arms to 90 degrees at the elbow and then to laterally raise the arms (Figure 2-9). These movements test the deltoid and supraspinatus muscles. Shoulder abduction should be viewed from the back and front since scapular elevation alone, can allow apparent shoulder abduction of 30 to 60 degrees. When a patient's movement suggests decreased abduction, scapular elevation is more visible from the back.

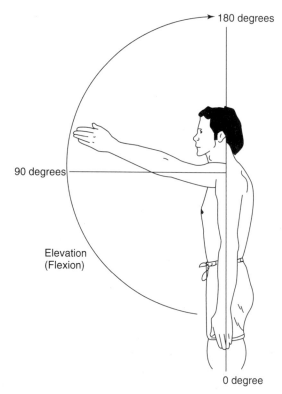

Figure 2-4   Normal ROM for forward flexion of the shoulder. (From American Academy of Orthopaedic Surgeons: *The clinical measurement of joint motion*, Rosemont, Ill, 1994, AAOS.)

Adduction assesses the AC joint and, in the case of clavicle fracture, the stability of the healing bone. The patient is asked to reach his or her hand and arm across the body toward the opposite shoulder. Normal adduction allows the individual to at least cup the opposite shoulder in his or her hand.

Internal rotation is evaluated by the inferior Apley "scratch" test (Figure 2-10). The patient is asked to reach as high as possible behind his or her back; normally the extended thumb reaches the T5 or T6 level. Since the inferior border of the scapula is usually at T7 or T8, the thumb should be higher than the bottom of the scapula.

External rotation of the shoulder is assessed by having the patient flex both elbows to 90 degrees; while keeping the elbows close to the body, the patient is asked to move

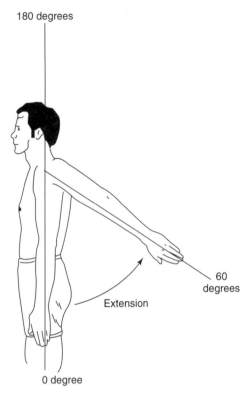

Figure 2-5 Normal ROM for extension. (From American Academy of Orthopaedic Surgeons: *The clinical measurement of joint motion*, Rosemont, Ill, 1994, AAOS.)

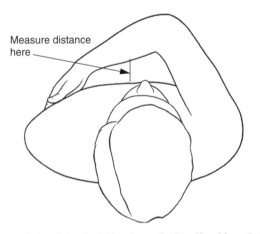

Figure 2-6 Normal Adduction of the Shoulder. Both shoulders should be evaluated, and the distance between the anterior chest wall and inner elbow should be compared on each side.

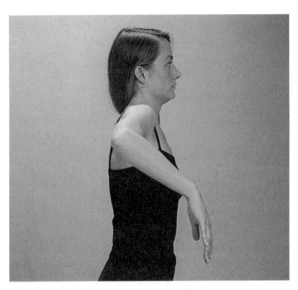

Figure 2-7 With 90 degrees of shoulder abduction, Normal internal rotation of the shoulder is 45 degrees. (From Reider B: *The orthopaedic physical examination*, Philadelphia, 1999, WB Saunders.)

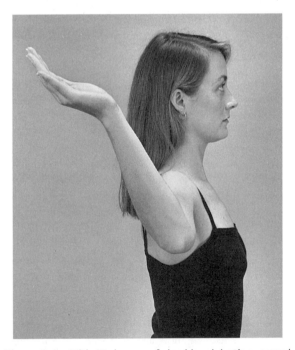

Figure 2-8 With 90 degrees of shoulder abduction, normal external rotation of the shoulder is at least 90 degrees. (From Reider B: *The Orthopaedic Physical Examination*, Philadelphia, 1999, WB Saunders.)

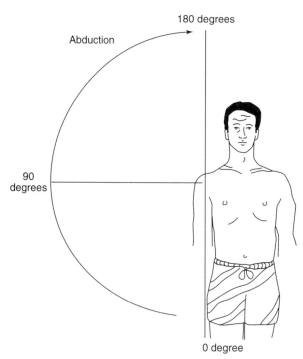

Figure 2-9 Testing Shoulder Abduction. The starting plane is 0 degrees with the arm at the side. Normal abduction is 170 to 180 degrees. (From American Academy of Orthopaedic Surgeons: *The clinical measurement of joint motion*, Rosemont, Ill, 1994, AAOS.)

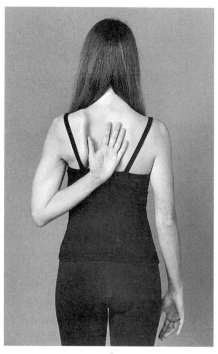

Figure 2-10   Apley "Scratch" Test (Inferior). This test is a combination of extension and internal rotation. (From Reider B: *The orthopaedic physical examination*, Philadelphia, 1999, WB Saunders.)

both hands laterally as far as possible (Figure 2-11). This tests the infraspinatus muscle. Once tested actively, resistance should then be applied to these movements. Pain with resisted movements or an inability to perform these motions is generally indicative of an abnormality. Table 2-1 summarizes specific muscle testing.

Palpation

Structures of the shoulder that easily lend themselves to palpation are scapula, acromion, clavicle, AC joint, greater and lesser tuberosities of the humeral head, and bicipital groove.

The scapula, suspended by various muscle groups, lies over the posterior thorax. The scapular spine is an oblique bony ridge that rises and becomes more prominent laterally. Its lateral end forms the acromion

process. The inferior two thirds of the scapula is most easily palpated along its medial border. The scapular borders may come into better definition with the patient's arms raised overhead. When the patient's arms are lying loosely at his or her side, the scapulae should be at the same level on the thorax.

Anteriorly the clavicle is usually easily palpated, beginning at the sternal notch and moving laterally. Because the clavicle is relatively superficial, defects such as fractures are not difficult to feel. At its lateral margin, the clavicle is joined to the acromion process by the AC ligament, which is felt as a small depression between the two bones. This area is normally tender to palpation. The AC joint is sometimes called the *arch of the shoulder*.

The greater tuberosity of the humerus lies below and lateral to the AC joint, beneath the deltoid muscle. Palpation is easiest when the patient's arms are hanging

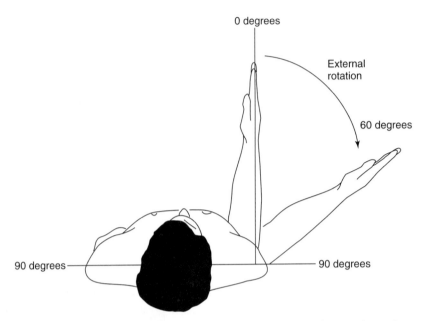

Figure 2-11   External Rotation of the Shoulder. With the arm at the side, normal external rotation to 60 degrees is the result of an intact infraspinatus muscle. (From American Academy of Orthopaedic Surgeons: *The clinical measurement of joint motion,* Rosemont, Ill, 1994, AAOS.)

TABLE 2-1	Testing Specific Shoulder Muscles
Structure	**Test**
Supraspinatus muscle	Resisted abduction "Empty can" test
AC joint	Cross-body adduction
Subscapularis muscle	Resisted internal rotation (Apley's "scratch" test—inferior)
Infraspinatus muscle	Resisted external rotation

AC, Acromioclavicular.

loosely by his or her side. Just medial to the greater tuberosity (again, anteriorly) is the lesser tuberosity. The bicipital groove, a longitudinal depression in the humeral head, separates these two projections. It can be felt by palpating the anterior humeral head while the patient straightens the elbow and internally and externally rotates the arm. The tendon of the long head of the biceps muscle lies in the bicipital groove.

PATHOLOGIC CONDITIONS AND TREATMENTS

Soft Tissues

Soft-tissue problems are among the most common shoulder complaints. They are usually classified as either an impingement type of problem or instability. Impingement problems include tendonitis, bursitis, and most rotator cuff problems. Instability generally refers to a problem of the GH joint, including its associated ligaments and muscles. Trauma can affect the soft tissues of and around the shoulder. Sprains of the AC and CC ligaments are commonly seen joint injuries.

Impingement Syndrome

Impingement syndrome, one of the most common shoulder complaints, refers to a collection of maladies whose primary pathologic condition involves varying degrees of wear and tear of the rotator cuff tendons and nearby tissues.[22] The subacromial area is the primary site of impingement on these tissues because the tendons and bursa become jammed between the humeral head and acromion. Impingement syndrome includes supraspinatus and bicipital tendonitis, as well as subacromial bursitis. Left untreated, impingement can eventually lead to tears of the rotator cuff.

Three distinct stages of impingement were described by Neer[23] and are still generally used to classify this syndrome. The stages are based on tissue damage and are clinically useful in predicting recovery with nonoperative or surgical treatment. Stages I and II usually respond to nonsurgical treatment, whereas stage III requires surgical repair.[3,12] Table 2-2 summarizes the stages of impingement.

History

Patients with impingement typically complain of pain associated with activities of the arm at or above shoulder level. There is usually no history of trauma. Pain tends to be described as aching and is often localized to the anterior shoulder but may extend to the middle portion of the deltoid.[1]

A painful arc, usually between 70 and 120 degrees, is the classic symptom of subacromial impingement (Figure 2-12). In spite of this painful arc, the patient usually has full ROM without any significant weakness.

Physical Examination

Inspection of the shoulder rarely reveals any obvious abnormality, except in the case of acute trauma. The large amount of soft tissue around the joint can often obscure swelling or joint effusion. The crucial aspect of inspection is evaluating ROM for the presence of a painful arc with active and passive abduction.

Increased pain with resisted shoulder abduction often occurs with supraspinatus strains. Degenerative changes of the AC joint contribute to impingement; pain with palpation of the AC joint is common in this syndrome.

Two common tests for impingement are the impingement sign and Jobe's, or the "empty can," test. If the patient experiences pain when the humerus is passively brought into full forward flexion, it is a positive sign of impingement. The "empty can" test (see Table 2-1), is performed by having the patient fully extend the elbow, abduct the shoulder to 90 degrees, turn the thumb toward the floor, and then raise the arm as if emptying a can of liquid (Figure 2-13). This test isolates function of the supraspinatus muscle. Pain during either active or resisted movement suggests supraspinatus impingement.

TABLE 2-2   Stages of Impingement Syndrome*

Stage	Abnormality	Cause	Symptoms
I	Subacromial edema and hemorrhage	Overuse	Normal ROM, no weakness Pain with provocative testing
II	Fibrosis and tendonitis; possible partial tear of rotator cuff	Repeated injury	Decreased ROM, esp. internal rotation May have mild weakness
III	Full-thickness rotator cuff tear	Trauma or degeneration of rotator cuff fibers	Positive impingement test True weakness Passive ROM greater than active ROM

*The earlier stages of impingement tend to affect younger patients; complete rotator cuff tears are more common in individuals older than ages 40 to 50.[8,29]

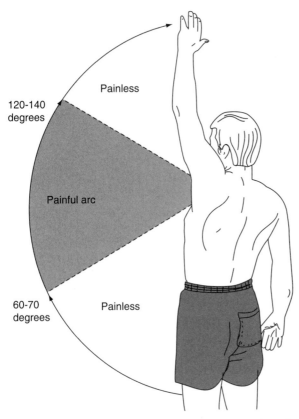

Figure 2-12 A painful arc with shoulder abduction is typical of subacromial impingement. (From Greenfield G, Stanish WD: Relieving shoulder pain without surgery, *Physician Sportsmedicine* 22:71, 1994.)

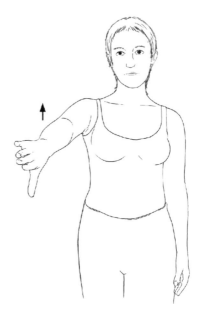

Figure 2-13 The isolated supraspinatus or empty can test—if pain occurs while raising the hand, impingement of the supraspinatus tendon is likely.

Diagnosis

A diagnosis of impingement syndrome is based primarily on history and clinical examination. Plain x-ray films may help evaluate bony abnormalities or other pathologic conditions that would make the diagnosis of impingement syndrome more likely. An x-ray study should include anteroposterior (AP) views with the shoulder in internal and external rotation, as well as a supraspinatus outlet (also called a lateral scapula Y) view. The latter view is critical in evaluating the shape of the acromion and estimating the subacromial space.[1,35] Subacromial spurring or a type III acromion can contribute to impingement, since the hook associated with a type III acromion further reduces the small subacromial space.[30]

The subacromial impingement test, which consists of an injection of a local anesthetic (usually 1% or 2% lidocaine without epinephrine) into the subacromial space, is frequently used to confirm a diagnosis of impingement.[12,33] This test can help differentiate between AC arthritis, shoulder instability or cervical radiculopathy, and impingement. If relief of symptoms occurs within 15 to 20 minutes after injection, the test is positive for impingement.

Treatment

Early treatment of impingement syndrome may help prevent its progression to a complete rotator cuff tear. Physical therapy is the mainstay of nonoperative treatment. Initially the patient should avoid activities that involve overhead movements of the arms. Once pain subsides, shoulder-strengthening exercises are initiated; as strength improves, activities designed to increase endurance are introduced. Therapy may be required for as long as 6 months before normal activity, including overhead movement, can be resumed.[3,11,22]

Ligamentous Injuries (Shoulder Separation)

History

Injuries to the AC joint and surrounding ligaments are common shoulder complaints. They result from trauma, such as a direct fall on the shoulder or on an outstretched arm. A direct blow to the joint or a traction injury of the humerus can also injure the AC joint. Injuries to the AC joint involve damage to the ligament joining the acromion and the clavicle; as with other ligamentous damage, these injuries are classified as sprains. In practice, AC sprains are most commonly referred to as shoulder separations.

Physical Examination and Diagnosis

Three grades of separations are frequently seen in primary care, although six types of AC injury have been classified.[30] Grade I injury consists of damage only to the AC ligament without injury to the joint capsule (Figure 2-14). There is little clinical abnormality revealed on physical examination other than tenderness to palpation of the AC joint. An x-ray (AP view) film shows normal position of the AC area. It is considered a grade II AC injury when the AC ligament and joint are disrupted and there is damage to the joint capsule (Figure 2-15). Physical examination may reveal a bump over the AC area, and bruising may be present. An x-ray study will show a widening of the AC joint, and the distal end of the clavicle may appear to be somewhat high riding. Sometimes a comparison view of the opposite shoulder is required for accurate evaluation of apparent widening of the AC joint.

Grade III AC injury refers to damage not only to the AC ligaments and capsule, but also to the CC ligament (Figure 2-16). With a grade III separation, there is obvious deformity of the shoulder, with the lateral end of the clavicle pointing upward; this is attributable to tearing and disruption of the CC ligament. Bruising is often present, and, in addition to AC tenderness, movement of the shoulder (especially adduction and forward flexion) is painful.[8]

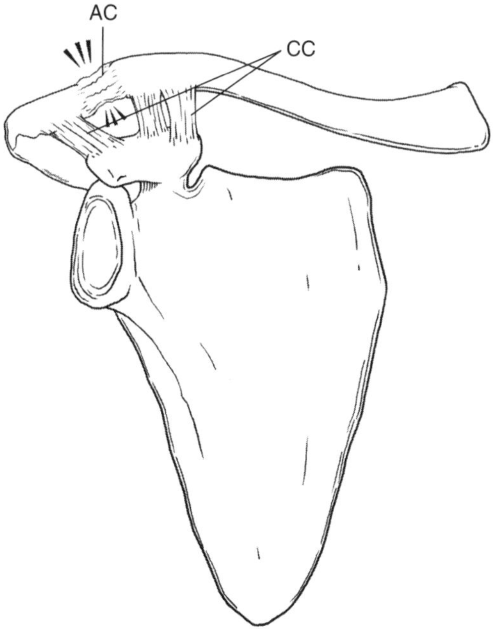

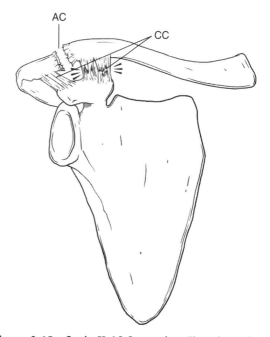

Figure 2-14   Grade I AC Separation. Both the AC and CC ligaments remain intact.

Figure 2-15   Grade II AC Separation. There is tearing of the AC ligament and stretching or partial tearing of the CC ligaments.

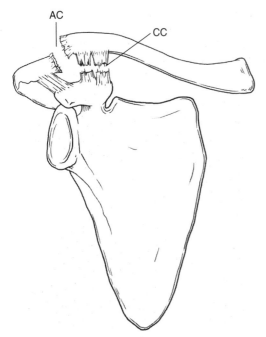

Figure 2-16   Grade III AC Separation. Both AC and CC ligaments are disrupted, resulting in some inferior displacement of the shoulder complex. The deltoid and trapezius muscles may be detached from the distal clavicle.

Treatment

Treatment of grade I through grade III separations includes application of ice, use of analgesics, and resting the shoulder, specifically by using a sling for 1 to 2 weeks. Initial ROM exercises are pendulum types of movements and are begun within a few days of injury. Grades I and II separations generally heal without sequelae within 6 to 8 weeks[27]; a patient with pain that persists for more than a few months should be referred to an orthopedic surgeon. Grade III AC separations involve dislocation of the AC joint and should be referred to an orthopedic surgeon. Although grade III AC separations heal with residual deformity (secondary to upward migration of the lateral clavicle), function is rarely affected.[21] Posttraumatic arthritis of the AC joint may develop with third-degree separations.

Sternoclavicular Injuries

The medial end of the clavicle, especially its articulation with the sternum, is rarely injured. When injury to this area occurs, it is often overlooked, even though it can occur with other serious injuries. Most sternoclavicular (SC) injuries are either sports related or attributable to motor vehicle accidents where a significant amount of force has been applied to the sternal area.

Considered the most serious injuries to this joint, SC dislocations can be either anterior or posterior. Posterior injuries pose a greater risk to the patient because of the potential for damage to underlying structures such as the trachea, esophagus, and great vessels.[36] Fortunately, anterior SC dislocations are more common than posterior ones.

History and Physical Examination

Patients usually relate a history of trauma or a fall, but atraumatic dislocation can also occur.[36] The patient may hold the arm of the affected side slightly forward and close to the body. Deformity is usually visible and may be accompanied by bruising. The SC area is tender to palpation and may be swollen. Patients should be referred to an orthopedic surgeon as soon as possible, since reduction of a SC dislocation can be difficult.

Diagnosis and Treatment

Any evidence of respiratory compromise or difficulty in swallowing is an emergency, and the patient should be transported to an emergency department. Plain x-ray films of the SC joint are difficult to obtain and interpret; computed tomography (CT) is the diagnostic modality of choice to evaluate the position of the injury and any resulting displacement of the clavicle.

Tendonitis

Tendonitis of the shoulder usually involves one of two structures: the rotator cuff or the biceps tendon. Although either can occur by itself, they frequently occur together.[24] Overusing or overstressing the shoulder are the predominant causes of tendonitis in this area. The supraspinatus tendon is the most commonly affected rotator cuff component.

Inflammation of the supraspinatus tendon can cause bursal inflammation and impingement. Chronic, untreated supraspinatus tendonitis can lead to rotator cuff rupture. When the supraspinatus tendon becomes inflamed, the already small area between the acromion and subacromial bursa through which it passes becomes even smaller. Pain occurs when, as a result, the tendon is compressed between the humerus and subacromial area.

Calcific tendonitis can also be the cause of shoulder pain. This condition can occur in patients with a history of significant shoulder use or repeated trauma to the shoulders (e.g., football players). However, most cases of calcific tendonitis are attributed to age-related wear-and-tear changes of the tendons. History and physical examination are similar to that seen in other forms of tendonitis, but x-ray studies typically reveal calcifications in the area of the supraspinatus tendon. The calcifications can be mistaken for avulsion fractures of the humeral head.

History

Patients generally recount a history of gradually worsening pain when performing overhead activities. Those prone to this problem include construction workers, plumbers, electricians, teachers, nurses, and pipe fitters. Pain is usually most severe over the supraspinatus insertion at the greater tuberosity of the humeral head; it is often sharp or aching and may radiate into the deltoid muscle or even down to the elbow. Pain does not extend below the elbow.

Weakness, numbness, and tingling of the hand do not generally occur; the presence of these symptoms is more indicative of a cervical spine problem. The patient frequently reports difficulty sleeping on the affected side.

Patients with bicipital tendonitis often relate similar symptoms and also report pain with heavy lifting. Differentiating between rotator cuff and bicipital tendonitis can be difficult on the basis of history alone.

Physical Examination

Tenderness over the supraspinatus tendon and the humeral head is common. Abduction of the shoulder may be uncomfortable and even painful. Resisted external rotation of the shoulder may be weak or painful. Isolated supraspinatus muscle testing (Jobe's test) is uncomfortable.

Bicipital tendonitis can be differentiated from rotator cuff tendonitis by the presence of tenderness in the bicipital groove.[24] Palpation of this area is made easier by having the patient allow the arm to hang loosely at his

or her side, then pronating and supinating the hand while the practitioner palpates the anterior portion of the humeral head. The groove is felt between the greater and lesser tuberosities.

Yergason's and Speed's tests are used to evaluate bicipital tendonitis. Yergason's test is performed by having the patient hold his or her arm close to the body and then flexing the elbow to 90 degrees while supinating the arm against resistance provided by the practitioner (Figure 2-17). Pain or tenderness in the bicipital groove is a positive test. Speed's test, which is more sensitive than Yergason's, is performed by having the patient fully extend the elbow, supinate the forearm, and forward flex the shoulder against resistance (Figure 2-18). Tenderness in the bicipital groove indicates bicipital tendonitis.

Diagnosis

History and physical examination are the prime factors in diagnosing tendonitis of the shoulder. An x-ray study may be helpful in gaining additional information regarding the relative size of the subacromial space or the presence of calcifications within the tendons. Some

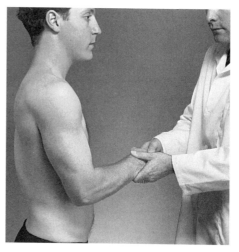

Figure 2-17 Yergason's Test. With the elbow flexed to 90 degrees, pain in the bicipital groove when the forearm is supinated against resistance can be indicative of biceps tendonitis. (From Reider B: *The orthopaedic physical examination,* Philadelphia, 1999, WB Saunders.)

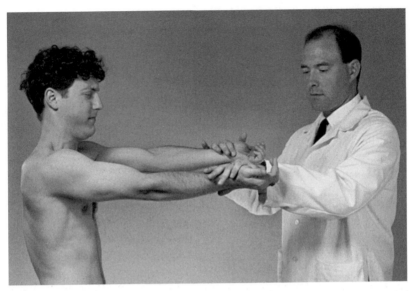

Figure 2-18   Speed's Test. While seated, the patient flexes the affected shoulder to 90 degrees, and the examiner provides resistance. While flexing the shoulder, the patient supinates the forearm, and completely extends the elbow. A positive test elicits increased tenderness in the bicipital groove and indicates bicipital tendinitis. (From Reider B: *The orthopaedic physical examination*, Philadelphia, 1999, WB Saunders.)

practitioners advocate waiting to obtain x-ray films until shoulder pain has been present for a minimum of 6 weeks.[24] Ultrasound, arthrogram, and magnetic resonance imaging (MRI) have also been used to diagnose tendonitis, but ordering these imaging studies should be left to the discretion of a specialist.

Treatment

Most cases of tendonitis will respond to conservative therapy: application of ice, nonsteroidal antiinflammatory drugs (NSAIDs), rest, and physical therapy. NSAIDs are usually prescribed for a 2- to 3-week course. Physical therapy modalities, including deep heat, ultrasound, and ROM exercises are generally helpful in alleviating symptoms. Individuals whose occupations require extensive overhead work, such as plumbers, electricians, fire sprinkler installers, and carpenters, often require a formal physical therapy program to regain strength and ROM, as well as to improve biomechanics of the shoulder. If the patient has an occupation in which shoulder activity is not prominent, ROM exercises can be performed at

home. Even though some patients may require 6 or more months of therapy, strengthening and endurance exercises should begin as soon as pain resolves and function begins to improve.[11] If there is no sign of improvement after 3 to 4 weeks of conservative therapy, the patient should be referred to an orthopedic surgeon.

Bursitis

Because of the proximity of the subacromial bursa to the insertion of the supraspinatus tendon within the relatively small subacromial space, inflammation of this bursa is frequently associated with other inflammatory conditions of the shoulder such as tendonitis. Bursitis tends to be an overuse type of abnormality and secondary to impingement or tendonitis.

History

Patients with bursitis have histories consistent with impingement syndrome or tendonitis. In practice, bursitis is usually considered a component of impingement syndrome.

Physical Examination and Diagnosis

There are no specific motions unique to bursitis. The best test for distinguishing bursitis from tendonitis is the injection of 5 to 10 ml of 1% lidocaine into the subacromial bursa. The test is positive when pain is relieved by the injection.

Treatment

Most bursitis responds to a course of NSAIDs, decreased overhead activity, and home exercises. Application of ice to the shoulder may alleviate acute pain. If the patient has no relief of symptoms within 2 to 3 weeks, a corticosteroid injection into the subacromial bursa may be indicated.

Rotator Cuff Injury

Rotator cuff injuries are considered to be more serious than other soft-tissue shoulder injuries However, most rotator cuff problems are the result of age-related wear on the muscles and tendons or untreated impingement that has progressed in severity.[3,12]

Rotator cuff injuries are rare in patients under age 40, but there is increasing evidence that aggressive physical activity or repeated trauma from contact sports may cause tears in younger patients.[3,11] Most full-thickness rotator cuff tears occur spontaneously in patients over age 50, presumably as the result of age-related tissue degeneration and changes in vascularity. The supraspinatus tendon is most often affected.

History

In patients over age 50, an acute, spontaneous onset of pain and an inability to abduct the shoulder are typical complaints associated with a degenerative tear of the rotator cuff. The patient may recount a history of reaching overhead (e.g., reaching into a cupboard, feeling "something give" in the shoulder, and then noticing that the ipsilateral arm dropped to the side). From that point on, the patient reports that it has been difficult and painful to abduct the arm. Pain frequently radiates laterally down the arm into the deltoid area; it may actually be worse when lowering the arm. Pain is almost always worse at night, and the patient is unable to sleep on the affected side. Some patients will experience decreased movement of the arm, rather than pain, as their primary complaint.

Physical Examination

Clinical signs associated with rotator cuff tears are essentially the same as those for impingement. Weakness with external rotation of the shoulder is a key finding of rotator cuff injury, since this is the only shoulder motion that involves only the rotator cuff muscles.

A visual examination of the posterior shoulder should assist the practitioner in assessing atrophy of the supraspinatus and infraspinatus muscles. Atrophy of these muscles, in combination with weak external rotation, is associated with chronic, large rotator cuff tears.

The drop arm test, in which the patient is asked to actively maintain the shoulder in 90 degrees of abduction and then to lower the arm slowly to the side, is considered a classic sign of a full-thickness rotator cuff tear if the arm falls to the side. In practice, a positive drop arm test is rarely seen, since most tears are relatively small. Most tears, particularly those that involve partial thickness tears of the muscle belly rather than the myotendinous region, will heal without surgical intervention.[18]

Diagnosis

In addition to the history and physical examination, several imaging studies are frequently employed to evaluate rotator cuff tears.

Plain x-ray films are still valuable in providing information regarding the subacromial space and the presence of subacromial spurring or soft-tissue calcifications that may contribute to impingement and tearing. When radiographing the shoulder, both a lateral scapular Y view and AP views should be ordered.

Ultrasound is gaining wider use as another noninvasive, lower-cost modality than MRI in evaluating partial-thickness rotator cuff tears. Depending on the expertise of the sonographer and the interpreting physician, ultrasound can be both highly sensitive and highly specific in determining the presence and size of tears.[29] As technique and technology improve, ultrasound may become the imaging study of choice for evaluating rotator cuff tears.

Arthrography, once considered the gold standard for diagnosing rotator cuff tears, has limited usefulness in visualizing the size of a tear. In addition, it is an invasive procedure that has the risk of introducing infection. In persons with metallic implants who cannot undergo MRI, arthrography may still be useful.

MRI has largely supplanted arthrography for diagnosing rotator cuff tears. Unlike arthrography, MRI can be used to evaluate the size of the tear, and it is noninvasive. It can also be used to differentiate tendonitis from bursitis. When a patient has ongoing pain and the clinical diagnosis is unclear, MRI is probably the diagnostic study of choice. Gadolinium-enhanced MRI provides greater sensitivity and specificity than noncontrast MRI. The greatest disadvantage of MRI is its expense.

Treatment

Conservative treatment of rotator cuff tears begins with the use of a sling for a few days and NSAID therapy for 1 to 2 weeks. During this period, subacromial injections are sometimes useful in reducing inflammation.[18] Maintaining shoulder motion is important; even in a sling, gentle pendulum-type exercises can be done. Physical therapy may improve ROM and strength. Although a massive tear of the rotator cuff will not be helped by conservative therapy, the clinical difficulty of differentiating tendonitis from a tear makes conservative treatment a reasonable first approach. Recommendations for the length of a conservative trial vary, but most practitioners advocate referral to an orthopedic surgeon and diagnostic testing if there is no improvement within 1 to 3 weeks. If surgical repair is performed, an adequate postoperative rehabilitation program is essential to regain optimal mobility and function. After surgery a return to normal function may require several months of therapy.

INSTABILITY

Shoulder instability is a frequent cause of the shoulder problems seen in the primary care setting. Impingement and instability may occur together. Normal GH stability is maintained by a number of complex biomechanical factors. Instability is the result of failure of the static stabilizers of the shoulder (primarily the three GH ligaments) to maintain the humeral head in the glenoid. Instability occurs with greater frequency in younger, athletic patients, particularly those who engage in overhead activity.[2,28]

Instability has been described as a continuum ranging from microinstability to complete dislocation. Multiple etiologies of instability exist. They include overuse, primary tendinitis, labral tears, generalized ligamentous laxity, traumatic and atraumatic instability, and posterosuperior glenoid impingement.[21] Most symptomatic instability is related to subluxation of the humeral head from the glenoid. Complete, acute dislocations are relatively rare and should be treated by an orthopedic surgeon.

Instability is generally classified according to direction, cause, and frequency of occurrence. Anterior instability is most frequently seen; other directions include inferior, posterior, and multidirectional. Ascertaining the cause of instability can help determine the most appropriate treatment and increase the likelihood of its success. For example, both a single episode of anterior instability after an acute trauma and instability caused by generalized ligamentous hyperlaxity tend to respond better to physical therapy than voluntary recurrent subluxation. The younger a patient is when the first episode of subluxation occurs, the greater the risk of recurrent subluxation; this is especially true of individuals under age 20.[33]

Anterior Instability

History

Anterior shoulder pain in athletes engaged in throwing sports or in patients who have a history of a "dead arm" in certain positions should be evaluated for anterior instability. Other common complaints include a sensation of the shoulder slipping out of the joint and a popping or clicking of the joint.[2] Some patients relate vague histories of discomfort and no real complaint of pain; in these cases, timing of symptoms and associated activity should be carefully determined.

Physical Examination, Diagnosis, and Treatment

Inspection may reveal that the individual holds the affected arm in a slightly abducted and externally rotated position. Examination should include the anterior apprehension test and the relocation test. The anterior apprehension test is performed by having the patient flex the elbow to 90 degrees, abduct the shoulder to 90 degrees, and then having the practitioner externally rotate the shoulder by raising the patient's hand (Figure 2-19). If the test is positive, the patient will have the sensation that the shoulder is about to subluxate again and will generally resist further external rotation.

While in this position, the relocation test can be done by applying posteriorly directed pressure on the anterior portion of the proximal humerus (Figure 2-20). This test is best performed with the patient lying supine on the examining table with the shoulder at the edge of the table. The patient with anterior subluxation will generally have a feeling of relief as the humeral head is relocated back in the glenoid. The test is positive if the patient's symptoms are relieved.

Inferior Instability

History

Patients with inferior instability may have few complaints other than pain when lifting light objects. Inferior instability is usually associated with either anterior or posterior instability; the most common direction for

subluxation to occur is anterior-inferior. On inspection no abnormality is noted, but a sulcus sign may be elicited on examination.

Physical Examination and Diagnosis

The sulcus sign is used to evaluate inferior instability. It is performed with the patient in a sitting position. With the patient's arm resting at the side, the practitioner pulls down on the humerus. An indentation, or sulcus, that appears between the acromion and humerus may indicate inferior instability (Figure 2-21). The distance between the acromion and the humeral head is then measured. A positive sulcus sign, by itself, does not indicate instability. The two shoulders must be compared, because there can be considerable normal variation in shoulder laxity.

Posterior Instability

Posterior instability of the shoulder is relatively rare; its incidence has been reported as between 2% and 5% of instabilities.[25] Patients may have a history of previous

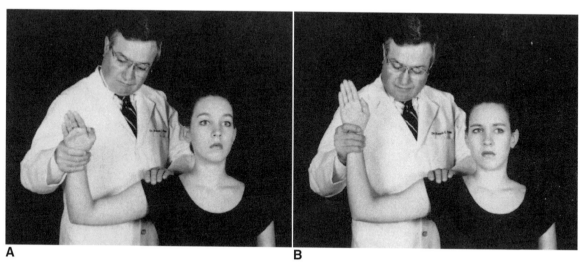

A   **B**

Figure 2-19   Apprehension Test. A, The patient is seated comfortably with the arms at the sides. The examiner slowly abducts and externally rotates the patient's affected shoulder. **B,** A positive test is indicated by a look or feeling of apprehension or alarm on the patient's face. The patient will usually resist further motion. The patient also may state that this maneuver duplicates the feeling of the previous dislocation. This test must be done slowly. If the test is done too quickly, there is a chance that the humerus will dislocate. A positive test indicates anterior shoulder dislocation trauma. (From Evans RC: *Illustrated orthopedic physical assessment,* ed 2, St Louis, 2001, Mosby.)

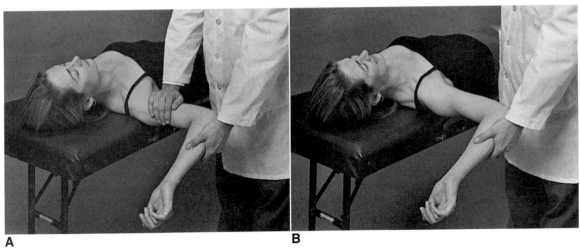

A   **B**

Figure 2-20   The relocation test is used to help confirm the diagnosis of anterior instability. **A,** While the arm is abducted and the elbow flexed to 90 degrees, posteriorly directed pressure over the proximal humerus is applied. **B,** Release of posteriorly directed pressure may cause return of pain or sensation of instability. (From Reider B: *The orthopaedic physical examination*, Philadelphia, 1999, WB Saunders.)

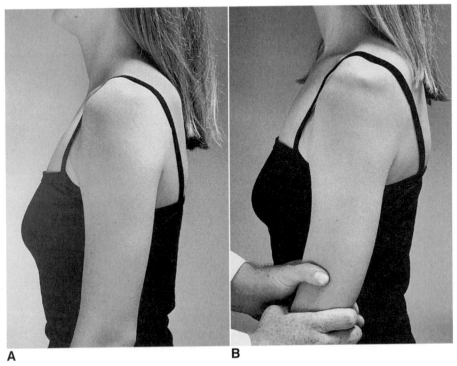

A   **B**

Figure 2-21   **A,** A downward-pulling force is applied to the patient's arm. **B,** An indentation (sulcus) at the acromiohumeral border may indicate inferior instability. (From Reider B: *The orthopaedic physical examination*, Philadelphia, 1999, WB Saunders.)

shoulder surgery, trauma, or generalized clonicotonic seizures.

History

Recurrent posterior subluxation of the shoulder is more commonly associated with patients who voluntarily sublux the shoulder. When obtaining a history, it is important to gain insight regarding possible secondary gain by the patient (i.e., sympathy or increased attention). Patients with incentives to voluntarily subluxate or dislocate the shoulder do poorly with either rehabilitation or surgery.[25]

Physical Examination and Diagnosis

On examination, internal rotation may be increased, and external rotation decreased. Inspection does not usually show any gross anatomic abnormality of the shoulder. Testing for posterior instability is performed by flexing the shoulder to 90 degrees and combining abduction with internal rotation while applying force to the humerus in an anterior-posterior direction[2] (Figure 2-22). If the test is positive, some patients will report feelings of instability; others may have only pain.

Multidirectional Instability

Instability in more than one plane is not uncommon. As previously noted, inferior instability is usually seen in association with either anterior or posterior instability.

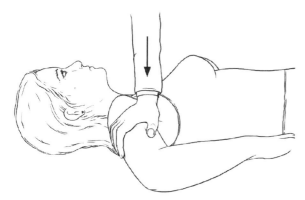

Figure 2-22   Testing for Posterior Instability. The shoulder is abducted and internally rotated while the practitioner applies posteriorly directed pressure to the proximal humerus.

This combination is termed multidirectional instability (MDI). If a patient has MDI but is diagnosed with only a unidirectional abnormality, rehabilitation is less likely to succeed. Overcorrection in one plane may actually precipitate problems in the opposite direction.

History

Clues to the presence of MDI include generalized ligamentous laxity, repetitive minor trauma associated with occupations requiring a great deal of overhead work, or sports requiring overhead throwing. Pain and feelings of the shoulder coming out of the socket, then popping or sliding back in are not uncommon.

Physical Examination and Diagnosis

In any case of instability, physical examination is crucial to making a correct diagnosis. Any pain or limitation of motion during both active and passive ROM should be noted. Tenderness of the anterior structures of the rotator cuff is not unusual. A neurologic assessment should be performed to rule out cervical disk or brachial plexus injury. Additional diagnostic testing includes x-ray studies, CT, and MRI.

A plain AP x-ray film of the shoulder in internal rotation may show a Hill-Sachs lesion of the humeral head. This lesion is seen as an indentation or divot on the posterior aspect of the humeral head. It may develop after repeated subluxations, but its absence does not exclude subluxation. The axillary Y-view can show an abnormality of the glenoid that may indicate wearing associated with subluxation.

Both CT and MRI should be ordered judiciously, because the expense of these imaging studies may not justify the amount of additional information they provide. However, CT and MRI, especially contrast studies, provide greater detail of the labrum than can be obtained with plain x-ray films. Caution should be used when ordering MRI in older patients, because age-related soft-tissue changes may mimic disorders of the glenoid and labrum.

Treatment

Physical therapy aimed at restoring strength and motion is the crux of initial treatment for shoulder instability. For acute subluxation, sling immobilization for a few days is indicated, followed by a formal physical therapy program. Therapy begins with activities designed to stretch the joint capsule. Once motion returns to a normal pattern, progressive strengthening exercises are begun.[2] If symptoms of instability continue after 3 to 6 weeks, the patient should be referred to an orthopedic surgeon.

Both arthroscopic and open repairs have been used to correct instability. At this time, open repair seems to have a lower incidence of recurrent instability. With advances in instrumentation and technique, arthroscopic repair may become the preferred surgical approach.

Superior Labrum Anterior and Posterior Lesions

History

Subluxation of the shoulder as a result of trauma may also result in injury to the labrum. A patient who has a history of a fall on an abducted arm with subsequent pain, locking, popping, snapping, or instability of the shoulder may have a labral tear. When the tear involves the superior aspect of the labrum and extends anteriorly and posteriorly, the injury is termed a superior labrum anterior and posterior (SLAP) lesion. SLAP tears are uncommon and are often associated with other problems, including instability and rotator cuff tears.[6,21,32] The superior portion of the labrum serves as an anchor for the long head of the biceps tendon on the glenoid; injuries in this area can cause significant disability.

Physical Examination, Diagnosis, and Treatment

The symptoms of SLAP lesions may mimic those of other shoulder complaints. Diagnosis is clinically difficult, and even with radiographic studies, arthroscopy is the primary mode of diagnosis.[6] Treatment of SLAP tears is surgical.

FRACTURES

Most shoulder fractures are the result of falls or direct blows to the shoulder area. As with all other fractures, any shoulder fracture should be referred to an orthopedic surgeon.

Clavicle Fractures

The most commonly broken bone in the body is the clavicle. The majority of these fractures involve the middle third of the bone, which overlies the brachial plexus. Fractures to the medial (proximal) third are the least common.

The major complications of a broken clavicle are associated injuries to the nervous or vascular systems and, occasionally, with a displaced clavicular fracture, to the pulmonary system.

History and Physical Examination

Patients typically relate a history of fall or other trauma. Movement of the shoulder or arm causes pain in the clavicular area. Deformity, usually swelling, is fairly obvious, and there is point tenderness over the fracture site. The ends of the fractured bone may be palpable. If the fracture is severely comminuted, tenting of the skin over the fracture may be visible.

Numbness and tingling of the fingers is not common; its presence may indicate associated injury to nerves of the brachial plexus. If it is present, the patient should be referred to an orthopedic surgeon. Ecchymosis over the anterior chest wall usually becomes evident several days after injury.

Diagnosis and Treatment

Plain x-ray films confirm the diagnosis. Two views, one an AP and another with the x-ray aimed 45 degrees cephalad, are usually ordered. Treatment consists of applying a clavicle strap, or a "figure-of-eight" shoulder bandage, for approximately 3 weeks. The use of a sling in addition to a clavicle strap may reduce discomfort. Even fractures that are displaced usually heal with this treatment. When healed, bony deformity at the site of the fracture is normal and permanent in adults. Functionally there is rarely any disability.

Distal or lateral clavicle fractures should be referred to an orthopedic surgeon, since attempts at immobilization of the bone using a clavicle strap are ineffective in stabilizing the bony fragments. The patient's arm should be placed in a sling before referral. These fractures are functionally similar to a separated shoulder and are treated with that in mind. Surgical repair may be indicated if the fragments are displaced.

Fractures to the medial clavicle (proximal third) are rare and often associated with other, severe trauma. A CT scan may be required to fully evaluate the extent of these injuries.

Proximal Humerus Fractures

Fractures to the proximal humerus involve the greater or lesser tuberosity or the anatomic or surgical neck. Cast immobilization of any of these is impractical. Because of frequent associated injury to surrounding structures, patients require referral to an orthopedic surgeon. Sling immobilization is appropriate in the primary care setting.

Proximal humerus fractures are often associated with osteoporosis. One result of an increasing elderly population is that proximal humerus fractures are being seen more frequently.[5] Most occur as a result of falling on an outstretched arm, but a proximal humerus fracture can also occur from a direct blow or a sudden, forced, hyperabduction injury to the shoulder.

Greater tuberosity fractures can be associated with rotator cuff tears and are sometimes the result of traumatic anterior shoulder dislocation. If the tuberosity fracture fragment is displaced by 1 cm or more, a rotator cuff tear is highly probable, since the greater tuberosity is the rotator cuff site of attachment. A displaced greater tuberosity fracture often requires surgical repair. Some orthopedic surgeons will surgically repair the fracture and the rotator cuff at the same time.

Lesser tuberosity fractures usually occur in conjunction with other fractures or posterior dislocation of the shoulder. If displaced, a lesser tuberosity fracture may indicate a tear in the subscapularis muscle. Fractures of the anatomic neck, which is more proximal than the surgical neck, are associated with the development of avascular necrosis of the humeral head. These fractures occur fairly often in association with tuberosity fractures, but they may be missed without careful radiologic examination and its expert interpretation.

The surgical neck is the most common site of proximal humerus fractures; usually these are easily seen on x-ray films. Associated damage to the axillary artery or the peripheral nerves is fairly common. Evidence of neurovascular injury requires immediate referral to an orthopedic surgeon for definitive treatment.

History and Physical Examination

The history of trauma can vary from a direct fall on the shoulder or a fall on an outstretched arm, to a motor vehicle accident or a sports-related injury. Some patients may recall feeling a pop, crack, or snap. Any report of numbness, tingling, or coolness of the fingers needs to be evaluated carefully to rule out nerve damage.

On examination the patient typically holds the affected arm close to the body and resists any movement. There may be soft-tissue swelling, but this can be difficult to assess in the shoulder clinically. Deformity is usually not significant, since the overlying muscles can obscure some bone displacement. Bruising may develop immediately or be delayed for hours or days.

A meticulous neurovascular examination is necessary for prompt identification and treatment of any associated injury. The presence of a peripheral pulse does not exclude axillary artery injury; consequently, even subtle signs of vascular compromise should be evaluated by a surgeon.

Diagnosis

Diagnosis of fractures to the proximal humerus depends on adequate x-ray examination. AP views of the shoulder in internal and external rotation and a lateral scapular Y view are the minimum. An additional film, the axillary view, is gaining increasing importance; it provides better information about both humeral alignment and glenoid integrity than other views.

Treatment

Most proximal humeral fractures can be successfully treated without surgery. A sling and swathe are used for approximately 2 weeks, and then early motion, consisting of pendulum exercises, is begun. Once the patient has started pendulum exercises, she or he should be instructed to perform them with the palm facing both front (external shoulder rotation) and back (internal rotation). A follow-up x-ray film is needed 4 to 6 weeks after injury; once the bone shows evidence of solid callus formation, active shoulder exercise can begin. Some patients may also require therapy to the elbow after it has been in a sling for 2 weeks. Most patients without associated rotator cuff injury will do well with this regimen.

Scapular Fractures

Overall, scapular fractures are quite rare; in a primary care setting they are rarer still. They occur primarily as the result of direct, high-energy injury and are often associated with other significant, even life-threatening injuries such as pneumothorax or pulmonary laceration.[20] Isolated scapular fractures can occur with lower-energy insult as a result of a direct blow or a heavy object landing on the posterior shoulder.

Because of the high incidence of associated severe injuries, which take precedence, diagnosis of scapular fractures is often delayed or even missed. Scapular fractures near the glenoid or acromion result in a greater degree of shoulder abnormality. Displaced scapular body fractures may result in suprascapular nerve injury and can also be associated with pulmonary injury. Fortunately most scapular fractures are nondisplaced because of the protection provided by the thick layers of muscular and soft tissues overlying the bone.

History and Physical Examination

Motor vehicle accidents, farm accidents, or falls from a significant height can all cause scapular injury, which is often signaled by posterior shoulder pain. Most of these patients will be evaluated and treated in a hospital setting. Persistent posterior shoulder pain, swelling, and decreased ROM without another cause may be attributable to a scapular fracture. Neurovascular symptoms are uncommon.

Examination may reveal soft-tissue swelling and tenderness over the scapula. Abduction of the shoulder may cause posterior shoulder pain. Deformity is not usually palpable. Suspected scapular fractures should be referred to an orthopedic surgeon after immobilizing the patient's arm in a sling and swathe.

Diagnosis

Lateral scapular, AP, and axillary x-ray films may show a fracture, but findings are generally very subtle and easily missed. The accepted radiographic tool for diagnosis is CT.

Treatment

Treatment is conservative; a sling and swathe is used for 1 to 2 weeks. As pain decreases, early passive ROM is started with pendulum types of exercises. Overhead, pushing, and lifting activities are restricted for about 6 weeks. A formal physical therapy program may be instituted to improve strength and motion, but many patients progress well with home exercises and gradual increases in activity.

MISCELLANEOUS SHOULDER PROBLEMS

Adhesive Capsulitis

Adhesive capsulitis, or frozen shoulder, is one of the more difficult shoulder problems to treat. Insidious in onset, it often progresses to a near-incapacitating level before treatment is sought. It most commonly affects patients older than age 50.

The usual cause is prolonged periods of disuse or immobilization. Immobilization may be the result of medical treatment such as use of a sling and swathe. Disuse is commonly the result of a patient's attempts to avoid painful movement. Thus a frozen shoulder can arise from conditions that cause painful shoulder movement, including bursitis, tendonitis, cervical spine disease, or muscle spasm; the patient first voluntarily avoids painful movement and then becomes progressively less able to move the shoulder. Other conditions, including diabetes, lung disease, and hyperthyroidism, have also been associated with adhesive capsulitis.[9] The patient's ROM progressively declines over a period of weeks to months.

History

Before seeking treatment, patients often experience decreased shoulder motion for several months. Sometimes they will be unable to recall an initial precipitating event. Pain does not necessarily accompany adhesive capsulitis, since the patient's ROM is limited so as to prevent any movement associated with pain. Pain is often worse at night, and the patient will be unable to sleep on the affected side.

Physical Examination

Examination reveals no gross deformity, but there may be atrophy of the deltoid or supraspinatus muscles. Atrophy of the supraspinatus and infraspinatus muscles may result in a prominent scapular spine on the affected side. There is no tenderness with palpation. The patient typically holds the arm close to the body. Decreased active and passive ROM is the cardinal finding noted on examination. Pain is present with ROM, most often with forward flexion and abduction. "Hiking up" of the scapula is common during abduction. Neurovascular involvement is indicated by any coolness, swelling, or tingling in the ipsilateral hand.

Diagnosis

Diagnosis is based primarily on history and physical examination. Plain x-ray films will help confirm the diagnosis by excluding the presence of a foreign body, significant AC degenerative joint disease, or dislocation.

Treatment

Adhesive capsulitis is difficult to treat. Aggressive physical therapy that concentrates on stretching and ROM may be required for up to 6 months. If no improvement is noted within 2 to 3 months of therapy, a manipulation under anesthesia may be necessary, followed by more physical therapy to rehabilitate the shoulder.

Prevention of adhesive capsulitis is important when treating the patient for other painful shoulder conditions. Early institution of pendulum exercises, moist heat, and the appropriate use of NSAIDs or analgesics will aid in maintaining shoulder mobility.

Thoracic Outlet Syndrome

Thoracic outlet syndrome (TOS) refers to a group of symptoms and complaints related to vascular or neurogenic compression of the subclavian artery or vein, or the brachial plexus. Compression can be either vascular or neurogenic in origin, but more often it is a combination of the two. The existence of the syndrome is still occasionally disputed, but most practitioners agree to its reality.

TOS has many synonyms, including first thoracic rib syndrome, cervical rib syndrome, Adson's syndrome, cervicothoracic outlet syndrome, pectoralis minor syndrome, Naffziger's syndrome, and neurovascular compression syndrome of the shoulder girdle.

TOS is generally classified into four categories: arterial, venous, classic neurogenic, and nonspecific neurogenic. Symptoms in any of these categories may be either functional or anatomic in origin. Functional TOS has symptoms that occur with specific activity; anatomic TOS symptoms are present regardless of activity.

Anatomy

The thoracic outlet is the area encompassed by the upper part of the sternum, the clavicle, the first rib, and the first thoracic vertebra. The blood vessels and nerves from the neck and mediastinum pass through the thoracic outlet on their way to the axilla. In addition to the thoracic duct, the vagus and phrenic nerves pass through the outlet, as does the sympathetic trunk.

The first rib has two grooves along its anterior surface. These grooves are separated by the insertion of the anterior scalene muscle. The subclavian vein lies in the more medial groove. The posterior groove, which lies behind the scalene muscle, contains the subclavian artery and the brachial plexus, which consists of the nerve roots of C5-T1. The first rib forms the floor of the opening and normally moves "like bird's wings" with inspiration and expiration.[17] The clavicle lies over the first rib just cranial to its posterior groove. The nerve roots of C8 and T1 pass laterally beneath the pectoralis minor muscle to reach the axilla; because of their anatomic position, these nerve roots can be readily affected by compression between the first rib and the clavicle. Because C8 and T1 further divide into the median and ulnar nerves, TOS symptoms may be similar to those of more peripheral ulnar and median neuropathy, and upper extremity complaints are common. Symptoms depend primarily on the location of the neurovascular compromise.

Functional TOS seems to be more common than anatomic TOS. It more often affects individuals in sedentary occupations or in certain jobs that stress the upper limbs. Construction and industrial workers whose jobs require repetitive movements, as well as secretaries, hairdressers, nursing staff, and cashiers, have an increased prevalence of TOS. Swimmers, professional or semiprofessional baseball pitchers, and quarterbacks are also at greater risk. Symptoms are generally unilateral.

Anatomic anomalies, such as cervical ribs or congenital bony or fibrous bands extending from a rudimentary cervical rib to the first rib, are less commonly associated with symptoms of TOS. It has been estimated that up to 50% of the population has cervical bands; therefore their usefulness in diagnosing TOS is limited. Entrapment of neurovascular structures in a narrowed costoclavicular space has also been proposed as the cause of symptoms.

Most cases of TOS are neurogenic in that symptoms of pain, weakness, paresthesia, and other complaints follow a C8-T1 nerve root distribution.[4] Pain may radiate into the anterior neck, upper chest, and even to the periorbital area.

Vascular TOS is usually attributable to venous obstruction, and patients may have symptoms typical of venous congestion, including swelling and cyanosis of the arm. Arterial TOS is the least common form, but its effects can be serious, leading to ischemia or even embolus formation of the upper extremity.

History

Pain, upper extremity tingling, sensory changes, weakness, coolness, and easy fatigability are typical TOS symptoms. Pain is most often described as a deep, dull, aching sensation that prevents normal usage. Overcompensation by the uninvolved extremity may cause pain, paresthesias, or other symptoms in the "good" side. There is some association of TOS with myofasciitis, whiplash injury, and bicipital and rotator cuff tendonitis.[4]

Physical Examination and Diagnosis

Diagnosis can be a challenge since characteristic changes in electromyography (EMG) or nerve conduction studies (NCS) are not always specific or present.[16] Neurologic examination of the upper extremity is important to rule out other types of neuropathy, such as ulnar nerve entrapment or carpal tunnel syndrome.

Three common tests used to evaluate TOS are Adson's test, Wright's test (or the hyperabduction test), and the abduction with exercise test (Roos' test). All three tests are provocative; they attempt to reproduce physiologic findings or symptoms, and none should be attempted for more than 1 to 2 minutes.

Adson's test is performed by having the patient extend and turn his or her neck toward the affected side and take a deep inspiration while the practitioner holds the patient's arm in a downward position and checks the radial pulse (Figure 2-23). The test is positive if the pulse is diminished or not felt at all. Unfortunately, the test is not an exceptionally specific one.

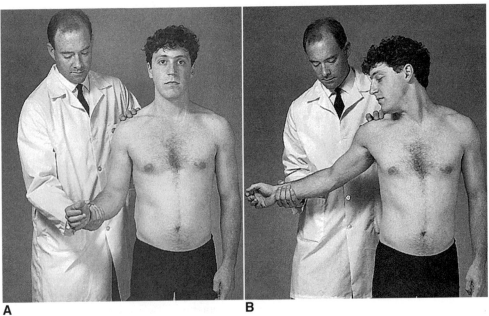

A   **B**

Figure 2-23   Adson's test is used to reproduce symptoms of thoracic outlet syndrome. **A,** Pulse quality is evaluated with the patient's arm resting at the side. **B,** The patient's shoulder is then abducted to 30 degrees and extended as far as possible while the head is turned toward the affected side. The practitioner palpates the radial pulse while the patient inhales deeply and holds the breath. A decrease or loss of pulse is considered a positive test. (From Reider B: *The orthopaedic physical examination*, Philadelphia, 1999, WB Saunders.)

Wright's test consists of having the patient hyperabduct the arm while externally rotating the shoulder. The practitioner notes any change in the radial pulse or any symptoms the patient has (Figure 2-24). If there is a change in the pulse and the patient has other TOS symptoms, the suggestion of TOS is increased.

Roos' test, abduction with exercise, is performed by having the patient abduct and externally rotate the shoulders to 90 degrees and then flex the elbows to 90 degrees while opening and closing the hands for 2 to 3 minutes (Figure 2-25). Any reproduction of symptoms, weakness, or neurovascular compromise indicates a positive test.

Treatment

Physical therapy is the initial treatment. It should be staged to progress from (1) postural training to (2) manual techniques to relax affected muscle groups, and then to (3) shoulder girdle muscle-strengthening exercises. Rest, heat, ice, muscle relaxants, NSAIDs, transcutaneous electrical nerve stimulation, and biofeedback are

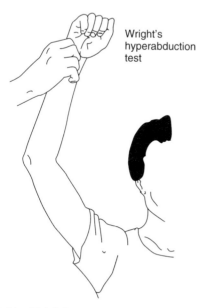

Figure 2-24 Wright's Test. Thoracic outlet syndrome may be present if the radial pulse quality diminishes while the shoulder is abducted. (From Atasoy E: Thoracic outlet compression syndrome, *Orthop Clin North Am* 27:285, 1996.)

often used in conjunction with physical therapy. If there is no improvement in symptoms after 2 to 4 months of physical therapy, referral for possible surgical intervention is indicated.

MISCELLANEOUS CAUSES OF SHOULDER ABNORMALITIES

Arthritis

Arthritis of the shoulder joint can be the result of trauma or of rheumatoid, osteoarthritic, or septic disease. Posttraumatic arthritis, which usually develops after age 40, can affect the AC or GH joints. Patients may or may not recall a specific traumatic event; a history of contact sports or a fracture or other significant trauma such as a motor vehicle accident increases the suggestion of this type of arthritis.[7] An x-ray study will confirm the diagnosis by showing degenerative changes and, often, evidence of previous fracture.

Rheumatoid arthritis of the shoulder is fairly uncommon. When it does occur, symptoms usually become noticeable later in the course of the disease; they are usually symmetric and follow a course typical of rheumatoid disease—morning stiffness with intermittent quiescence and flares. An erythrocyte sedimentation rate (ESR), antinuclear antibodies, and rheumatoid factor should be serologically evaluated if there is evidence of recurrent shoulder bursitis or other joint involvement.

Osteoarthritis (OA) typically affects older patients and may be more associated with crepitus than with pain. Adhesions may develop, which result in painful, decreased ROM. When OA is left untreated, muscle atrophy and adhesive capsulitis may develop. When accompanied by bony spurring, OA may be associated with tendonitis, impingement, and even rotator cuff tears. Diagnosis is confirmed on x-ray films.

Treatment of arthritis begins with ROM exercises, moist heat, and medication. Pain with OA is not always caused by inflammation; therefore a mild analgesic such as acetaminophen is an appropriate starting point. NSAIDs, including cyclooxygenase-2 (COX-2)–specific inhibitors are also appropriate. Most ROM exercises concentrate on stretching and can be performed at home. Moist heat is applied twice daily for symptomatic

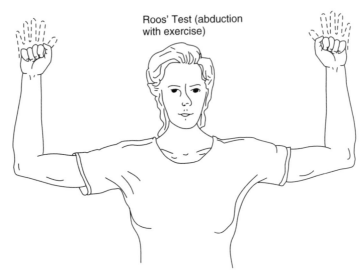

Roos' Test (abduction
with exercise)

Figure 2-25   Abduction with exercise test (Roos' test) is used to reproduce symptoms of thoracic outlet syndrome. (From Atasoy E: Thoracic outlet compression syndrome, *Orthop Clin North Am* 27:285, 1996.)

reduction of stiffness. If symptoms do not improve with 3 to 4 weeks of conservative treatment, referral to an appropriate specialist should be made.

Gout

The shoulder is an unusual initial site for gouty arthritis, but it can occur; gout is typically a monoarticular disease. An acute onset of a red, hot, painful joint in a patient with a history of hyperuricemia or a family history of gout should suggest to the practitioner the possibility of gout. Diagnosis is made by joint aspiration. Microscopic analysis reveals the presence of monosodium urate crystals in the joint fluid. Differentiating between gout and a septic joint is crucial for appropriate treatment of each. Treatment of gout in the shoulder is the same as the treatment of gout in other joints.

Infection

Septic arthritis of the shoulder joint is fairly uncommon. Elderly patients and those with chronic diseases or immune deficiencies are more prone to septic joint disease. Infection can be introduced by direct contamination from improper injection techniques, hematogenous spread, or inoculation from infected adjoining tissue. In

the shoulder, onset is often insidious, and symptoms may not be dramatic, but infection of any joint is an emergency. A history that includes fever, chills, nausea, vomiting, and lethargy in the presence of shoulder joint swelling (effusion) without other obvious pathologic conditions should suggest infection.[26]

Any patient who has an acutely inflamed, tender, erythematous joint accompanied by signs of systemic infection should be immediately referred to an orthopedic surgeon or emergency department. If facilities are available, blood work, specifically complete blood count with differential, blood cultures, and an ESR evaluation, need not be delayed until after referral. Joint aspiration with Gram's stain and culture provides the definitive diagnosis, but antibiotics may need to be started empirically before final culture results are available.

Neurologic Problems

Cervical radiculopathy and degenerative disk disease, especially of levels C4 through C6, can cause shoulder pain. If careful history and examination do not reveal any shoulder abnormality, cervical spine evaluation and x-ray studies should be performed. Cervical compression testing is the most sensitive indicator of cervical radiculopathy and is an important clinical test to help differentiate shoulder from radicular pain. Having the patient turn the head and slightly flex the neck while the practitioner applies downward pressure over the vertex of the skull (Spurling's maneuver, see Figures 1-14 and 1-15) is the most important clinical test for cervical radiculopathy. The presence of pain in the neck, shoulder, or arm is indicative of cervical disk disease; NCS and EMG will help differentiate pain sources.

Isolated nerve injuries can also affect shoulder function. The subscapularis nerve, which innervates the supraspinatus and infraspinatus muscles, can be damaged by overstretching or by nerve compression as a result of vigorous physical activity. The patient usually has no history of a single precipitating event. Typical complaints are a deep, aching pain and shoulder or arm weakness associated with specific planes of movement. A physical examination will usually reveal decreased ROM and weakness of specific muscle groups during resisted motion. If the clinical examination is inconclusive, diagnosis is confirmed by the results of EMG and NCS. Brachial plexus damage can result from traction types of injury to the upper extremity.

Injury to the suprascapular nerve may mimic cervical disk disease or rotator cuff pathology. Its symptoms are usually a dull aching over the lateral shoulder. Weakness of external rotation and abduction may be present.[31] Long thoracic nerve palsy has been associated with viral illnesses and immunizations and as a complication of surgical procedures performed near the axilla. Damage to the spinal accessory nerve can also occur with surgical procedures in the shoulder area.[16]

Ideally, treatment of neurologic pain is directed at correcting the underlying problem, but in reality most care is symptomatic. Physical therapy, directed at stretching and strengthening the appropriate muscle groups, combined with rest, NSAIDs, and moist heat, may diminish or eliminate symptoms. Referral to a neurologist, physiatrist, orthopedic surgeon, or neurosurgeon may be necessary if a course of conservative therapy is ineffectual.

Tumors

Benign and malignant tumors of both bone and soft tissue can affect the shoulder. Malignant bone tumors may be either primary or metastatic, the latter most commonly the result of primary sites of the thyroid, lung, breast, kidney, and prostate. A malignant apical tumor that infiltrates the brachial plexus and nearby vertebrae (Pancoast's tumor) can initially present symptoms similar to a rotator cuff tendonitis or shoulder strain.

Deep, unrelenting pain, particularly of an expanding nature, is suggestive of a tumor. An x-ray differentiation of benign and malignant tumors is extremely difficult and may not be possible in some instances. Any patient with evidence of bone tumor should be referred to an orthopedic surgeon or an oncologist if there is a history of malignancy.

INDICATIONS FOR REFERRAL

See the Red Flags box for referral information.

Red Flags *for Shoulder Disorders*

Patients with these findings may need to be referred for more extensive work-up.

Red Flags for Shoulder Disorders	Action
Bruising; AC joint tenderness; painful shoulder movement (especially adduction and forward flexion); obvious deformity of the shoulder (the lateral end of the clavicle pointing upward)	Possible grade III AC separation or dislocation of AC joint; refer to orthopedic surgeon
Arm of affected side slightly forward and close to body; sternoclavicular area tender to palpation and may be swollen; possible visible deformity and bruising	Possible sternoclavicular dislocation; refer to orthopedic surgeon as soon as possible; if evidence of difficulty in breathing or swallowing, refer patient to emergency department
No improvement of rotator cuff injury after 1 to 3 weeks of treatment	Possible need for surgery or further diagnostic testing; refer to orthopedic surgeon
Continued symptoms of multidirectional shoulder instability after 3 to 6 weeks	Arthroscopy and open repairs may be necessary; refer to orthopedic surgeon
A history of fall on abducted arm with subsequent pain, locking, popping, snapping, or instability of shoulder; may mimic other shoulder complaints	Possible SLAP lesion or lateral tear; refer to orthopedic surgeon
Any shoulder fracture	Refer to an orthopedic surgeon
No improvement in symptoms of TOS after 2 to 4 months of physical therapy	Refer to orthopedic surgeon for possible surgical intervention
No improvement in symptoms of arthritis within 3 to 4 weeks of conservative treatment	Refer to appropriate specialist
Acutely inflamed, tender, erythematous joint with signs of systemic infection	Immediately refer to orthopedic surgeon or emergency department; blood work, especially CBC with differential, blood cultures, and ESR need not be delayed until after referral
Course of conservative therapy for possible nerve injuries is ineffectual	Refer to neurologist, physiatrist, orthopedic surgeon, or neurosurgeon
Deep, expanding, unrelenting pain; radiographic presence of tumor	Possible bone tumor; refer to orthopedic surgeon or oncologist, if history of malignancies exists

AC, Acromioclavicular; *CBC,* complete blood count; *ESR,* erythrocyte sedimentation rate; *SLAP,* superior labrum anterior and posterior; *TOS,* thoracic outlet syndrome.

REFERENCES

1. Almekinders LC: Impingement syndrome, *Clin Sports Med* 20:491, 2001.

2. An YH, Friedman RJ: Multidirectional instability of the glenohumeral joint, *Orthop Clin North Am* 31:275, 2000.

3. Arcuni SE: Rotator cuff pathology and subacromial impingement, *Nurse Practitioner* 25:58, 2000.

4. Atasoy E: Thoracic outlet compression syndrome, *Orthop Clin North Am* 27:265, 1996.

5. Blaisier R et al: "Shoulder trauma: bone." In Beaty JH, editor: *Orthopaedic knowledge update 6*, Rosemont, Ill, 1999, American Academy of Orthopaedic Surgeons.

6. Burkhart SS, Morgan C: SLAP lesions in the overhead athlete, *Orthop Clin North Am* 32:431, 2001.

7. Carfagno DG, Ellenbecker TS: Osteoarthritis of the glenohumeral joint: nonsurgical treatment options, *Phys Sportsmedicine* 30:19, 2002.

8. Clarke HD, McCann PD: Acromioclavicular joint injuries, *Orthop Clin North Am* 31:177, 2000.

9. Connolly JF: Unfreezing the frozen shoulder, *J Musculoskel Med* 15:47, 1998.

10. Ebraheim NA and others: Quantitative anatomy of the scapula, *Am J Orthop* 29:287, 2000.

11. Evans PJ, Miniaci A: Rotator cuff tendinopathy: many causes, many solutions, *J Musculoskel Med* 15:32, 1998.

12. Faber KJ, Singleton SB, Hawkins RJ: Rotator cuff disease: diagnosing a common cause of shoulder pain, *J Musculoskel Med* 15:15, 1998.

13. Guanche C et al: The synergistic action of the capsule and the shoulder muscles, *Am J Sports Med* 23:301, 1995.

14. Halder AM, Itoi E, An K-N: Anatomy and biomechanics of the shoulder, *Orthop Clin North Am* 31:159, 2000.

15. Lazarus MD and others: Effect of chondral-labral defect on glenoid concavity and glenohumeral stability, *J Bone Joint Surg Am* 78(A):94, 1996.

16. Leffert RD: Nerve lesions about the shoulder, *Orthop Clin North Am* 31:331, 2000.

17. Lindgren KA: Thoracic outlet syndrome: A functional disturbance, *Muscle Nerve* 18:528, 1995.

18. Mantone JK, Burkhead WZ Jr, Noonan J Jr: Non-operative treatment of rotator cuff tears, *Orthop Clin North Am* 31:295, 2000.

19. Matsen FA et al: *Practical evaluation and management of the shoulder*, Philadelphia, 1994, WB Saunders.

20. McKoy BE, Bensen CV, Hartsock LA: Fractures about the shoulder, *Orthop Clin North Am* 31:205, 2001.

21. Meister K: Injuries to the shoulder in the throwing athlete. Part One: Biomechanics/pathophysiology/classification, *Am J Sports Med* 28:265, 2000.

22. Morrison DS, Greenbaum BS, Einhorn A: Shoulder impingement, *Orthop Clin North Am* 31:285, 2000.

23. Neer CS: Impingement lesions, *Clin Orthop* 173:70, 1983.

24. Patton WC, McCluskey GM: Biceps tendinitis and subluxation, *Clin Sports Med* 20:505, 2001.

25. Petersen SA: Posterior shoulder instability, *Orthop Clin North Am* 31:263, 2000.

26. Pommering TL, Wroble RR: Septic arthritis of the shoulder: treating an atypical case, *Phys Sportsmedicine* 24:75, 1996.

27. Rawes ML, Dias JJ: Long-term results of conservative treatment for acromioclavicular dislocation, *J Bone Joint Surg Br* 78(B):410, 1996.

28. Rizio L, Uribe JW: Overuse injuries of the upper extremity in baseball, *Clin Sports Med* 20:453, 2001.

29. Roberts CS, Walker JA II, Seligson D: Diagnostic capabilities of shoulder ultrasonography in the detection of complete and partial rotator cuff tears, *Am J Orthop* 30:159, 2001.

30. Rockwood CA Jr, Williams GR, Young DC: Injuries to the acromioclavicular joint. In Rockwood CA Jr et al, editors: *Rockwood and Green's fractures in adults*, ed 4, Philadelphia, 1996, Lippincott-Raven.

31. Romeo AA, Rotenberg DD, Bach BR Jr: Suprascapular neuropathy, *J Amer Acad Orthop Surg* 7:358, 1999.

32. Schulte KR, Warner JJP: Uncommon causes of shoulder pain in the athlete, *Orthop Clin North Am* 26:505, 1995.

33. Ticker JB, Fealy S, Fu FH: Instability and impingement in the athlete's shoulder, *Sports Med* 19:418, 1995.

34. Vanathros WJ, Monu JUV: Type 4 acromion: a new classification, *Contemp Orthop* 30:227, 1995.

35. Wang JC, Hatch JD, Shapiro MS: Comparison of MRI and radiographs in evaluation of acromial morphology, *Orthopedics* 23:1269, 2000.

36. Yeh GL, Williams GR: Conservative management of sternoclavicular injuries, *Orthop Clin North Am* 31:189, 2000.

Chapter 3

Arm and Elbow

The elbow joint is one of the most stable joints in the human body. The anatomy and biomechanics of the elbow are presented first, after which common soft-tissue injuries and frequently missed radial head and neck fractures are discussed. All these conditions can be diagnosed and treated in the primary care setting.

ANATOMY

Bony Structures

The elbow is a relatively stable hinge joint with three articulations: the ulnohumeral joint, the humeroradial joint, and the radioulnar joint. The distal humerus broadens to form the medial and lateral condyles. Adjacent to the medial and lateral condyles are the larger medial epicondyle and smaller lateral epicondyle. The epicondyles are the bony prominences that serve as the bony attachments for many of the forearm muscles (Figure 3-1).

Contained in the medial condyle is the trochlea, which articulates with the proximal ulna, forming the ulnohumeral joint. The capitellum, which articulates with the radial head and forms the humeroradial joint, is contained in the lateral epicondyle. The proximal radioulnar joint allows the radius to roll over the ulna, providing pronation and supination.

The superior aspect of the proximal ulna is concave to form a congruent articulation with the trochlea. This concavity is known as the trochlear notch. Anterior to the trochlear notch is the coronoid process. Just posterior to the trochlear notch is the olecranon, the prominent posterior tip of the elbow.

The proximal radius contains the radial head and neck with its tuberosity. The radial head is rather flattened and articulates with the capitellum. Just distal to the head is a section, smaller in diameter, known as the neck. A small bony prominence, the radial tuberosity, is where the biceps tendon inserts.

The elbow is always described from the anatomic viewpoint (palms facing anteriorly). The joint in that position has a normal valgus axis (Figure 3-2) and a range of motion (ROM) in four planes: flexion and extension (Figure 3-3, *A*) and supination and pronation (Figure 3-3, *B*).

Soft-Tissue Structures

The medial (ulnar) collateral and lateral (radial) collateral ligament complexes supply ligamentous support to the elbow. Each ligament originates from its respective condyle and then spreads in a triangular fashion to attach to the forearm bones. The medial collateral ligament is made up of the anterior and posterior bundles, and the oblique part. It is the primary constraint against valgus stress to the joint.[8,13] The Y-shaped lateral collateral ligament complex is composed of superior, anterior, and posterior bands. In addition to stabilizing the ulnohumeral joint, these bands maintain elbow stability against varus and external rotational forces.[24]

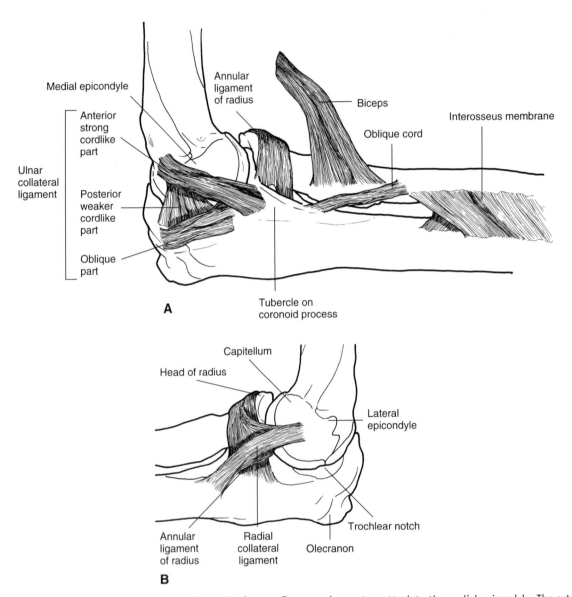

Figure 3-1   Basic Bony Anatomy of the Elbow. The forearm flexors and pronators attach to the medial epicondyle. The extensors and supinators primarily attach to the lateral epicondyle.

In women the estrogen effect on ligaments may cause a normal hyperextension of the elbow in full extension. On examination, this hyperextension will be found to be bilateral.

Muscles

There are two muscle compartments on the upper arm, the anterior and posterior. The anterior compartment contains the coracobrachialis, biceps brachii, and

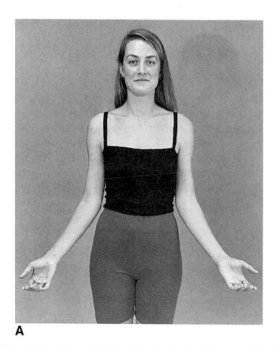

A

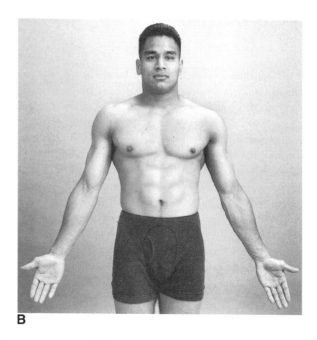

B

Figure 3-2   Normal Valgus Angle of the Elbow. This is also known as the "carrying" angle. A, Women tend to have a greater angle than B, men. (From Reider B: *The orthopaedic physical examination*, Philadelphia, 1999, WB Saunders.)

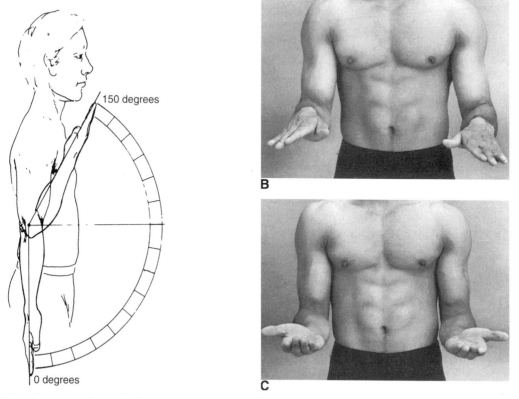

150 degrees

0 degrees

A

B

C

Figure 3-3   Four basic planes of elbow range of motion. A, flexion and extension; B, pronation; C, supination.

brachialis muscles. The triceps brachii and anconeus muscles are contained in the posterior compartment. The triceps attaches to the olecranon, the biceps attaches to the radius, and the brachialis inserts onto the ulna.

The muscles of the anterior compartment are best described as elbow flexors. In fact, the brachialis muscle acts solely as an elbow flexor. The brachioradialis and extensor carpi radialis muscles also assist in elbow flexion.[1] The biceps brachii helps flex the elbow but is also a powerful supinator of the forearm.[15] The musculocutaneous nerve innervates all these muscles. The pronator muscles of the forearm, the pronator teres and pronator quadratus, originate from the medial epicondyle and the distal ulna, respectively.

The radial nerve innervates the posterior compartment. The triceps brachii, as its name implies, has three heads; this muscle is the primary elbow extensor. The anconeus assists with initiating and maintaining extension. The extensor-supinator muscles of the forearm originate from a common tendon that attaches to the lateral epicondyle.

Neurovascular Structures

The median, radial, and ulnar nerves all cross the elbow joint. In the upper arm the median nerve courses anteriorly to the distal humerus and lies medially to the brachial artery. It then enters the antecubital fossa medially to the brachialis muscle and the biceps tendon. After crossing the elbow joint, the nerve passes between the humeral and ulnar heads of the pronator teres muscle; then it runs distally to the forearm beneath its flexor muscles.

Starting posteriorly in the proximal humerus, the radial nerve spirals around the bone, lying in the radial groove before it passes anteriorly, piercing the lateral intermuscular septum. The radial nerve lies anteriorly between the brachialis muscle, and the brachioradialis muscle bellies at the lateral elbow. Before crossing the elbow, the radial nerve divides into its superficial and deep branches. The nerve provides sensory innervation to the dorsoradial aspect of the hand and the extensor muscles of the finger and thumb.

The ulnar nerve (commonly referred to as the "funny bone") runs along the posterior upper arm, along the muscle belly of the triceps. It traverses the elbow just posterior to the medial epicondyle, lying in the cubital tunnel. At this point the nerve is very superficial. It then pierces the humeral and ulnar heads of the flexor carpi ulnaris muscle as it enters the forearm.

The brachial artery, a continuation of the axillary artery, provides blood supply to the arm. In the upper arm the brachial artery lies medial to the anterior muscle compartment. At the level of the elbow the brachial artery branches into the radial and ulnar arteries.

Physical Examination

The examination of the elbow begins with an inspection for symmetry, contour, alignment, and bony or soft-tissue enlargements. When inspecting the elbow, the practitioner should view both the anterior and posterior aspects of the joint. It is often helpful to compare the symptomatic side with the unaffected one. Bilateral comparison is helpful when assessing the normal "carrying angle" of the elbow. Normally, when the patient extends the elbows with the palms facing forward, as if carrying a bucket, valgus alignment is about 10 degrees in men and 13 degrees in women.[1] An increased angle may be attributable to previous trauma; it may also predispose the patient to ulnar nerve irritation.

The practitioner continues the examination by palpating three bony landmarks: the olecranon and the lateral and medial epicondyles. These three prominences should form a straight transverse line when the elbow is fully extended and an isosceles triangle when the elbow is flexed. Just distal to the lateral epicondyle is the radial head. The radial head, lateral epicondyle, and olecranon also form a triangle on the lateral aspect of the elbow (Figure 3-4).

The medial and lateral epicondyles are easy structures to palpate. They are very painful in conditions such as epicondylitis. After palpating the lateral epicondyle, the practitioner should move the examining finger distally approximately 1.5 cm to palpate the radial head. While pronating and supinating the patient's forearm, the radial head should be easily palpable. Exquisite pain at this site is typical of a radial head fracture. Posteriorly the prominent olecranon is also easily palpated; defects can often be felt with fracture or bursitis.

The patient should be asked to perform as much active ROM as is comfortable. Normal ROM is between

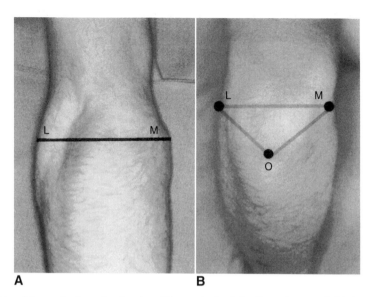

Figure 3-4　Relationship of the major bony landmarks of the posterior left elbow, **A**, extended joint and **B**, showing *L*, lateral epicondyle; *M*, medial epicondyle; and *O*, the olecranon. (From Colman WW, Strauch RJ: Physical examination of the elbow, *Orthop Clin North Am* 30[1]:18, 1999.)

0 degrees extension and 130 to 150 degrees of flexion. Pronation and supination are usually 90 degrees, 70 to 80 degrees at a minimum. Once again, bilateral comparison can be helpful in identifying any deficit. When there is a history of trauma, it is best not to perform passive ROM, since further injury may result.

Full extension is the most clinically relevant measure of motion. Limitation of full extension may suggest presence of an effusion, which can mechanically block full extension.[10,12] In addition, full extension of the elbow should elicit a "hard-end feel" and come to an abrupt end point at full extension. If the end point is soft and springy, an effusion may be present.

DISORDERS OF THE BONE

Radial Head or Neck Fractures

Fractures of the radial head or neck occur most often from falling on the outstretched hand, which transmits force to the elbow. Patients who fall and sustain a wrist injury MUST be examined for a concomitant radial head or neck fracture.

There are four basic types of radial head fractures. Three of the four types are illustrated in Figure 3-5. Type I fractures are the result of an impacting force onto the radial head. In adults, radial head fractures are almost always nondisplaced and can be easily missed on routine x-ray films. A type II radial head fracture involves the base of the radial head or the head itself and is displaced, impacted, or angulated. A type III fracture is comminuted, displaced, and involves the entire head. A type IV fracture involves dislocation of the radial head and capitellum. Any of these types of fractures require urgent orthopedic surgery referral.

History

A fall onto an outstretched arm is the most frequent history of a patient with a radial head fracture. In this type of injury, either the elbow or wrist may take the brunt of the force. Pain is usually immediate, and swelling occurs rapidly. An inability to move the elbow joint normally may be noticed by the patient before elbow swelling. Some patients wait to seek treatment, believing they have sprained the arm.

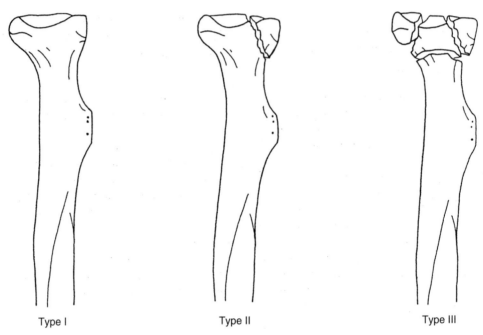

Type I   Type II   Type III

Figure 3-5   Three of the four most common types of radial head fractures. Type I fractures are common and can be treated in the primary care setting. (From Brown DE, Neumann RD, editors: *Orthopedic secrets,* ed 2, Philadelphia 1999, Hanley & Belfus.)

Physical Examination

Symptoms are characterized by swelling and exquisite point tenderness over the radial head or neck and an inability to fully extend the arm. Supination of the forearm is limited by pain. Flexion is limited secondary to accompanying joint effusion. Extension may be decreased due to mechanical blockage from a bone fragment or soft tissue. The presence of a joint effusion suggests an occult fracture, but this finding is more often true for adults than children.[21] Neurovascular status of the hand and fingers should be evaluated to rule out any associated nerve injury. If a patient has a history of trauma and has point tenderness over the radial head or neck, an anteroposterior (AP) and lateral x-ray study of the elbow is warranted.

Diagnosis

History and physical examination provide the basis for an accurate diagnosis but are insufficient alone. Even plain radiographic studies may not provide enough information to identify a radial head fracture accurately.

Because the most common types of radial head fractures are nondisplaced, they are often missed on initial x-ray films. This is attributable to the nature of the impaction fracture, since the bones run into one another and the fracture line is never seen. Sometimes a radial head fracture does not become apparent on x-ray films until several days after the injury. As a result the presence of soft-tissue findings on initial films can be useful in identifying the presence of a fracture.

One specific finding is known as a fat pad or sail sign. When a fracture occurs, the resulting hemarthrosis displaces the normal anterior and posterior distal humeral fat pads. It is important to look for a fat pad sign on the initial x-ray film; this sign indicates an effusion in the elbow and suggests that a fracture is likely (Figure 3-6). On a lateral x-ray film, this sign appears as a dark bulge that somewhat resembles a sail. Clinically the presence of a posterior fat pad sign is more important than an anterior fat pad.

Treatment

Nondisplaced radial head or neck fractures (see Figure 3-5) can be managed comfortably in the primary care setting. Treatment consists of a sling for 10 to 14 days

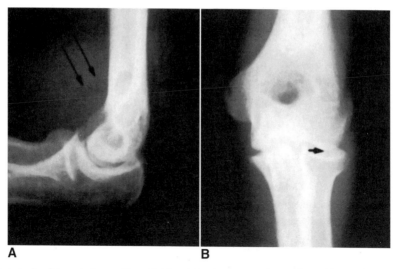

A   **B**

Figure 3-6   Positive anterior fat pad sign, with radial head fracture as seen on a lateral x-ray film. (From Mercier LR: *Practical orthopedics*, ed 5, St Louis, 2000, Mosby.)

and a course of nonsteroidal antiinflammatory drugs (NSAIDs). After 2 weeks the x-ray films should be repeated since new callus (bone) formation will be evident, indicating healing is occurring. At the 1- to 2-week mark the practitioner should prescribe gentle ROM exercises of the elbow, emphasizing elbow extension. Although return of full ROM is the goal of therapy, it is not unusual to have some residual loss of a few degrees of full extension if exercises are delayed or not practiced. Fortunately, however, the lack of a couple of degrees of extension is usually functionally insignificant.

Although most nondisplaced radial head fractures heal with a short course of immobilization and early ROM, if the practitioner is unfamiliar with radial head fractures, it is prudent to refer the patient to an orthopedic surgeon. Fractures other than types I or II may require surgical intervention.

Other Fractures Near the Elbow and Forearm

The practitioner should be familiar with a few additional types of fractures and injuries near the elbow and the proximal forearm. These typically require orthopedic referral and surgical stabilization.

Isolated fractures of the distal humerus are fairly uncommon in the adult seeking primary care. Fractures of the epicondyles usually occur in conjunction with an elbow dislocation. Most require surgical fixation. Supracondylar fractures are most often the result of a forced extension injury, usually forcing the distal humerus posteriorly.

Although a Monteggia fracture is more common in children, it can occur in adults. This fracture consists of a dislocation of the radial head combined with a fracture or the proximal ulna. Only 1% to 2% of forearm fractures are Monteggia fractures.[7]

Galeazzi fractures occur when the distal radial shaft is fractured and the distal radioulnar joint is dislocated. Other names for this injury include the "fracture of necessity," "reverse Monteggia" fracture, or "Piedmont" fracture. These fractures account for 3% to 6% of forearm fractures.

A "nightstick" fracture refers to an isolated ulnar shaft fracture. The term comes from its original description of victims of nightstick beatings, since they used their arms in an attempt to shield themselves from the blows. These fractures can be either displaced or nondisplaced. In either case, the fracture is notoriously unstable and often requires surgical stabilization or cast immobilization for up to 6 weeks or more.

SOFT-TISSUE DISORDERS

Lateral Epicondylitis (Tennis Elbow)

Lateral epicondylitis, commonly referred to as "tennis elbow," is not confined to tennis players. The name is associated with strong extensor action of backhand shots in racquet sports. It is quite common on the dominant extremity and in patients whose occupations or hobbies demand repetitive, rotary movements of the forearm.[6] It typically affects persons in their fourth and fifth decades. The specific pathogenesis of tennis elbow is degeneration of the tendon fibers at their insertion over the epicondyle. The presence of microtears of the tendon along with altered biomechanics and repair, rather than inflammation, has led some clinicians to use the terms epicondylagia or tendinosis when describing this pathology.[6,23]

History

Typically patients note the gradual onset of a dull ache along the outer aspect of the elbow, worsened by grasping and twisting motions. The pain is normally localized, but in severe cases it may radiate down the forearm and patients may complain of weakness in the arm and hand. Numbness and tingling are not associated with tennis elbow; if present, a neurologic problem may be the cause of pain or may be a coexistent condition.

Physical Examination

On physical examination, soft-tissue swelling may be present over the lateral epicondyle, but usually the elbow looks completely normal. There is exquisite point tenderness with palpation of the lateral elbow. Pain is typically most severe about 5 mm distal and anterior to the lateral epicondyle.[6] Resisted wrist extension typically exacerbates the pain; this provocative maneuver is diagnostic for lateral epicondylitis (Figure 3-7). Resisted extension of the long finger stresses the extensor comminus digitorum tendon that originates at the lateral epicondyle; this maneuver may also increase pain.

Sometimes combining supination of the forearm with resisted wrist extension elicits a greater pain response than resisted extension alone.

Medial Epicondylitis (Golfer's Elbow)

The abnormality of medial epicondylitis is similar to lateral epicondylitis; however, it is much less common and occurs at the flexor origin. Repeated flexion activities of the forearm, such as swinging a golf club, cause a localized periostitis over the medial epicondyle. On physical examination there is exquisite point tenderness over the medial epicondyle, and the pain is exacerbated by resisted wrist flexion. Maximal tenderness is about 5 mm anterior and distal to the medial epicondyle.

Diagnosis

The history and physical examination are generally all that are required to diagnose lateral and medial epicondylitis. Provocative testing is fairly specific for these problems. Disability and pain tend to be more severe in chronic lateral epicondylitis than in medial epicondylitis.[22] Before diagnosing medial epicondylitis, the practitioner should make certain that symptoms are not the result of an ulnar neuropathy. Clinically this differentiation can be made by tapping the ulnar nerve at the cubital tunnel (Tinel's test). Tinel's test is positive for ulnar nerve irritation if the patient experiences tingling and numbness in the little finger. An x-ray study is not usually necessary, but may be useful in ruling out soft tissue calcifications or osteochondral lesions.

Treatment

Initial treatment consists of measures to reduce pain and the avoidance of all aggravating activities. Applying ice to the affected epicondyle twice a day will reduce local inflammation. A tennis elbow band is helpful in many instances. The band acts as a biomechanical counterforce, relieving the tension from the epicondyle and transferring it to the band. Correct positioning of the band is crucial for maximal effectiveness (Figure 3-8). The band should be applied approximately two finger widths below the lateral epicondyle.

If symptoms do not improve within 6 weeks, a course of physical therapy that includes ultrasound, deep massage, phonophoresis, and other modalities can be pre-

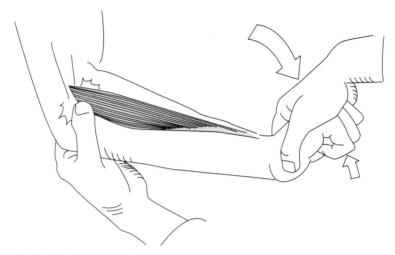

Figure 3-7   Provocative Testing for Lateral Epicondylitis. The patient attempts to extend the wrist against resistance. Pain over the lateral epicondyle is a positive test.

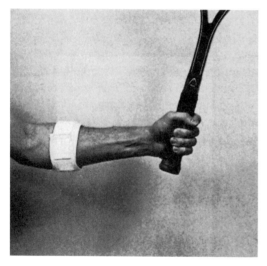

Figure 3-8   Correct Positioning of a Tennis Elbow Band. The band is worn over the proximal forearm, approximately the width of two fingers below the lateral epicondyle. (From Mercier LR: *Practical orthopedics*, ed 5, St Louis, 2000, Mosby.)

scribed to reduce inflammation. Once pain has lessened, the patient should be instructed to perform gentle wrist flexion-extension exercise with the elbow fully extended (Figure 3-9, *A, B*). If the symptoms persist after

6 weeks of physical therapy, other options should be considered. Corticosteroid injections remain somewhat controversial.[11,25,26] Injection of a local anesthetic, combined with a corticosteroid, often provides relief of symptoms.[3] Using aseptic technique, 2 ml of solution is injected into the peritenon area of the lateral epicondyle. One or two repeated injections at 6-week intervals may be necessary to provide relief. More than three injections rarely increase the likelihood of symptom remission.

If the patient is still symptomatic after three injections or 3 months after treatment and conservative measures have been exhausted, the patient should be referred to an orthopedic surgeon for evaluation and possible surgical treatment.

Olecranon Bursitis

Two clinically important bursae overlie the olecranon process, a point that is highly vulnerable to trauma. The bursa most often affected by inflammation lies between the skin and the attachment of the triceps muscle. Olecranon bursitis develops as the bursa sac fills with fluid secondary to a traumatic blow directly over the point of the elbow or with repeated trauma to the elbow (Figure 3-10). Bursitis can also develop secondary to other disease processes such as rheumatoid arthritis or

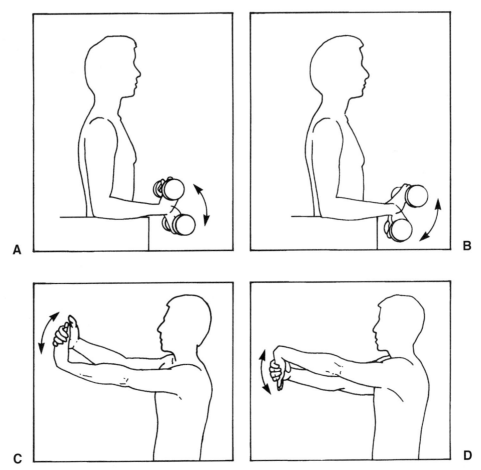

Figure 3-9   Exercises for Tennis Elbow. A and **B**, Wrist flexion and extension exercises should be performed with the forearm supported and using very light weights. **C** and **D**, Forearm stretching exercises with the elbow in extension. Stretches should be held for 5 to 10 seconds and repeated 10-20 times daily. (From Mercier LR: *Practical orthopedics*, ed 5, St Louis, 2000, Mosby.)

gout. Infection can also cause bursal swelling and pain. *Staphylococcus aureus* is the most commonly identified organism.[4] Many cases of olecranon bursitis are often misdiagnosed as nonseptic.

A patient with septic bursitis is more likely to have a fever, and he or she is more likely to have pain or tenderness over the bursa than the patient with nonseptic bursitis.[19] At least partially because of greater pain, these patients tend to seek treatment sooner than persons with nonseptic bursitis. Some degree of surround-

ing cellulitis is also more common with a septic bursa. Purulent bursitis requires incision and drainage in an operating room.

History

Localized swelling at the point of the elbow may follow a relatively minor trauma, such as bumping the elbow against a hard object. People who have desk jobs and frequently rest their elbows on the hard arms of a chair or on a desktop may develop chronic bursitis. Chronic bur-

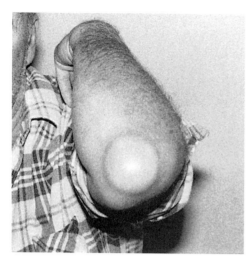

Figure 3-10 Clinical appearance of chronic olecranon bursitis. (From Mercier LR: *Practical orthopedics*, ed 5, St Louis, 2000, Mosby.)

sitis tends to present as a boggy, nontender area over the olecranon. Dry skin over the olecranon can be seen in patients with either acute or chronic bursitis.

Initially pain is relatively minor. As swelling progresses, the area becomes increasingly tender. In chronic bursitis the bursa may be painful with any pressure, even in the absence of significant swelling. Often the patient will report a feeling of "sponginess" or "bogginess" that is accompanied by swelling of the posterior elbow. Erythema tends to remain localized to the olecranon; spreading erythema may indicate cellulitis or a septic bursa.

Physical Examination

On physical examination there is marked localized swelling and fluctuation of the posterior aspect of the elbow. The area may be erythematous and warm. Tenderness is almost always present by the time a patient comes for evaluation, but it varies in intensity. The patient's ROM, particularly extension, is usually not affected; this helps differentiate bursitis from a joint effusion. If there is any skin breakdown or drainage (Figure 3-11), the patient may have a septic bursa or joint and should be immediately referred to an orthopedic surgeon.

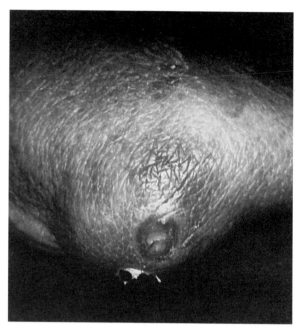

Figure 3-11 Clinical appearance of septic olecranon bursitis. Note the skin lesion and cellulitis. (From Noble J, editor: *Textbook of primary care medicine*, ed 3, St Louis, 2001, Mosby.)

Diagnosis and Treatment

The most important diagnostic challenge is to differentiate between bursitis and a septic joint. Patients with septic arthritis will have painful ROM along with erythema and effusion. In addition, a patient with a septic joint often appears acutely ill.

Aspiration (with an 18-gauge needle) of the bursa allows the clinician to examine the fluid (Figure 3-12). Aspiration should be performed under aseptic conditions, and fluid should be sent for Gram's stain, culture, crystals, and cell count if it is cloudy or purulent. If purulent, immediate referral to an orthopedic surgeon for operative drainage is necessary. Although injections are controversial, if the fluid is clear or bloody, the injection of a corticosteroid combined with a local anesthetic may prevent recurrence. After aspiration, a compression dressing can be applied over the site. Immobilization in a sling for 1 week may also be beneficial. *It is imperative that **no** corticosteroid medication be injected if there is any possibility of infection.*

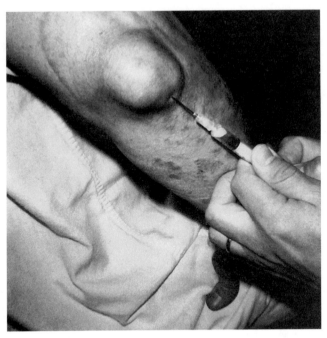

Figure 3-12 Technique of aspirating olecranon bursitis using a large bore needle. (From Noble J, editor: *Textbook of primary care medicine*, ed 3, St Louis, 2001, Mosby.)

If symptoms recur, an x-ray study is indicated to rule out exostosis (bone spurs), which may be causing the recurrent bursitis. If bone spurs are present, referral to an orthopedic surgeon is indicated to have the calcium deposits excised.

Elbow Sprains

Ligamentous injury to the elbow most often involves the medial collateral ligament. This type of injury is not uncommon in people who participate in overhead throwing activities.[5] As with other sprains the initial insult can be the result of repetitive microtrauma or an acute event. An acute trauma can result in an avulsion of a small bone fragment from the medial epicondyle.

History

The patient may recall a distinct event that precipitated the onset of pain, or he or she may just relate progressive pain along the medial aspect of the elbow. Pain tends to be aggravated by any activity that involves overhead throwing. Swelling may be "felt" rather than seen by the patient. Usually there is no significant decrease in ROM.

Physical Examination

When examining the patient, there is usually no significant discoloration around the joint. The medial aspect of the elbow is usually tender to palpation. Application of valgus stress to the joint in 30 degrees of flexion causes increased pain or instability. Application of valgus stress can be accomplished by the "milking maneuver." This test involves asking the patient to flex the affected elbow. With the hand of the "well" side, the patient reaches beneath the affected arm and grabs the thumb of the symptomatic side. This results in flexion of the wrist and valgus stress of the elbow and specifically tests the posterior band of the anterior bundle.[5]

Diagnosis

Diagnosis is based on the patient's history and physical examination. Stress radiographs can show joint widening.

Plain AP, lateral, and oblique radiographs may demonstrate tissue calcifications that indicate chronic or repetitive trauma.

Treatment

Treatment begins with resting the affected elbow by avoiding overhead throwing or other activities known to aggravate symptoms. NSAIDs may be helpful in reducing inflammation. A course of physical therapy directed at improving throwing biomechanics and promoting tissue healing is frequently helpful. Corticosteroid injection into the area between the epicondyle and tendon sheath may resolve symptoms. A throwing and reconditioning program begins once the individual has regained full ROM and strength. Full recovery from a medial collateral ligament injury can take up to 6 months. If the patient is a competitive athlete, he or she should be referred to an orthopedic surgeon or sports medicine physician for possible surgical intervention.

Tendonitis

Inflammation of the triceps tendon is a relatively rare cause of elbow pain, but it can occur in patients who engage in repetitive activities requiring forceful elbow extension, such as baseball pitching, tennis, or weight lifting. Pain tends to be localized to the posterior aspect of the distal humerus and is aggravated by resisted elbow extension. Treatment involves reducing inflammation and avoiding activities that cause pain.

Occasionally the triceps tendon can rupture, causing acute pain, localized ecchymosis, and weakness of elbow extension. This type of injury is usually the result of a fall onto an outstretched hand or a direct blow to the tendon. Sometimes there is a defect or a small loose body palpable at the site of the tear. Up to 80% of triceps tendon ruptures are associated with a bony avulsion fracture. If limitation of extension is great or an abnormality is noted on examination, the patient should be referred to an orthopedic surgeon for repair.

Biceps Rupture

Tearing of the biceps tendon can occur either at the proximal head or, less commonly, at the distal insertion. Regardless of location the basic cause is a sudden, eccentric load to the contracted muscle. One of the most common mechanisms for this injury occurs when a patient is carrying a heavy load that suddenly shifts. As the patient attempts to catch the load, the biceps cannot recover quickly enough to support the additional strain, and it tears. The use of anabolic steroids is associated with an increased risk of tendon rupture. Weight lifters, movers, body builders, and even snowboarders may be at increased risk for this injury. Men between ages 40 and 60 are most likely to sustain a distal biceps rupture.

Most patients can easily recall a single specific event associated with sudden, significant pain. Usually they will also recall hearing or feeling a pop in the upper arm immediately before the onset of pain. Pain generally subsides and becomes a deep, aching sensation. Ecchymosis and swelling occur soon after injury.

On examination, ecchymosis and a palpable (and sometimes visible) defect are discovered over the belly of the biceps. A palpable mass will be present distally if the proximal head of the biceps ruptures as the musculotendinous unit "falls" distally (Figure 3-13). A proximal mass indicates a distal biceps rupture. Pain and ecchymosis are present at the site of rupture. Weakness of elbow flexion and supination are typical.

Treatment can be conservative, consisting of rest, ice, and analgesic medication until acute pain subsides, but surgical repair tends to have a better outcome with regard to pain relief and function.[2,27] Residual weakness

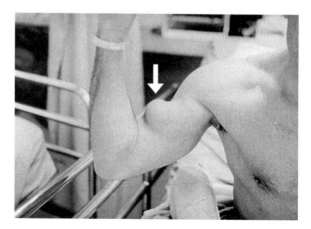

Figure 3-13 Clinical appearance of ruptured long head of biceps tendon. (From Reider B: *The orthopaedic physical examination*, Philadelphia, 1999, WB Saunders.)

is common; if the patient is athletic, young, or works in an occupation that requires strong elbow flexion or supination, surgical repair may be indicated. In these cases, patients should be referred to an orthopedic surgeon.

Dislocations

A fall onto an outstretched arm with the elbow extended can result in a fracture, dislocation, or both. The majority of elbow dislocations cause the forearm to dislocate posteriorly to the distal humerus (Figure 3-14). Almost invariably, an elbow dislocation also causes disruption of the medial and lateral collateral ligaments of the joint.[16]

A dislocation without an associated fracture is known as a simple dislocation; complex dislocations are associated with a fracture. Even simple dislocations can be complicated by neurovascular damage, especially to the median and ulnar nerves or to the brachial artery. Careful neurovascular assessment of the upper extremity is necessary.[9]

Simple elbow dislocations are generally first seen and managed in an emergency department. They can be difficult to reduce and are often manipulated under general anesthesia. After reduction, the elbow is rested in a sling, and gentle ROM exercises are started within 2 weeks of the injury. Surgery is rarely necessary to achieve adequate reduction. However, complex elbow dislocations often require surgical repair.

Cubital Tunnel Syndrome

Compression of the ulnar nerve at the elbow is commonly referred to as cubital tunnel syndrome. As noted earlier, the ulnar nerve is fairly superficial at the elbow and is therefore subject to traumatic forces. Normally the nerve lies within a tunnel on the posterior medial epicondyle. In some persons the nerve subluxates or dislocates over the medial elbow with elbow flexion; this dislocation is believed to make the nerve more susceptible to trauma.[18] Compression of the nerve can occur at the arcade of Struthers (a fibrous band of tissue that connects part of the medial humerus with the medial epicondyle), a frequent site of entrapment. Other causes of ulnar nerve injury at the elbow include traction, friction, and repetitive stretching.[17]

History

A patient with cubital tunnel syndrome typically reports a progressive, aching pain that begins on the medial side of the elbow and the proximal forearm. Symptoms tend to become more constant and may wake the patient at night. As symptoms increase, arm weakness may be noted. Numbness and tingling along the ulnar nerve distribution occur; the ring and little fingers are commonly affected. Since these two fingers are considered "grasping" digits, weakness may manifest itself as difficulty grasping or holding objects.

Physical Examination

Inspection of the upper extremity does not usually reveal any gross abnormality unless symptoms have been present for some time and there is muscle atrophy. Weakness of the intrinsic muscles of the hand is common; this is manifested by weakness of finger flexion, adduction, and abduction. Tinel's test is one of the most commonly used tools to evaluate cubital tunnel syndrome. If the patient experiences numbness and tingling along the course of the ulnar nerve when the examiner taps the ulnar nerve at the cubital tunnel, the result is a positive Tinel's test. However, it should be noted that up to 20% of the normal population has a positive Tinel's test without any evidence of cubital tunnel syndrome.[18]

Diagnosis

Diagnosis is based on clinical examination and the results of electromyographic and nerve conduction studies (NCSs). The practitioner should remember that NCSs are generally not helpful until symptoms have been present for at least 4 to 6 weeks.

Treatment

Conservative therapy involving splinting, medication, and avoidance of aggravating factors is helpful in many instances. A long arm splint (with the elbow in approximately 45 degrees of flexion), worn for 1 to 2 weeks with periodic removal for ROM exercises, may reduce inflammation or stretching of the nerve. Repetitive flexion of the elbow should be avoided, as should any activity that places direct pressure on the elbow.

If symptoms persist or worsen after a 3- or 4-week trial period, the patient should be referred to an ortho-

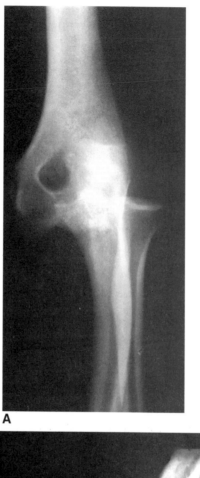

A

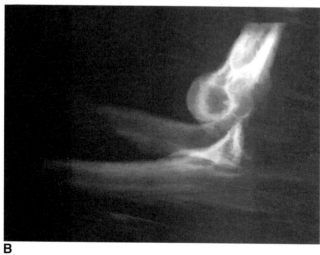

B

Figure 3-14   X-ray appearance of simple posterior elbow dislocation. **A**, AP view. **B**, Lateral view. (From Mercier LR: *Practical orthopedics*, ed 5, St Louis, 2000, Mosby.)

pedic specialist for surgical treatment. Although ulnar nerve transposition is the most commonly used technique, direct decompression of the nerve is sometimes performed.[14,20]

DIFFERENTIAL DIAGNOSIS

When evaluating elbow complaints, both the wrist and shoulder should also be assessed for abnormalities since either of these sites can cause referred pain to the elbow. Referred pain from the cervical spine can also cause elbow pain. The C5 dermatome supplies the lateral aspect of the elbow, C6 supplies the anterior portion, and C7 affects the posterior elbow.

INDICATIONS FOR REFERRAL

See the Red Flags box for referral information.

Red Flags *for Elbow Disorders*

Patients with these findings may need to be referred for more extensive work-up.

Red Flags for Elbow Disorders	Actions
Impacting force on radial head fracturing base of radial head or head itself; head is displaced, impacted, or angulated	Possible type I or type II radial head fracture; if practitioner is unfamiliar with radial head fractures, refer to orthopedic surgeon
Fracture is comminuted and involves entire radial head	Possible type III radial head fracture; refer to orthopedic surgeon; may require surgical intervention
Fracture involves dislocation of radial head and capitellum	Possible type IV radial head fracture; refer to orthopedic surgeon; may require surgical intervention
Forced extension injury, forcing distal humerus posteriorly	Possible fracture of the epicondyle; refer to orthopedic surgeon; possible surgical fixation required
Dislocation of radial head combined with ulnar shaft fracture	Possible Monteggia fracture; refer to orthopedic surgeon
Fractured radial shaft and dislocated distal radioulnar joint	Possible Galeazzi fracture; refer to orthopedic surgeon
Displaced or nondisplaced isolated ulnar shaft fracture	Possible "night stick" fracture; refer to orthopedic surgeon
Tennis elbow; symptomatic after three corticosteroid injections or 3 months' treatment; all conservative measures taken	Refer to an orthopedic surgeon for possible surgical treatment
Cloudy, purulent fluid aspirated from inflamed and swollen bursa joint	Possible septic joint; refer to orthopedic surgeon for operative drainage; *do not inject corticosteroid if infection is possible*
Recurring bursitis symptoms	Bone spur may be present; refer to orthopedic surgeon to have calcium deposits excised
Pain along medial aspect of the elbow; sometimes tender to palpation; application of valgus stress to joint in 30 degrees of flexion causes increased pain or instability	Possible elbow sprain; if patient is an athlete, refer to an orthopedic surgeon or sports medicine physician for possible surgical intervention
Inflammation of triceps tendon; acute pain, localized ecchymosis, and weakness of elbow extension; sometimes a defect or small body loose at site of tear	Possible triceps tendon rupture, if limitation of extension is marked or an abnormality is noted on examination; refer to orthopedic surgeon for repair
Biceps rupture in a young athlete, or in one who works in occupation requiring elbow flexion or supination	Refer to orthopedic surgeon; surgical repair may be indicated
Symptoms of cubital tunnel syndrome persist or worsen after 3 to 4 months of conservative therapy	Refer to orthopedic surgeon for ulnar nerve transposition, direct decompression, or other surgical intervention

REFERENCES

1. Bernstein AD et al: Elbow joint biomechanics: basic science and clinical applications, *Orthopedics* 23:1293, 2000.

2. Bernstein AD and others: Distal biceps tendon ruptures: a historical perspective and current concepts, *Am J Orthop* 30:193, 2001.

3. Bowen RE and others: Efficacy of nonoperative treatment for lateral epicondylitis, *Am J Orthop* 9:642, 2001.

4. Cea-Pereiro JC and others: A comparison between septic bursitis caused by *Staphylococcus aureus* and those caused by other organisms, *Clin Rheum* 20:10, 2001.

5. Chen FS, Rokito AS, Jobe FW: Medial elbow problems in the overhead-throwing athlete, *J Am Acad Orthop Surg* 9:99, 2001.

6. Ciccotti MG, Charlton WPH: Epicondylitis in the athlete, *Clin Sports Med* 20:77, 2001.

7. Clare DJ, Corley FG, Wirth MA: Ipsilateral combination Monteggia and Galeazzi injuries in an adult patient: a case report, *J Orthop Trauma* 16:130, 2002.

8. Cohen MS, Bruno RJ: The collateral ligaments of the elbow: anatomy and clinical correlation, *Clin Orthop* 383:123, 2001.

9. Cohen MS, Hastings HA II: Acute elbow dislocation: evaluation and management, *J Am Acad Orthop Surg* 6(1):15, 1998.

10. Colman WW, Strauch RJ: Physical examination of the elbow, *Orthop Clin North Am* 30:15, 1999.

11. Crowther MA and others: A prospective randomised study to compare extracorporeal shock-wave therapy and injection of steroid for the treatment of tennis elbow, *J Bone Joint Surg Br* 84:678, 2002.

12. Docherty MA, Schwab RA, Ma J: Can elbow extension be used as a test of clinically significant injury? *Southern Med J* 95:539, 2002.

13. Eygendaal D and others: Biomechanical evaluation of the elbow using roentgen stereophotogrammetric analysis, *Clin Orthop* 396:100, 2002.

14. Filippi R and others: Recurrent cubital tunnel syndrome: etiology and treatment, *Minim Invasive Neurosurg* 44:197, 2001.

15. Haugstvedt JR, Berger RA, Berglund LJ: A mechanical study of the moment-forces of the supinators and pronators of the forearm, *Acta Orthop Scand* 72:629, 2001.

16. Hildebrand KA, Patterson SD, King GJW: Acute elbow dislocations, *Orthop Clin North Am* 30:63, 1999.

17. Izzi J et al: Nerve injuries of the elbow, wrist, and hand in athletes, *Clin Sports Med* 20:203, 2001.

18. Khoo D, Carmichael SW, Spinner RJ: Ulnar nerve anatomy and compression, *Orthop Clin North Am* 27:317, 1996.

19. Laupland KB, Davies HD: Olecranon septic bursitis managed in an ambulatory setting: the Calgary Home Parenteral Therapy Program, *Clin Invest Med* 24:171, 2001.

20. Lowe JB III et al: Current approach to cubital tunnel syndrome, *Neurosurg Clin North Am* 12:267, 2001.

21. Major NM, Crawford ST: Elbow effusions in trauma in adults and children: is there an occult fracture? *Am J Roentgenology* 178:413, 2002.

22. Pienemaki TT, Siira PT, Vanharanta H: Chronic medial and lateral epicondylitis: a comparison of pain, disability, and function, *Arch Phys Med Rehabil* 83:317, 2002.

23. Runeson L, Haker E: Iontophoresis with cortisone in the treatment of lateral epicondylitis (tennis elbow): a double blind study, *Scand J Med Sci Sports* 12:136, 2002.

24. Seki A, Olsen BS and others: Functional anatomy of the lateral collateral ligament complex of the elbow: configuration of Y and its role, *J Shoulder Elbow Surg* 11:53, 2002.

25. Smidt N and others: Corticosteroid injections for lateral epicondylitis: a systematic review, *Pain* 96:23, 2002.

26. Speed CA: Corticosteroid injections in tendon lesions, *BMJ* 323:382, 2001.

27. Vardakas DG and others: Partial rupture of the distal biceps tendon, *J Shoulder Elbow Surg* 10:377, 2001.

Wrist and Hand

The human hand and wrist, with its remarkably complex anatomy, has evolved to permit the individual an unparalleled interaction with the environment. The interaction of nerves, tendons, ligaments, and bones and their nutritional blood supply provide the hand with an amazing capacity for maneuvering, strength, flexibility, and perception. The sum of this complex anatomy conveys to our species a mastery of our environment and the ability to generate limitless forms of art, music, communication, labor and much more. In fact, there are few activities specific to humans that do not involve the hand. The tremendous importance and function of the hand, in as much as it depends on the intricate balance of all its anatomy, requires a formidable level of *prompt* and *diligent* care to prevent disability.

ANATOMY

Bony Structures

The bony anatomy of the wrist joint consists, in part, of the articulation between the distal radius and the distal ulna. Known as the distal radioulnar joint, it allows pronation and supination of the forearm as the distal radius rolls over the distal ulna. The radiocarpal joint, or what most people consider the wrist joint, is the articulation between the distal radius and ulna and the proximal row of carpal bones (Figure 4-1).

The proximal carpal row consists, from radial to ulnar, of the scaphoid, the lunate, and the triquetrum.

The scaphoid is the largest of the proximal carpals. Lying next to it is the lunate, named for its resemblance on a lateral x-ray to a crescent moon. Both the scaphoid and the lunate articulate directly with the distal radius. On the ulnar aspect of the proximal row is the triquetrum (derived from the Latin word, triquetrus, or three-cornered). This bone is shaped somewhat like a pyramid. The triquetrum does not articulate directly with either the radius or ulna, but it shares joint surfaces with the lunate, the hamate, and the pisiform bones. The pisiform bone lies within the flexor carpi ulnaris (FCU) tendon and has an articulation with the triquetrum.

The wrist joint is not made up solely of the radiocarpal joint. The intercarpal joints form the remainder of this articulation. The intercarpal joints include the articulations between the proximal and distal carpal rows of bones.

Moving from the radial to the ulnar side of the wrist, the distal carpal bones are the trapezium, the trapezoid, the capitate, and the hamate. The trapezium lies between the scaphoid and the base of the first metacarpal; remembering that "the trapezium is under the thumb" helps distinguish its position from that of the trapezoid. The trapezoid somewhat resembles a wedge; it articulates with the scaphoid, the capitate, and the base of the second metacarpal. In the center of the row is the largest of all the carpal bones, the capitate. This bone articulates with the scaphoid, the lunate, the hamate, the trapezoid, and the bases of the second and third metacarpals. On the ulnar side is the hamate, most notable for its

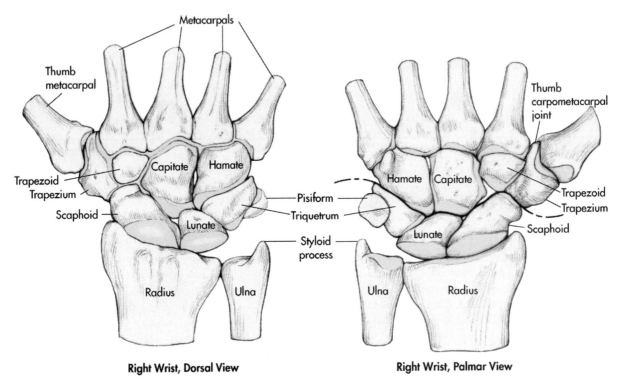

Figure 4-1   Dorsal and palmar views of right wrist and carpal bone. (From C.L.A.S.S.: *Clinical anatomy study system*, St Louis, 1996, Mosby.)

hooklike process. This carpal bone articulates with the capitate, the triquetrum, and the bases of the fourth and fifth metacarpals. The hamate is also important because it serves as an attachment for the flexor retinaculum and the insertion of the FCU muscle.

The distal row of carpal bones articulates with the metacarpal bones, thereby forming the carpometacarpal (CMC) joints. Traditionally the metacarpals and phalanges are numbered one through five, starting with the thumb as number one. The CMC joints of the index (second) and long (third) fingers are rather rigid and do not have much functional range of motion (ROM). The CMC joints of the fourth and fifth fingers, however, have much more motion. One can demonstrate this by grasping the heads of the fourth and fifth metacarpals and pushing them in a palmar or dorsal direction. Next, compare their degree of translation to those of the sec-

ond and third metacarpals by repeating this maneuver. This mobility is significant when one considers treatment of fractures and dislocations of these metacarpals. Figure 4-2 shows the anatomic relationship of the wrist and hand bones.

The metacarpal bones make up the breadth of the hand, whereas the phalangeal bones provide structure to the fingers. The proximal phalanges articulate with the metacarpals, forming the metacarpophalangeal (MCP) joints. Next, the bases of the middle phalanges form the proximal interphalangeal (PIP) joints by articulating with the distal ends of the proximal phalanges. Finally, the distal phalanges articulate with the distal ends of the middle phalanges, forming the distal interphalangeal (DIP) joints of the hand.

The articulations of the thumb are different from those of the other digits. The thumb's CMC joint (the

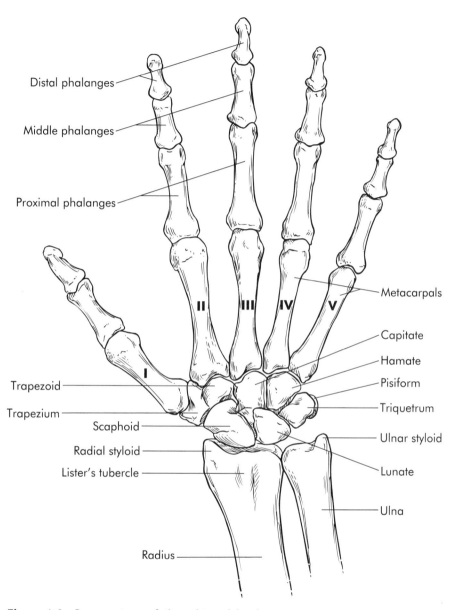

Figure 4-2 Bony anatomy of the wrist and hand. (From C.L.A.S.S.: *Clinical anatomy study system*, St Louis, 1996, Mosby.)

proximal phalanx on the trapezium) is a saddle joint, which allows for great ROM of the digit and allows the thumb to oppose the other digits, but predisposes this joint to premature arthritis.

Next is the MCP joint of the thumb, which comes into play in trauma of the ulnar collateral ligament. The thumb does not have a middle phalanx; therefore, only an interphalangeal (IP) joint is present.

Ligaments

Both the wrist and hand benefit from abundant ligamentous support. The joints of the wrist are strengthened by broad dorsal and palmar radiocarpal ligaments that connect the distal radius to the carpal bones. The palmar ligaments are named for their bony connections (Figure 4-3) and are more important clinically because of their role in preventing wrist instability.[22] The distal radioulnar joint has both dorsal and palmar ligaments.

An ulnocarpal ligament extends from the ulnar styloid into the carpal bones. Radial and ulnar collateral ligaments begin at their respective styloid processes and attach to the carpal bones.

In the carpal area of the wrist, there are dorsal and palmar intercarpal ligaments that run transversely and reinforce the connections between the bones of each carpal row. These ligaments connect the scaphoid and the lunate, the lunate and the triquetrum, the trapezium and the trapezoid, the trapezoid and the capitate, and finally the capitate and the hamate bones. The scapholunate ligament is very important in maintaining the normal stability between these adjacent carpal bones. Disruption of the scapholunate ligament can lead to pain, crepitus and accelerated degenerative changes of the wrist joint.[28]

Intercarpal interosseous ligaments also join and strengthen the articulations between the proximal carpal row and the radiocarpal joint. Small ligaments, called short collateral ligaments, further reinforce the radial and ulnar sides of the wrist.

Interosseous, palmar, and dorsal ligaments connect and help stabilize the intermetacarpal area and the CMC joints. The metacarpal heads of the second through fifth digits are connected by the deep transverse metacarpal ligaments.

Each of the joints of the hand is reinforced and protected by a number of ligaments. At the MCP, PIP, and

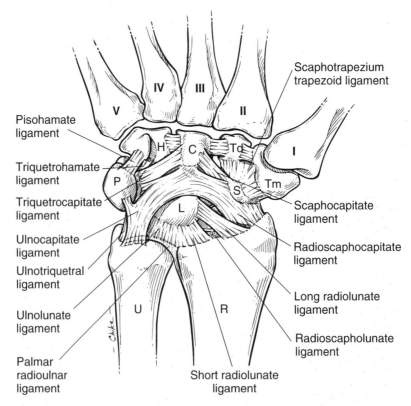

Figure 4-3   The palmar carpal tunnel ligaments of the right wrist. (From Mackin EJ et al, editors: *Rehabilitation of the hand and upper extremity*, ed 5, vol 1, St Louis, 2002, Mosby.)

DIP joints, both the palmar plate and collateral ligaments are present. The palmar plate serves to enlarge
the articular surface at the joints. The collateral ligaments, which are named for either the radial or ulnar
side of the digit on which they lie, provide stability of the
joints during flexion and extension. Injury to the collateral ligaments during strenuous manual activity or contact sports is not uncommon and can lead to permanent
disability.

Muscles

The muscular anatomy of the wrist area comprises the tendons of the forearm muscles that pass over the wrist joint.
There are six dorsal compartments on the extensor side of
the wrist that hold nine extensor muscles. A transverse
fibrous band of tissue, called the *extensor retinaculum*, defines
the borders of each of the six compartments (Figure 4-4).

   The first dorsal compartment, found over the radial
styloid, contains the extensor pollicis brevis and the

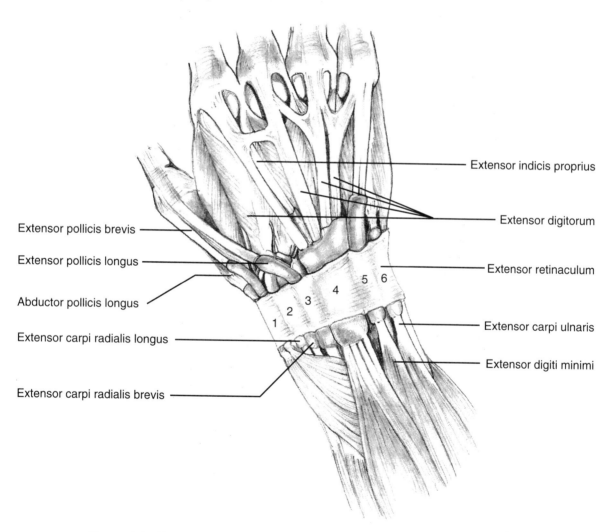

Extensor indicis proprius

Extensor digitorum

Extensor pollicis brevis

Extensor pollicis longus

Abductor pollicis longus

Extensor retinaculum

Extensor carpi radialis longus

Extensor carpi ulnaris

Extensor digiti minimi

Extensor carpi radialis brevis

Figure 4-4 The extensor retinaculum on the dorsum of the wrist. Each extensor
compartment is numbered. (From Mackin EJ et al, editors: *Rehabilitation of the hand and upper
extremity*, ed 5, vol 1, St Louis, 2002, Mosby.)

abductor pollicis longus. These muscles extend and abduct the thumb. Moving toward the dorsal side of the radius, the second dorsal compartment contains the extensor carpi radialis longus and the extensor carpi radialis brevis, which primarily extend the wrist and deviate it radially. The third dorsal compartment contains the extensor pollicis longus as it passes around Lister's tubercle on the dorsum of the distal radius. The fourth dorsal compartment contains the extensor digitorum communis (made up of four tendons) and the extensor indicis proprius. The fifth dorsal compartment, located over the distal radioulnar joint, contains the extensor digiti quinti proprius. The sixth and final dorsal compartment holds the extensor carpi ulnaris (ECU). Clinically, these compartments come into play in various pathologic conditions, such as DeQuervain's tenosynovitis, an inflammation of the first dorsal compartment.

On the palmar side of the wrist is the carpal canal, which contains all the flexor tendons to the digits and the thumb, as well as the median nerve. Like the dorsal aspect of the wrist, the palmar side has a deep fascial band, named the *transverse carpal ligament*, that maintains the position of the tendons when they contract. In total, nine tendons lie in the carpal canal. Other important tendons that cross the wrist but are not contained in the carpal canal are the FCU and flexor carpi radialis (FCR) tendons. Finally, the palmaris longus with its broad insertion into the palmar fascia also crosses the wrist, although it is absent in up to 15% to 20% of the normal population (Figure 4-5).[36]

The muscular anatomy of the hand includes those muscles which are contained and function solely within the hand, aptly named the *intrinsic* muscles of the hand. These intrinsic muscles can be divided into four groups: the lumbricals, the interossei, the thenar musculature, and the hypothenar musculature. The ulnar or median nerve provides innervation to each of the intrinsic groups.

Located at the base of the thumb, the thenar muscles are supplied by the recurrent branch of the median nerve, with the exception of the deep head of the flexor pollicis brevis, which is supplied by the deep branch of the ulnar nerve. These muscles include the adductor pollicis, flexor pollicis brevis, abductor pollicis, and opponens pollicis. The wad of soft tissue on the palmar

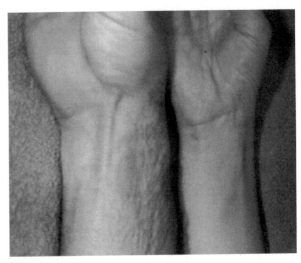

Figure 4-5 Presence *(left)* and absence *(right)* of palmaris longus tendon. (Courtesy Mara Dinits, MD, University of Maryland School of Medicine.)

side of the thumb represents this group of strong, bulky musculature.

Other muscles in the hand include the lumbricals and the interossei. The lumbricals basically allow simultaneous flexion of the metacarpal joint with extension of the PIP joint and DIP joints. The lumbrical muscles originate from the flexor digitorum profundus tendons near the distal end of the flexor retinaculum and combine to insert in the extensor mechanism of the PIP and DIP joints. The lumbricals lie along the radial aspect of the index, middle, ring, and little fingers (Figure 4-6). The two most ulnar lumbricals take innervation from the ulnar nerve; whereas the two most radial are supplied by the median nerve.

There are four dorsal and three palmar, or volar, interossei that act as flexors of the MCP joints with a direct insertion into the sagittal bands and palmar plate by the proximal phalanx. The dorsal interossei abduct the fingers away from the midline; the palmar interossei adduct the digits (Figure 4-7). All the interossei are innervated by the deep branch of the ulnar nerve.

Finally, the hypothenar pad is comprised of the abductor digiti minimi, flexor digiti minimi, and

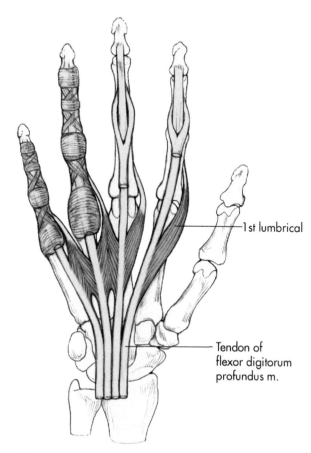

1st lumbrical

Tendon of
flexor digitorum
profundus m.

Figure 4-6 Palmar view of the left hand lumbrical muscles. (From C.L.A.S.S: *Clinical anatomy study system*, St Louis, 1996, Mosby.)

opponens digiti minimi muscles. These muscles are all supplied by the ulnar nerve.

Tendons

Tendons play a significant role in the complex movements of the digits. Both extensor and flexor tendons can be affected by trauma and disease. Some basic understanding of the extensor and flexor mechanisms is useful when clinically evaluating hand and finger problems.

The anatomy of the extensor mechanism of the digits is quite complex and beyond the scope of this text. Briefly, however, it is important to note that the extensor digitorum muscle of the forearm gives rise to the extensor tendons of the fingers. The extensor tendons,

which lie on the dorsum of the hand, tightly attach to the joint capsules of the digits. At each joint, fibers from the tendons pass from dorsal to palmar, forming an envelope type of structure around each joint called the extensor hood. Each finger's extensor tendon is divided into three portions: two lateral bands and one central slip. The central slip, which attaches on the dorsum of the middle phalanx of each digit, is important in that it allows and maintains normal extension of the joint. The reader is referred to hand anatomy texts and to the ongoing detailed description for an explanation of the extensor mechanism.[12,27]

A few details of flexor tendon anatomy must be understood. After entering the central area of the palm, the flexor tendons of the hand fan out toward their associated digits. Each digit has a pair of flexor tendons, one superficial (flexor digitorum superficialis) and one deep (flexor digitorum profundus). The superficial flexor tendons attach to the shaft of the middle phalanges (in the case of the thumb, to that of the proximal phalanx). The flexor digitorum profundus tendons attach to the base of the distal phalanges.

The flexor tendons pass through a closed retinaculum, which has occasional reinforcements called pulleys (Figure 4-8). Of importance is the A1 pulley, which occurs just proximal to the MCP joint of the digits. The A1 pulley is important in trigger finger abnormalities that are discussed in a later section. Clinically the A2 and A4 pulleys are the most important. The A2 overlies the proximal phalanx, and the A4 overlies the middle phalanx. These pulleys prevent a phenomenon called bowstringing, a process that reduces the mechanical efficacy of the flexor tendon.[2]

Neuroanatomy

Motor function to the hand is supplied by branches from the median and ulnar nerves. The radial nerve provides no motor (muscle) innervation in the hand. Sensation is supplied by the radial, median, and ulnar nerves (Figure 4-9); these three nerves arise from the lower cervical or first thoracic nerve roots (C7, C8, T1).

The median nerve is contained within the carpal canal at the wrist (Figure 4-10). The median nerve supplies sensation to the palmar aspect of the hand and thumb and of the index and middle fingers, as well as of

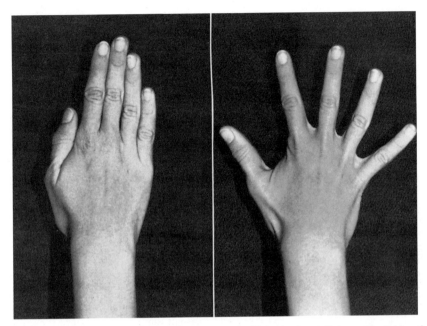

Figure 4-7   Testing Function of the Interossei. With the hand flat on the table, the patient is asked to spread the fingers apart. Abduction and adduction are assessed from the relationship of the digits to the axis of the third metacarpal. (From Mackin EJ et al, editors: *Rehabilitation of the hand and upper extremity*, ed 5, vol 1, St Louis, 2002, Mosby.)

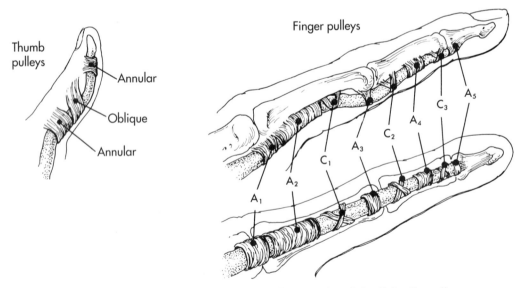

Figure 4-8   The extensive pulley system of the flexor tendon of the digits. The pulleys are designated A for annular or C for cruciate. (From Mackin EJ et al, editors: *Rehabilitation of the hand and upper extremity*, ed 5, vol 1, St Louis, 2002, Mosby.)

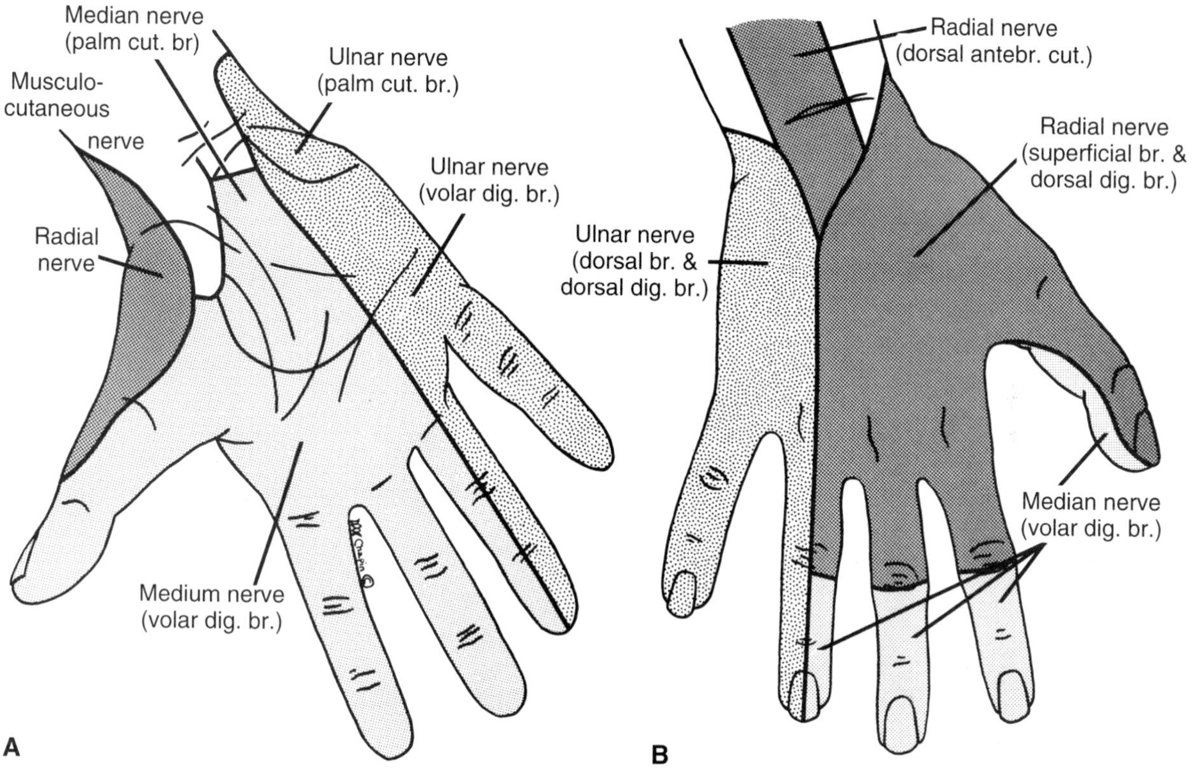

Figure 4-9   Sensorimotor Innervation of the Hand. A, Volar (or palmar) aspect. **B,** Dorsal aspect. (From Noble J, editor: *Textbook of primary care medicine,* ed 3, St Louis, 2001, Mosby.)

the radial half of the ring finger; dorsally it innervates the middle and distal phalanges of the index and middle fingers, as well as the radial half of the ring finger. The deep recurrent branch of the median nerve innervates the thenar musculature (except for the deep head of the flexor pollicis brevis).

At the wrist the ulnar nerve travels under the FCU, crossing the wrist into the hand via Guyon's canal. The ulnar nerve supplies sensation to the ulnar aspect of the hand, both dorsal and palmar, including the small finger and the ulnar half of the ring finger. The dorsal radial side of the wrist is innervated by the dorsal sensory branch of the radial nerve, where it exits near the first dorsal compartment.

The digital nerves, which are divisions of the ulnar and median nerves, provide sensation to the fingers. The digital nerves send cutaneous branches dorsally near the PIP joint to provide sensation to the dorsal fingertip. The more proximal dorsum receives some innervation from cutaneous branches of median, radial, and ulnar nerves, depending on the digit.

EXAMINATION OF THE HAND

General History

An experienced clinician will often note that a diagnosis can be made in the majority of cases simply by obtaining a detailed account from the patient of the inciting events. The location, timing, character, and alleviating factors of pain all must be described. The specific location and progression of numbness, tingling, popping or clicking, as well as the position of the hand or arm when these symptoms occur, is extremely important.

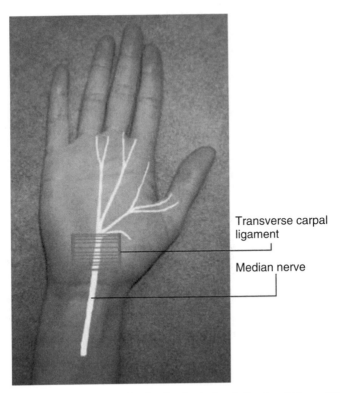

Transverse carpal
ligament

Median nerve

Figure 4-10 Typical median nerve distribution in the hand. (Courtesy RA Pensy, MD, University of Maryland Department of Orthopedics.)

Describing previous treatment efforts will often help a patient report the underlying pathology. Finally, a quick, general past medical history is important when considering diseases such as gout, rheumatoid arthritis, peripheral vascular disease, diabetes, and so on.

Questions regarding trauma are generally straightforward. However, certain injury patterns deserve special mention. For example, paint gun injuries can be especially misleading because an innocuous appearing pinpoint entry wound may belie the tremendous amount of tissue destruction that has tracked through the finger and into the palm.[21] Electrical burns in this area, as in other parts of the musculoskeletal system, should be treated with respect because of the amount of tissue damage throughout the course taken by the electrical current. Chemical injuries or splashes will often require a specific treatment protocol, and this history should be given to a poison control center and the physician to

whom the patient has been referred. An important distinction must be made between crush versus laceration injury mechanisms. Elements to consider are where the injury may have been sustained – whether in fresh, salt, or swamp water, on a farm or in handling animals – or, if a bite has occurred, what species of reptile or mammal may have been involved. Finally, a large risk of joint infection and resultant osteomyelitis is carried by a benign-appearing laceration overlying an MCP joint that is the result of an altercation in which the MCP has struck an opponent's mouth.[24]

Physical Examination

In general, examination of the wrist should include at least a cursory evaluation of the elbow. Many problems that are expressed at the wrist, particularly those of a neurologic nature, may actually start at the elbow. Initial examination of the wrist and hand should always include

Box 4-1	*Normal ROM for the Wrist and Hand*
Wrist extension	at least 80 degrees
Wrist flexion	20 degrees
Ulnar deviation	30 degrees (usually exceeds radiation by 10 degrees)
Radial deviation	20 degrees
Supination	80 degrees
Bronation	80 degrees
Thumb flexion (MCP joint)	approximately 60 degrees
Thumb extension	0 degrees (but the thumb can have extension of 10 to 40 degrees)
Thumb flexion(IP joint)	0 to 80 degrees
Thumb abduction	at least 50 degrees
Thumb opposition	is measured as the largest possible distance, in centimeters, from the flexor crease of the thumb IP joint to the distal palmar crease directly over the middle finger MCP joint
Lesser digits (MCP joints)	from 0 to 90 degrees
PIP joints	from 0 to 100 degrees
DIP joints	from 0 to 70 degrees

DIP, Distal metaphalangeal; *IP,* Interphalangeal, *MCP,* metacarpophalangeal; *PIP,* proximal Interphalangeal; ROM, range of motion.

an evaluation of ROM. Having the patient make a clenched fist will often demonstrate the location of pathology quickly. Box 4-1 summarizes normal ROM.

Examination of the hand and wrist first entails inspection. Look for any obvious deformity in the bony structure, such as the "silver fork" deformity (i.e., when the distal radius fracture is angulated, the wrist has the appearance of the curve of a fork) classically associated with a Colles' type of wrist fracture (described in the section "Distal Forearm Fractures"). Note any rotational deformity of the digits by comparing the orientation of the nail beds and the orientation of the digits with flexion of the MCP and PIP joints. Occasionally metacarpal and phalangeal fractures result in rotational abnormalities that manifest themselves most readily in the disruption of the normal "cascade" of the fingernails.

Obvious swelling is a good indication of trauma, but intercarpal dislocations can be accompanied by subtle degrees of swelling and minimal deformity. To more accurately assess swelling and evaluate for local injury, the next step is palpation. Gently palpate the wrist and the digits, looking for any crepitus or tenderness; either may indicate underlying bony abnormalities. Some fractures of the hand and wrist are difficult to visualize on x-ray films; consequently, delineating exact points of maximal tenderness, although potentially uncomfortable for the patient, will allow the astute examiner a better chance of arriving at the correct diagnosis.

Neurologic Examination

Figure 4-9 illustrates the sensory distributions of the median, radial, and ulnar nerves. The most accurate test of the *sensory* function of the median nerve is done at the tip of the index finger, that of the radial nerve at the dorsal first web space, and that of the ulnar nerve at the tip of the small finger. The *motor* function of the median nerve can be evaluated most accurately by having the patient make the "OK" sign, that of the ulnar nerve by

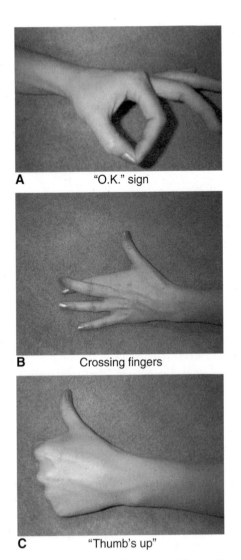

Figure 4-11 Testing motor function of the median nerve **(A)**, ulnar nerve **(B)**, and radial nerve **(C)**. (Courtesy RA Pensy, MD, University of Maryland Department of Orthopedics.)

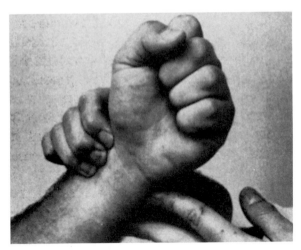

Figure 4-12 Allen's Test. Both the radial and ulnar arteries are manually occluded at the wrist, then the ulnar artery is released while radial artery compression continues. A normal response (negative test) occurs when circulation is restored to the hand. (From Mercier LR: *Practical orthopedics*, ed 5, St Louis, 2000, Mosby.)

having the patient cross the fingers, and that of the radial nerve by having the patient give the "thumbs-up" sign (Figure 4-11).

The vascular examination of the hand is also important. The radial and ulnar artery pulses should be palpable on the palmar side of the wrist just proximal to the wrist flexion crease. Allen's test should be performed if any occlusive disorder is suggested or if there are lacer-ations over the wrist (Figures 4-12 and 4-13). This test involves elevating the affected hand, having the patient make several successive clenched fists, then compressing both the ulnar and radial arteries at the wrist. After releasing pressure over the radial *or* ulnar arteries, a competent arterial tree will allow complete return of flow through the released artery, and the hand should regain its pink hue.

Occlusive disorders can be embolic phenomena, for instance those that occur from the mural thrombi sometimes seen with an atrial septal defect. An unusual but troublesome problem is Buerger's disease, an inflammation of the blood vessels that can arise in male cigarette smokers, who often develop severe occlusive problems.

Soft-tissue examination of the hand and wrist should always include an inspection and evaluation of any areas of swelling. Color can be quite important, especially in vascular occlusive problems.

It is often helpful to palpate soft tissue around the wrist and hand, especially if tenosynovitis is present. Boggy tenosynovitis can be seen in rheumatoid arthritis (RA) or infection and can occur around either the extensor tendons or flexor tendons. Palpation can also

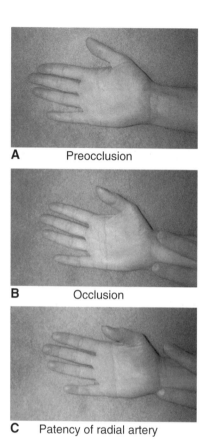

A   Preocclusion

B   Occlusion

C   Patency of radial artery

Figure 4-13 Allen's Test. Allen's test is performed by **A,** evaluating preocclusion circulation to the hand; **B,** occluding the radial and ulnar arteries; and **C,** releasing the occlusion of one of the arteries and observing return of circulation. (Courtesy RA Pensy, MD, University of Maryland Department of Orthopedics.)

help to eliciting tenderness over areas where there are soft-tissue problems, such as over the A1 pulley in the trigger finger. The snapping of the flexor tenosynovium through the A1 pulley can often be palpated.

ABNORMALITIES AND TREATMENT

Phalangeal Fractures

Phalangeal fractures are among the most common hand fractures seen in primary care. They are often concusing a crush injury or a direct blow. A fracture to any of the phalanges creates its own specific set of potential complications.

The proximal phalanx is more commonly fractured from a direct blow than either the middle or distal phalanges. Proximal phalanx fractures can cause damage to the flexor or extensor tendons. Fractures of the middle phalanx, especially near the base, can also result in flexor or extensor tendon damage. Injury to the palmar plate is not uncommon with a fracture to the palmar aspect of the base of the middle phalanx. Since this is the area where the flexor tendon inserts, loss of function may occur if the injury is not properly treated. Distal phalanx fractures are most frequently associated with a crush injury, such as being struck with a hammer or caught between two heavy objects.

Sometimes a fracture sustained during an altercation can be attributed to a rotational force that also causes a rotated digit. These injuries are usually unstable, and the patient should be referred to an orthopedic hand surgeon.

History. Most patients are able to recall a specific event that caused the trauma. Immediate onset of either pain or numbness is typical. The patient may recall hearing or feeling a pop or crack, and swelling develops rapidly. The patient may apply ice to the digit soon after injury. A patient with a phalangeal fracture may relate that he or she did not believe the digit was broken "because I could still move it." In an unstable fracture, any attempt to move the digit may result in crepitus and increased pain.

Physical Examination. Almost universally, swelling of the affected digit is present. Fractures around joints often have greater local edema than those in the shaft of the bone. Ecchymosis is not always present, depending on how soon after injury the patient is seen. Movement is usually limited and painful. Point tenderness over the site of fracture is typical. Any evidence of rotational, ulnar, or radial deviation indicates a displaced fracture that will likely require reduction.

Diagnosis. History and examination provide the basis for diagnosing a finger fracture. Radiographic (x-ray) studies are usually all that are necessary to confirm the diagnosis. Simple anteroposterior (AP), lateral, and oblique views are the standard projections. These views will generally provide sufficient information to evaluate the presence, orientation, and any displacement of the fracture.

Treatment. Treatment of phalangeal fractures deserves special attention. Splinting the hand can be fraught with pitfalls. A poorly designed splint worn too long will often result in stiffness that far surpasses the original injury's impact on function.

A distal phalanx fracture often involves a subungual hematoma; if this involves more than 50% of the underlying nail bed, it is an indication to have the nail removed and the nail bed repaired by a hand surgeon to prevent long-term nail deformity.[13] Often relief of the intense pressure and pain from a subungual hematoma can be obtained by boring a small hole through the nail with a sterile 18-gauge needle. The fracture itself is usually amenable to splinting with a prefabricated Stax or Alumifoam splint that crosses the DIP joint only.

Middle and proximal phalanx fractures, if nondisplaced, can often be splinted to good result. However, splints need to be applied carefully to only the affected digit, or at most to one adjacent digit for stability, to prevent stiffness to other, noninvolved digits. In general, the fingers should be splinted in the "intrinsic plus," or the function/protection position: with the MCP joints flexed at or near 90 degrees, and near full extension at the PIP and DIP joints (Figure 4-14). Anatomically this keeps the collateral ligaments of the respective joints stretched, preventing them from scarring in a shortened state and thus decreasing mobility of the joint. Extensive rehabilitation will be required for the unfortunate patient who has been placed in a splint that is ill fashioned and worn longer than 2 to 3 weeks. Therefore, most if not all fractures of the phalanges should be referred to a hand specialist for definitive care, and they should be seen promptly for follow-up to prevent stiffness.

Avulsion Fractures

A commonly seen injury is an avulsion fracture off the base of the middle phalanx at the PIP joint (Figure 4-15). It is very important for the examiner to rule out instability of the PIP joint. Often the injury causes a joint to dislocate and then spontaneously reduce.

It is important to assess the competency of the radial and ulnar collateral ligaments to allow the injury to be treated appropriately. The practitioner needs to look for subluxation of the PIP joint on x-ray films. If no subluxation is noted and the joint is stable on examination, "buddy taping" for a period of 2 to 3 weeks is an appropriate treatment. If the joint demonstrates instability on ROM testing, the joint should be splinted in a reduced position and the patient urgently referred to a hand surgeon.

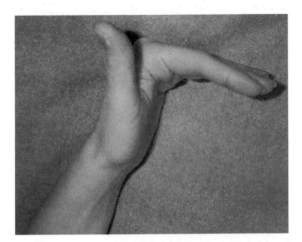

Figure 4-14 Intrinsic Plus Position. Splinting in this position helps maintain function of the collateral ligaments of the digits. (Courtesy RA Pensy, MD, University of Maryland Department of Orthopedics.)

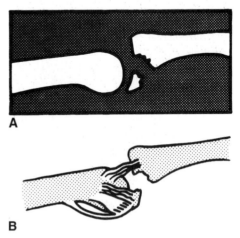

Figure 4-15 Diagrammatic X-ray Representation. A, An unstable fracture of the base of the middle phalanx. **B,** A pull of flexor tendon and collateral ligament that causes a fracture displacement. (From Noble J, editor: *Textbook of primary care medicine,* ed 3, St Louis, 2001, Mosby.)

Metacarpal Fractures

Fractures of the metacarpals, especially the fifth, are usually the result of a direct blow to the hand. One of the most commonly seen injuries is an apex dorsal angulated fracture of the distal portion (neck) of the fifth metacarpal (Figure 4-16). Called the boxer's fracture, this injury is often the result of punching a relatively immovable object (e.g., a wall or a head). Similar fractures can occur in any of the lesser digits. A rotational component to these fractures is not unusual. The patient with a rotated fracture should be referred to an orthopedic surgeon.

A fracture of the distal fifth metacarpal does not always require complete anatomic reduction to provide a return to normal function. The acceptable degree of angulation varies according to which metacarpal is affected. Angulation up to thirty degrees is acceptable in the fifth metacarpal, because, as mentioned earlier, this metacarpal has the greatest arc of motion at its articulation with the carpal bones. Fractures of the first, second, and third metacarpals have less tolerance to angulation because of the more limited motion of their respective CMC joints. Residual angulation of the metacarpal fracture will often generate an extensor lag, a loss of the ability to completely extend the digit (Figure 4-17).

History. The usual history of a metacarpal fracture involves a direct blow to the bone. Fights, falls, and motor vehicle accidents are all common causes. Pain and swelling are almost immediate. Normal extension of the finger is usually impossible soon after injury, but it may improve to varying degrees over the first few days. Numbness and tingling of the finger are common but usually resolve. Ecchymosis over the base of the finger and over both the palm and dorsum of the hand is common.

Immediate referral to an emergency department or a hand surgeon should be made for any lacerations over a joint that result from an impact with another individual's mouth or teeth. High rates of infection and associated

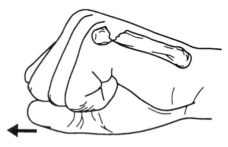

Direction of hand

Figure 4-16 Boxer's Fracture. Fracture of the distal fifth metacarpal angulates in a volar direction. (From Hartley A: *Practical joint assessment: upper quadrant*, ed 2, St Louis, 1995, Mosby.)

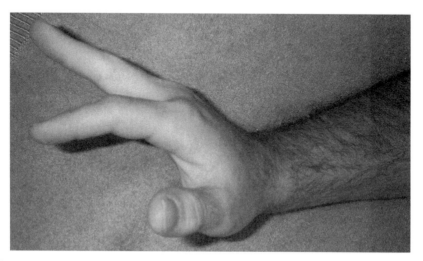

Figure 4-17 Extensor Lag. Inability to fully extend the index finger due to an angulated metacarpal neck fracture. (Courtesy RA Pensy, MD, University of Maryland Department of Orthopedics.)

morbidity are associated with the inoculation of virulent oral human flora that reproduce rapidly and quickly within the joint, destroying articular cartilage and sometimes resulting in osteomyelitis.[24]

Physical Examination. Examination usually confirms the history described by the patient. The fingers should be carefully inspected for evidence of any rotational deformity (Figure 4-18). ROM may reveal an inability to fully extend the MCP joint of the affected digit. Pain and palpable deformity over the fracture site are the rule.

Diagnosis. X-ray films will confirm the practitioner's clinical diagnosis. It is important to obtain AP, lateral, and oblique views of the hand to determine metacarpal alignment and the extent of any displacement.

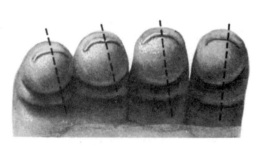

Normal alignment of fingernails

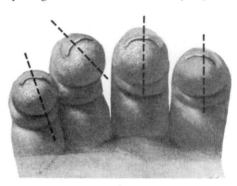

Alignment of fingernails with malrotation of ring finger

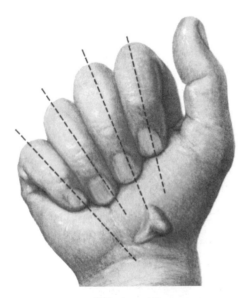

Normal flexion of fingers

A

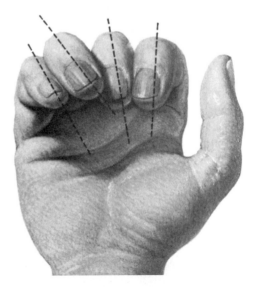

Flexion of fingers with malrotation of ring finger

B

Figure 4-18   Two Methods of Observing Finger Malrotation. A, Normal alignment of the nail beds and digits. **B,** Malrotation attributable to fracture. (From Canale ST, editor: *Campbell's operative orthopedics*, ed 10, vol 1, St Louis, 2003, Mosby.)

Treatment

Ideally, metacarpal fractures are treated by an orthopedic hand surgeon, who can manage displacement and rotational problems. Treatment may require surgical stabilization of the fracture (Figure 4-19). However, it is important for the practitioner to be able to recognize a metacarpal fracture.

A well-molded splint will usually keep the patient comfortable and protected until he or she can obtain definitive medical care. The splint may be a commercial wrist splint or a simple palmar splint; it is only necessary for it to extend from the middle of the proximal phalanx to the palmar side of the forearm. Analgesic medications and nonsteroidal antiinflammatory drugs (NSAIDs) can improve the patient's comfort.

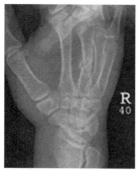

A

Metacarpal fracture

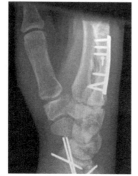

B

Metacarpal status postfixation

Figure 4-19   Unstable metacarpal fracture. **A,** Comminuted third metacarpal shaft fracture. **B,** Same fracture after plate and screw fixation.

Fractures Involving the Thumb

Fractures of the first (thumb) metacarpal deserve special attention because of the thumb's unique function. In addition to direct trauma, a cause of first metacarpal fractures can be forced abduction of the thumb, such as a fall on an outstretched hand.

A rather uncommon but important fracture is the Rolando fracture, which is a comminuted, intraarticular fracture of the base of the first metacarpal. Usually there are three main fracture fragments. This type of injury should be splinted and the patient immediately referred to an orthopedic surgeon. A Rolando fracture is very difficult to stabilize, even with surgery.

Bennett's Fractures

One of the clinically most important fractures is a noncomminuted intraarticular fracture of the base of the metacarpal. Known as a Bennett's fracture, this type of injury is often displaced because the abductor pollicis longus pulls the shaft radially (Figure 4-20). The remaining piece of bone can then be rotated by the pull of its capsular attachment. Anatomic reduction of the fracture must be accomplished to prevent long-term MCP joint problems.

Examination reveals ecchymosis, edema, and pain at the MCP joint of the thumb. ROM of the IP joint is usually intact but may be painful. Plain x-ray films will confirm the diagnosis (Figure 4-21). The best primary care treatment is to splint the entire thumb and refer the patient to an orthopedic surgeon, since these fractures frequently require operative stabilization.

Carpal Fractures

Carpal fractures are less common than other fractures of the hand, are often missed on initial evaluation, and can be harder to treat.

Scaphoid Fracture

One of the most important and most often missed carpal injuries is a scaphoid fracture. The scaphoid is the most frequently fractured carpal bone, and, as mentioned earlier, an intact scaphoid is crucial to normal wrist function (Figure 4-22). The scaphoid bone is divided into proximal and distal poles; an area known as the *scaphoid*

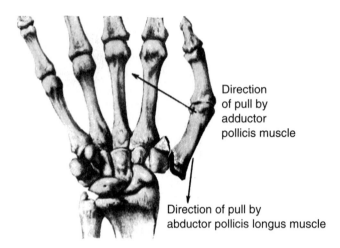

Figure 4-20   Bennett's Fracture. The metacarpal shaft can be displaced by the divergent pull of its muscles. (From Canale ST, editor: *Campbell's operative orthopedics*, ed 10, vol 1, St Louis, 2003, Mosby.)

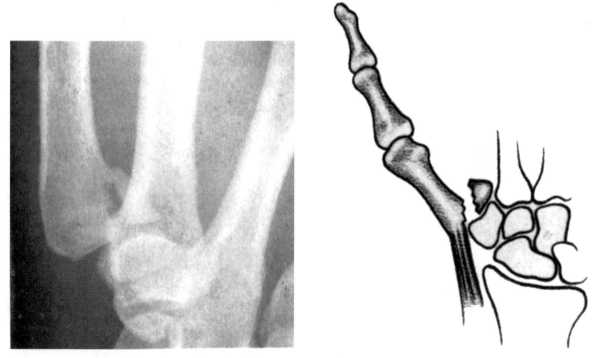

Figure 4-21   Bennett's Fracture. Radiographic and diagrammatic appearance. (From Mercier LR: *Practical orthopedics*, ed 5, St Louis, 2000, Mosby.)

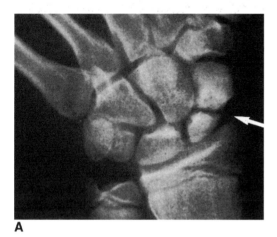

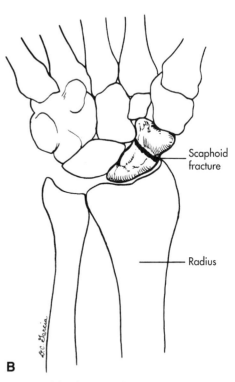

A   **B**

Figure 4-22 Scaphoid Fracture. The scaphoid waist, an area lying between the proximal and distal poles, is the most common site of fracture. (**A,** From Mercier LR: *Practical orthopedics,* ed 5, St Louis, 2000, Mosby. **B,** From Mackin EJ et al, editors: *Rehabilitation of the hand and upper extremity,* ed 5, vol 1, St Louis, 2002, Mosby.)

waist lies between the two. Fractures of any of these areas can occur (Figure 4-23); complications tend to be more frequent with proximal pole fractures.[14] Undiagnosed and untreated scaphoid fractures can cause chronic wrist pain, loss of grip strength, and an acceleration of degenerative changes of the wrist joint.[20]

History. A fall on an outstretched hand is the classic history of a scaphoid fracture (Figure 4-24). Initially there may be little pain, and the patient may continue to use the wrist. Pain, often described as a deep, dull aching near the base of the thumb, may increase in severity as the wrist is used. As with other carpal injuries there may not be a great deal of swelling.[10] The patient may consider the injury "only a sprain" and delay seeking treatment. Numbness and tingling in the digits are fairly uncommon.

Physical Examination. Inspection may not reveal any significant abnormality. Palpation is one of the key diagnostic tools in identifying a scaphoid fracture. Tenderness of the anatomic snuff-box is highly suggestive of a fracture of the scaphoid even in the presence of x-rays that are negative (Figure 4-25). The anatomic snuff-box is a triangular depression on the dorsal-radial aspect of the wrist at the base of the thumb.

A classic test is to ask the patient to slightly ulnarly deviate the wrist; the examiner then palpates the anatomic snuff-box to check for tenderness. If a scaphoid fracture is present, resisted pronation of the wrist may also elicit pain at the anatomic snuff-box. Any patient with tenderness in this area should be treated as one with a scaphoid fracture, regardless of x-ray findings.

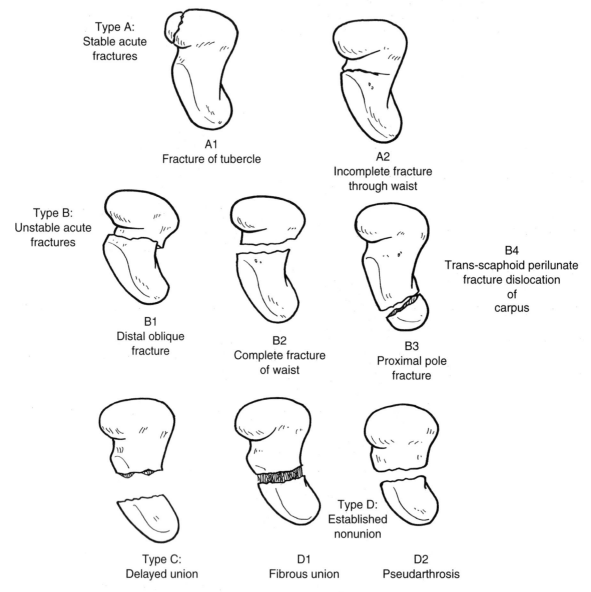

Type A:
Stable acute
fractures

A1
Fracture of tubercle

A2
Incomplete fracture
through waist

Type B:
Unstable acute
fractures

B1
Distal oblique
fracture

B2
Complete fracture
of waist

B3
Proximal pole
fracture

B4
Trans-scaphoid perilunate
fracture dislocation
of
carpus

Type C:
Delayed union

D1
Fibrous union

Type D:
Established
nonunion

D2
Pseudarthrosis

Figure 4-23   Types of scaphoid fractures. (From Bucholz RW: *Orthopaedic decision making*, ed 2, St Louis, 1996, Mosby.)

Diagnosis. History and physical examination are the critical factors in diagnosing scaphoid fractures. An x-ray study is usually helpful, but fractures can be missed even with good films.[20] Any patient with a suggested scaphoid fracture should be referred to an orthopedic physician, preferably a hand surgeon.

Because fractures are often difficult to visualize on x-ray films, a suspected scaphoid fracture should be

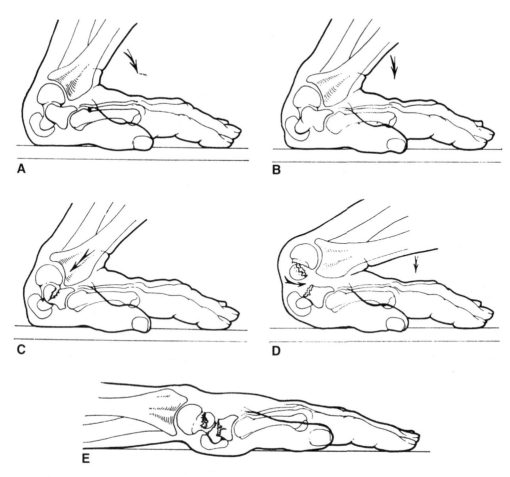

Figure 4-24 Events Causing Carpal Bone Fractures. A, Forced hyperextension of the wrist. **B,** Scaphoid fracture. **C,** Capitate bone fracture. **D,** Rotation of the capitate fracture after injury. **E,** Wrist in neutral position with fractured carpal bones. (From Canale ST, editor: *Campbell's operative orthopedics,* ed 10, vol 1, St Louis, 2003, Mosby.)

splinted for at least 10 to 14 days and then x-rayed again to establish definitively whether a scaphoid fracture is present. The inflammatory phase of bone healing, which occurs during the initial 7 to 10 days after a fracture, often generates a radiolucent line at the fracture site, allowing the clinician to make the diagnosis with repeat radiographs. A bone scan has been shown to be 100% reliable in detecting scaphoid fracture.[32] Some authors recommend computed tomography (CT) or magnetic resonance imaging (MRI) to evaluate displaced fractures.[20,26]

Treatment. Treatment of a scaphoid waist fracture should include a short-arm thumb spica cast with the wrist held in slight flexion and slight radial deviation. Fracture of the proximal pole may necessitate use of a long-arm thumb spica cast for 6 weeks, which is followed by use of a short-arm thumb spica cast.[9] Casting may have to continue for as long as 3 months, depending on patient age, smoking history, clinical exam, and follow-up radiographic findings. Scaphoid fractures should be followed by a hand surgeon because of their high rate of complications, including a high rate of nonunion.

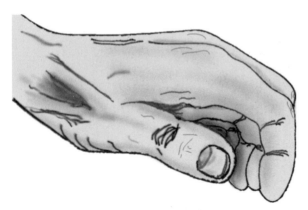

Figure 4-25 Anatomic Snuff-Box. A roughly triangular indentation on the radial side of the wrist. Palpation of this area should be performed with a single digit to elicit point tenderness. Until proven otherwise, tenderness in the anatomic snuff-box should be treated as a scaphoid fracture. (From Mackin EJ et al, editors: *Rehabilitation of the hand and upper extremity*, ed 5, vol 1, St Louis, 2002, Mosby.)

Displaced scaphoid fractures require operative intervention to prevent nonunion and progressive arthritis; new techniques are being developed to minimize surgical trauma, such as arthroscopically assisted screw fixation.[28]

Triquetrum Fracture

Another common carpal fracture is an avulsion fracture off the dorsal aspect of the triquetrum. This injury occurs after a fall or when the wrist is forcibly hyperextended. The patient typically reports pain over the dorsum of the wrist. Swelling and bruising on the back of the hand usually occur. Finger motion and strength are rarely, if ever, affected.

Physical Examination. On examination, hyperextension of the wrist may cause pain. With palpation, point tenderness can usually be elicited over the ulnar side of the proximal carpal row.

Diagnosis. Diagnosis is based primarily on x-ray findings and clinical evaluation. An avulsion fracture is often visualized only on the lateral view, where small avulsion fragments are noted (Figure 4-26). These injuries are successfully treated with immobilization, but patients can experience dorsal wrist pain for 3 to 4 months after injury.

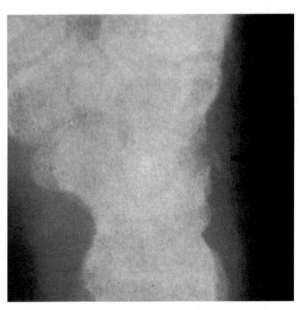

Figure 4-26 Avulsion Fracture of the Triquetrum. This fracture is often visible only on a lateral x-ray view as shown here. (From Mercier LR: *Practical orthopedics*, ed 5, St Louis, 2000, Mosby.)

Hamate Fracture

A hamate fracture represents one of the least common bony problems in the wrist. This fracture is usually seen in someone who has fallen directly on the hand. Also, many golfers or baseball players who incorrectly hit the ball report pain and tenderness in the palm of the hand because of a fracture of the hamate.

On examination, tenderness in the hypothenar eminence usually represents a fracture of the hook of the hamate bone.

A hamate fracture is hard to visualize on x-ray film unless a carpal tunnel view can be obtained. A CT scan is the current recommendation to rule out a fracture of the hook of the hamate bone.

Distal Forearm Fractures

Fractures of the distal radius or ulna can result from a multitude of types of traumatic force. Most of these fractures are easily diagnosed by history, clinical examination, and x-ray evaluation. Generally they should be treated by an orthopedic surgeon, especially if the

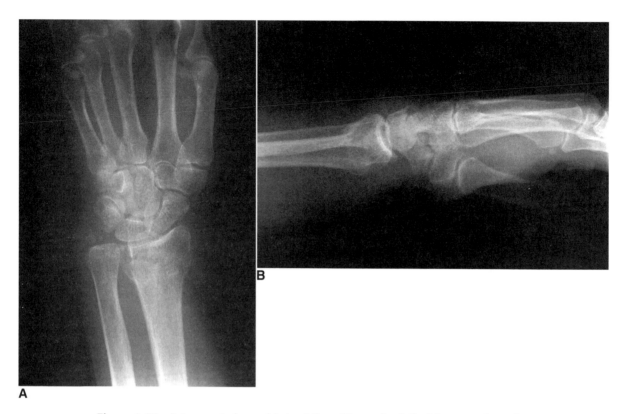

Figure 4-27   Anteroposterior and Lateral X-ray Views of a Colles' Fracture. Impaction **(A)** and dorsal angulation **(B)** of the distal fracture segment. This fracture should be reduced as soon as possible to prevent damage to the neurovascular structures around the wrist. (From Mercier LR: *Practical orthopedics*, ed 5, St Louis, 2000, Mosby.)

fractures are displaced. Primary care treatment consists of diagnosing the fracture, immobilizing it, and referring the patient to an orthopedic surgeon.

A general knowledge of common wrist fractures is useful when communicating with the orthopedic surgeon. Knowledge of the basic treatments of wrist fractures can help the practitioner prepare the patient for what to expect from the orthopedic surgeon.

A simple distal radius fracture is usually nondisplaced and does not involve the articular surface. This fracture is treated with a short-arm cast for approximately 4 weeks.

A Colles' fracture is typically the result of a fall, often with a significant amount of force placed on the wrist. In

this fracture there is dorsal angulation and often some radial deviation of the distal fragment (Figure 4-27). This fracture may involve the articular surface (Figure 4-28). A Colles' fracture must be reduced to restore realignment. Treatment options include short- or long-arm casting, open reduction and internal fixation, (Figure 4-29) or closed reduction with casting or placement of an external fixator.

A Smith's fracture (Figure 4-30) is essentially an injury that occurs in the opposite direction of a Colles' fracture. Treatment options are similar to those for a Colles' fracture.

A Barton's fracture is a fracture through the articular surface of the dorsal aspect of the distal radius

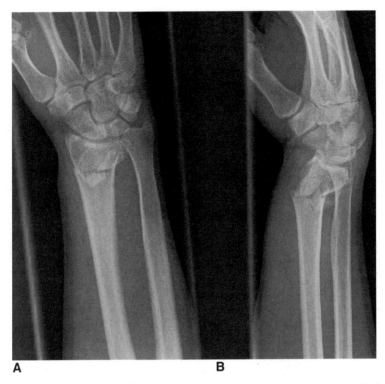

A   **B**

Figure 4-28   Intraarticular Colles' Fracture. A, Anteroposterior view shows multiple fragments. **B,** Oblique view demonstrates marked dorsal angulation of the distal fragments.

(Figure 4-31) or, in the case of a reverse Barton's, through the palmar aspect (Figure 4-32). The distal fracture fragment is displaced volarly and proximally and requires operative treatment.

A chauffeur's fracture is an intraarticular fracture of the radial styloid. It is named for its frequency during the early 1900s when a car would backfire on starting, causing the starting crank to swing back and strike the distal radius (Figure 4-33).[5] This fracture can occur when the wrist is forcefully wrenched backward, such as when a person holds onto a steering wheel during a head-on collision. The distal fragment displaces distally (toward the carpal bones) and may be rotated. Pinning the distal fragment may be necessary.

Dislocations

Dislocations of the wrist and hand result from a number of types of injury; causes include contact sports, falls, motor vehicle accidents, and altercations. Dislocations

occur at various joints, resulting in pain, deformity, and decreased movement. Neurovascular structures may be affected by the malalignment of the joint.

Patients usually have an idea of the specific event that caused the dislocation. Symptoms generally depend on the location of the injury, but decreased ability to move the joint is nearly universal. Pain may be variable; it tends to be worse when the joint is moved. Swelling, too, is variable. Tenderness of the joint to palpation is typical. Neurovascular changes can be seen with significant dislocations. Diagnosis is based on history, physical examination, and x-ray evaluation. Additional diagnostic tests such as CT and MRI studies are unnecessary unless significant associated soft-tissue or vascular injury is suggested.

Radiocarpal Joints

Dislocations of the radiocarpal joints are uncommon but severe. A dislocation of the distal radioulnar joint can

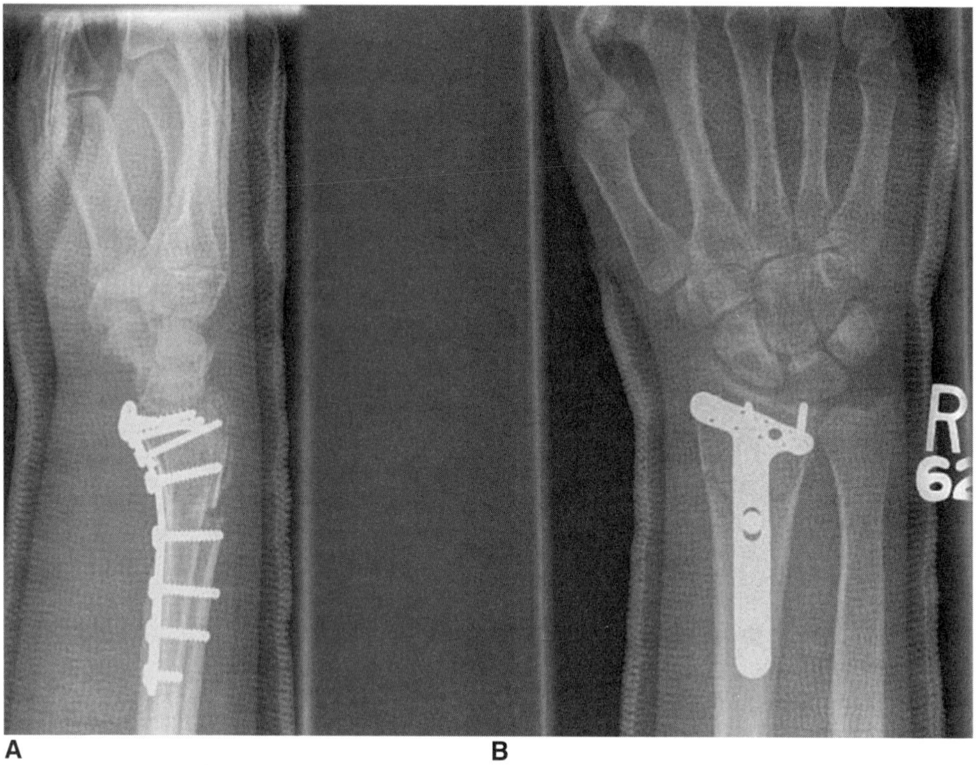

A   **B**

Figure 4-29   Intraarticular Colles' Fracture After Open Reduction and Internal Fixation.
A, Lateral, and **B,** anteroposterior views of repaired comminuted Colles fracture.

occur from significant stress to the joint, such as that caused by a fall from a height or by a motor vehicle crash. A dislocation of the radiocarpal joint is often mistaken for a simple wrist sprain and treated as such. It is only after pain continues beyond 6 to 8 weeks that the patient may return for reexamination. At this point the patient should be referred to a hand surgeon. An MRI is useful in diagnosing dislocations attributed to ligamentous disruptions.

Carpal Joints

Fractures can be associated with dislocations of the carpal joints. There are variations of these injuries where the lunate dislocates from the distal radius. The mechanism for most of these dislocations is a fall on an outstretched hand with resultant hyperextension of the wrist. Since carpal dislocation alters the relationship between carpal bones, these injuries are usually significant and require the attention of a hand surgeon. (Most carpal dislocations are the result of ligamentous disruption and are discussed under "Ligamentous Injuries" later in this chapter.)

Carpometacarpal Joints

Dislocations of the CMC joints most frequently occur at the ring and little fingers. Often there is an associated fracture. It is appropriate that the practitioner reduce and splint these injuries.

After the administration of appropriate anesthesia, such as a local nerve block, reduction is easily obtained by hanging the patient in finger trap traction with applied countertraction. It is important to remember that countertraction (i.e., pushing the displaced bone) is the force that reduces the dislocation. Using only a

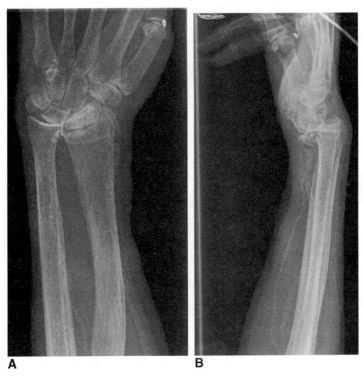

A   **B**

Figure 4-30   Smith's Fracture. These fractures are inherently unstable because of shear forces across the fracture from the flexor muscles of the wrist.

pulling force can turn a simple dislocation into a complex one.

Reducing the dislocation is not absolutely necessary before referring the patient to an orthopedic hand surgeon, but the hand should always be splinted. After splinting, the patient should be referred, because the unstable nature of these injuries usually necessitates surgical treatment.

Metacarpophalangeal Joints

Dislocations of the MCP joints are most commonly seen at the thumb. This dislocation is often the result of a sports-related injury where the digit is forced into hyperextension. Both simple and complex dislocations occur. Simple dislocations can be manually reduced; complex dislocations involve soft-tissue interposition in the joint (Figure 4-34). With x-ray films, a sesamoid bone may be seen to be interposed between the metacarpal and the proximal phalanx. Tenting of the skin

is often present at the joint. Complex dislocations need to be treated surgically.

Proximal Interphalangeal Joints

Dislocations at the PIP joints occur when there is disruption of the palmar plate and usually of the radial or ulnar collateral ligament. Gentle manipulation can be attempted to reduce these dislocations after x-ray films have confirmed there is no associated fracture, and digital block anesthesia has been performed (Figure 4-35). Splinting the PIP joint at approximately 45 degrees of flexion is appropriate before referring the patient to an orthopedic hand surgeon.

LIGAMENTOUS INJURIES

Ligamentous injuries around the hand and wrist are quite common. Left untreated, these injuries can cause wrist instability, resulting in chronic pain, loss of ROM, weakness, and degenerative changes.

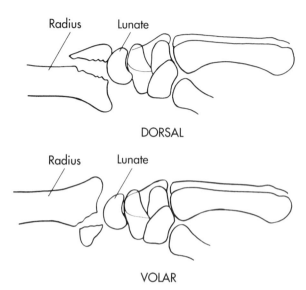

Figure 4-31 **Barton's Fracture.** The distal fracture fragment is displaced in a dorsal direction. (From Mackin EJ et al, editors: *Rehabilitation of the hand and upper extremity*, ed 5, vol 1, St Louis, 2002, Mosby.)

Scapholunate Ligament

One of the most commonly seen ligamentous injuries in the wrist is to the scapholunate ligament. Like most others, this ligamentous injury is most often the result of a traumatic force being applied to the joint. It can cause the patient to develop pain and a dorsal intercalated segment instability deformity.[28]

History. A fall onto an outstretched arm with the wrist supinated and ulnarly deviated is the most common history for an injury to the scapholunate ligament.[22] Pain occurs almost immediately, and the patient may report that "something just doesn't feel right" in the wrist. Weakness, clicking, or snapping in the wrist may also be noted by the patient, especially with repetitive motion. Dorsal wrist and hand swelling frequently occur. Bruising tends to develop within hours to 1 or 2 days after injury.

Physical Examination. Inspection of the wrist usually reveals swelling and discoloration over the dorsum of the hand. Palpation may elicit tenderness just medially to the anatomic snuff-box. Movement of the

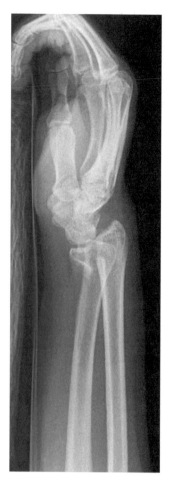

Figure 4-32 **Palmar (or volar) Barton's Fracture.** This intraarticular fracture of the distal radius results in volar displacement of the distal fracture fragment.

fingers is usually normal, but making a tight fist or hyperextending the wrist can increase pain.

Diagnosis. Injury to the scapholunate ligament can be difficult to diagnose, but Watson's test and certain x-ray studies can help. Watson's test is designed to elicit symptomatic clicking and sometimes a palpable clunk over the scaphoid. To perform this test the examiner applies pressure upward against the volar pole of the scaphoid as the wrist is taken from a ulnarly deviated direction to a radially deviated position. In effect, this reduces the scaphoid back to the lunate, and usually a distinctive clunk is felt or heard.

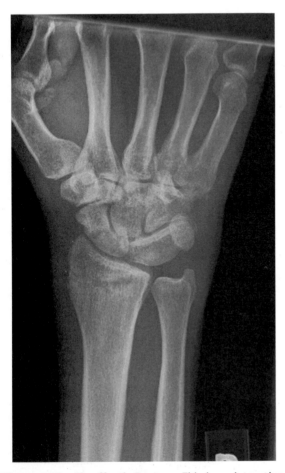

Figure 4-33 Chauffeur's Fracture. This is an intraarticular fracture of the radial styloid.

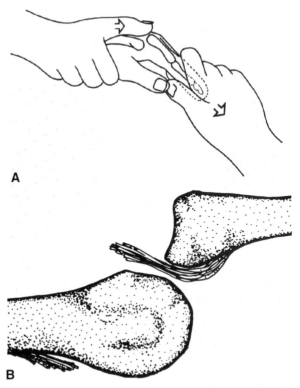

Figure 4-34   A, Method of reducing a simple posterior dislocation of the metacarpophalangeal joint. While applying gentle traction to the digit, the practitioner pushes the dislocated phalanx distally, back into its anatomic position. **B,** The presence of soft tissue in the joint may prevent reduction. (From Mercier LR: *Practical orthopedics*, ed 5, St Louis, 2000, Mosby.)

X-ray films should be taken with both PA and lateral views, as well as a supinated clenched-fist view. The AP x-ray film usually shows an increased space between the scaphoid and lunate bones (Figure 4-36). This space can be accentuated on a supinated clenched-fist view; when clenching the fist, the capitate is pushed toward the proximal carpal row and acts, in the presence of a ligament disruption, something like a wedge. As previously mentioned, fractures of the carpus can be accompanied by dislocations resulting from disruption of the carpal ligaments. The posteroanterior (PA) radiograph in Figure 4-37 (see Figure 4-37, *A*) demonstrates a fracture of the scaphoid. The lateral x-ray film shows the scapholunate

angle to be greater than the normal 60 to 70 degrees (see Figure 4-37, *B*); the lunate is completely dislocated and flexed out of the proximal row of the carpus.

Treatment.   There are several options for treatment of an injury to the scapholunate ligament. Depending on the patient's functional status, it may be appropriate to prescribe a period of immobilization. The patient can then be observed to see how symptomatic the wrist is, despite the injured ligament. Many patients will heal with this treatment. Other treatments include surgical ligament reconstruction; several procedures have been shown to be effective and should be performed by qualified hand surgeons (Figure 4-38).

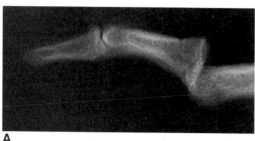

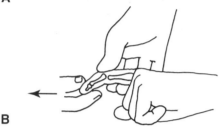

B

Figure 4-35 Simple Proximal Interphalangeal Joint Dislocation and Method of Reduction. A, Lateral x-ray film showing posterior displacement of the middle phalanx. **B,** A combination of gentle manual traction and pushing is used to reduce the dislocation. (From Mercier LR: *Practical orthopedics,* ed 5, St Louis, 2000, Mosby.)

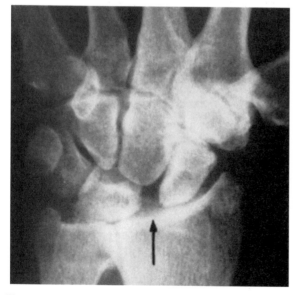

Figure 4-36 Radiographic Appearance of Scapholunate Disruption. Arrow indicates area of abnormal widening of the intercarpal space. (From Mercier LR: *Practical orthopedics,* ed 5, St Louis, 2000, Mosby.)

Lunotriquetral Ligament

Another, less common carpal instability is a lunotriquetral dissociation, which can result in a volar intercalated segment instability deformity.[15] An AP x-ray film may visualize an increased lunotriquetral space. On the lateral view the lunate is in a palmarly displaced direction in line with the scaphoid.

Triangular Fibrocartilage Complex

On the ulnar side of the wrist the triangular fibrocartilage complex (TFCC) is an important stabilizer of the wrist joint. The complex itself is made up of the palmar ulnocarpal ligaments, the ulnocarpal meniscus homologue, the ulnar collateral ligament, the transverse fibrous or distal radioulnar ligament, and the base of the ECU.[8] The TFCC separates the distal ulna from the carpal bones and helps support the triquetrum.

TFCC tears usually occur with a twisting injury of the wrist. The diagnosis of TFCC tears can be difficult. In most cases the examination elicits exquisite tenderness between the ECU and FCU tendons. Localized swelling may be present over the ulnocarpal area.

A TFCC tear can be confused with tendonitis of the ECU or the FCU. Pain with the latter conditions primarily occurs with movement of the wrist and is not as severe as that associated with a TFCC tear.

An arthrogram can be helpful and will demonstrate the leakage of dye proximally (Figure 4-39). However, radiologists have recently improved their ability to read MRIs; consequently, the MRI is slowly replacing arthrography.[34]

Treatment of TFCC injuries can be difficult; options include casting in supination, injections, joint leveling procedures, and arthroscopic débridement or reconstruction of the tear. Once the diagnosis has been confirmed, or if the underlying diagnosis of wrist pain on the ulnar side remains elusive, referral to a hand surgeon is appropriate.

Ulnar Collateral Ligament

Another commonly seen ligamentous injury of the hand is to the ulnar collateral ligament of the thumb, and is known as gamekeeper's or skier's thumb. This injury is usually the result of a fall on the thumb that forcibly deviates it radially, rupturing the ulnar collateral ligament.

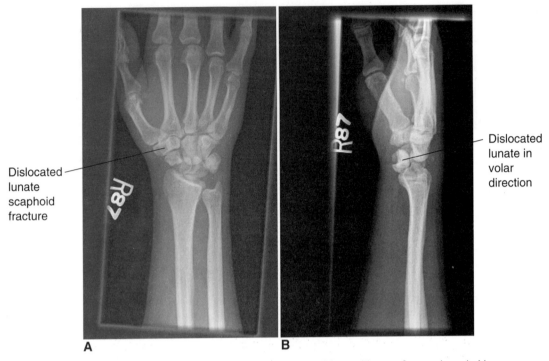

Dislocated
lunate
scaphoid
fracture

Dislocated
lunate in
volar
direction

A   B

Figure 4-37   Perilunate Fracture and Dislocation. A, Dislocated lunate, fractured scaphoid; B, dislocated lunate in volar direction.

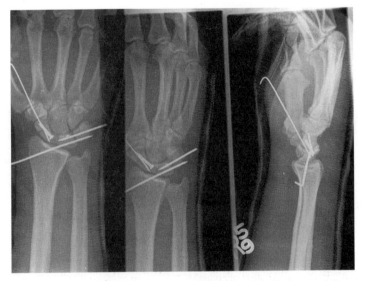

Figure 4-38   Perilunate Dislocation Status After Open Reduction and Percutaneous Fixation. A series of pins stabilize the lunate dislocation and scaphoid fraction.

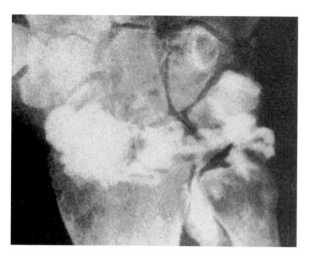

Figure 4-39   Tear of the Triangular Fibrocartilage Complex. Abnormal arthrogram of the wrist showing leakage of contrast material into the distal radiocarpal joint because of a tear of the TFCC. (From Firooznia H et al, editors: *MRI and CT of the musculoskeletal system*, St Louis, 1992, Mosby.)

Often this ligament will rupture and lie above the adductor aponeurosis, a condition known as Stener's lesion[15] (Figure 4-40). As the thumb phalanx is radially deviated, its ulnar collateral ligament may rupture and pull from under the adductor covering. As the joint then realigns, this ligament then comes to rest on top of the adductor hood and remains separated from its normal insertion, thus preventing healing. It is important to recognize this injury promptly so that surgical treatment can be initiated.

History. A fall onto an outstretched thumb is the most common history. Pain and swelling occur soon after impact. The patient will often complain of an unstable thumb and weakness when trying to twist open a bottle top. Weakness with pinching the thumb and index finger can also be present (Figure 4-41).

Physical Examination and Diagnosis. The predominant findings on inspection are swelling and pain on the ulnar side of the MCP joint of the thumb. A weak pinch may be noted. There may be varying degrees of ligament instability.

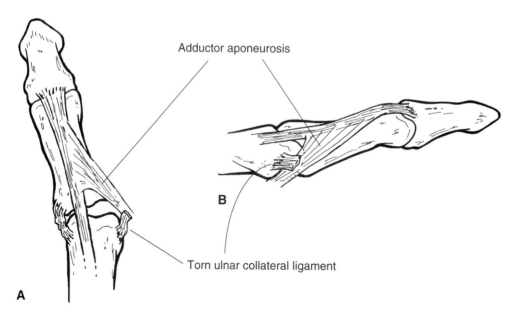

Adductor aponeurosis

B

Torn ulnar collateral ligament

A

Figure 4-40   Stener's Lesion of the Thumb. A, Dorsal view showing rupture of ligament and interposition of adductor aponeurosis. **B,** Lateral view showing relationship of torn ulnar ligament and adductor aponeurosis that prevents healing of ligament. (From Bucholz RW: *Orthopaedic decision making*, ed 2, St Louis, 1996, Mosby.)

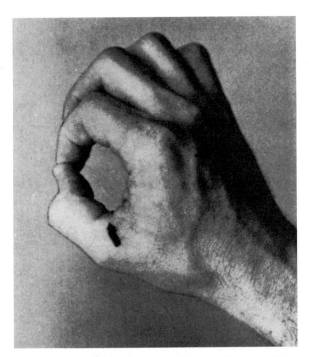

Figure 4-41   Testing the Ulnar Collateral Ligament of the Thumb. The ulnar collateral ligament of the thumb *(marked)* provides stability when pinching the thumb and index finger. (From Mercier LR: *Practical orthopedics*, ed 5, St Louis, 2000, Mosby.)

X-ray films should be obtained to identify and protect a possible displaced fracture, before stressing the joint.[19] Once films are reviewed and no fracture is found to be present, the joint can be stressed to assess ligament stability. One method is to hold the thumb flexed to approximately 30 degrees and then radially deviate the joint. Complete rupture of the ulnar collateral ligament of the thumb is demonstrated by a complete lack of an end point when compared with the other side. Many times the phalanx is seen on an AP x-ray view to deviate radially when stressing the joint (Figure 4-42). On the lateral x-ray view there may be palmar subluxation of the proximal phalanx on the metacarpal head.

Treatment. If there is complete rupture of the ulnar collateral ligament, the patient should be referred to an orthopedic hand surgeon for surgical repair. If the ligament has some intact fibers, prolonged immobilization (i.e., a minimum of 4 to 6 weeks) with a thumb spica splint or cast may be all that is necessary. Physical therapy may be indicated after immobilization to restore normal ROM.

Other Collateral Ligament Injuries

Finger sprains are typically the result of either radial or ulnar collateral ligament injuries to the PIP or, less commonly, to the DIP joints of the digits. Sports, falls, work-related trauma, and direct blows can cause stretching or tearing of these ligaments. As with other sprains, collateral ligament injuries of the digits are graded on a scale of one to three, depending on the severity.

Grade I injuries involve damage to the ligament but no joint instability. On examination there may be swelling and tenderness with palpation, but no functional abnormality. Grade II injuries involve stretching or partial tearing of the ligament. Swelling tends to be accompanied by bruising, and some joint laxity is evident when it is stressed. Pain with palpation is present. The result of a grade III injury is complete disruption of the ligament. There is no end point when the ligament is stressed, and the joint is painful and feels unstable to the patient. A grade III injury should be buddy taped, and the patient should be referred to an orthopedic surgeon for definitive treatment.

Grades I and II injuries can be treated by taping the injured finger to an adjacent finger without taping over the joints. Buddy taping provides support to the injured finger while allowing protected flexion and extension. The use of NSAIDs can increase patient comfort. The patient should be advised of the long recovery period (i.e., up to 4 or more months) until the joint is free of pain. Persistent, even permanent, enlargement of the joint is not unusual.

Another less common injury is the disruption of the radial or ulnar collateral ligament of an MCP joint. To clinically evaluate this injury, the examiner should ask the patient to gently flex and then extend the wrist. The digits will rotate away from the side of the torn collateral ligament. Treatment is best performed by an orthopedic hand surgeon.

TENDON INJURIES

Extensor Tendon

Pain may be the only presenting symptom of extensor tendon injuries, especially in proximal lacerations.

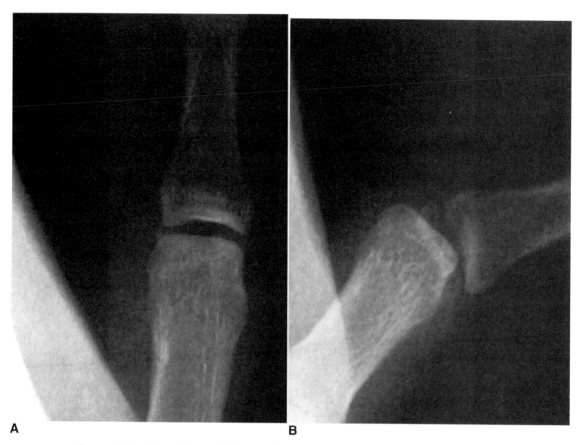

A   **B**

Figure 4-42   Ulnar Collateral Ligament Rupture. A radiographic view of the thumb showing metacarpophalangeal instability when nonstressed **(A)** and stressed **(B)**. (From Mercier LR: *Practical orthopedics*, ed 5, St Louis, 2000, Mosby.)

Because of multiple contributions to the extensor system, there can be some function to extend the digit despite laceration to an individual area of an extensor tendon. Lacerations that involve less than 50% of the tendon do not need to be repaired.

Surprisingly, complete disruptions of a tendon may be accompanied by little pain. The primary finding on examination, regardless of location, is an inability to extend the digit distal to the site of tendon injury (Figure 4-43).

Extensor tendon injuries are described as occurring in zones (Figure 4-44). Zone 1 includes the central slip

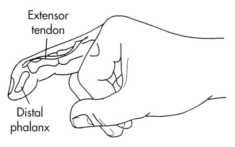

Figure 4-43   Mallet finger deformity caused by rupture of the extensor tendon at the distal interphalangeal joint. (From Hartley A: *Practical joint assessment: upper quadrant*, ed 2, St Louis, 1995, Mosby.)

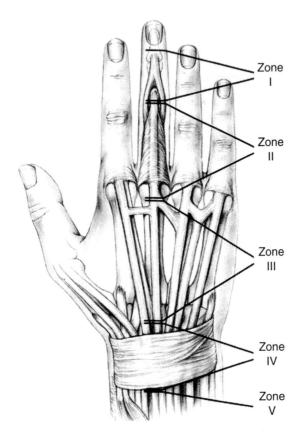

Figure 4-44 Extensor tendon zones of the hand and wrist. (From Canale ST, editor: *Campbell's operative orthopedics*, ed 10, vol 1, St Louis, 2003, Mosby.)

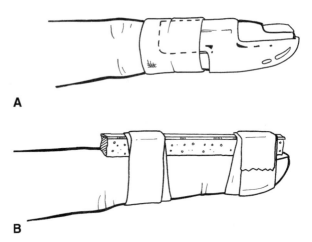

Figure 4-45 Two Types of Distal Phalanx Splints. A, Commercially available Stax splint. **B,** Padded aluminum splint cut and taped to finger. (From Bucholz RW: *Orthopedic decision making*, ed 2, St Louis, 1996, Mosby.)

insertion distally and extends from the area of the digit just before the PIP joint to the tip of the finger. Zone I injuries are usually mallet injuries or a disruption of the terminal tendon; these can usually be treated nonsurgically with splinting of the DIP joint in extension. A padded aluminum dorsal splint worn full time for 6 to 8 weeks (Figure 4-45) will usually allow the tendon to heal sufficiently to regain normal finger extension.

Zone II extends from the MCP joint to the central slip insertion at the base of the middle phalanx. Left unrecognized, injuries in this zone can lead to a boutonnière deformity. A boutonnière deformity consists of flexion of the PIP joint and hyperextension of the DIP joint. This deformity can be successfully treated by having the patient perform flexion exercises of the DIP joint

with the PIP joint in full extension. Injuries in zone II usually take at least 8 weeks to heal.

Patients with tendon injuries in zones III through V should be referred to a hand surgeon or a qualified orthopedic or plastic surgeon. Zone III comprises the distal end of the extensor retinaculum to the MCP joint of the hand; basically this area encompasses the back of the hand. In zone III the tendons are relatively free and have no ligamentous attachment. Injuries to tendons in zone 3 should be sutured. Zone IV injuries occur under the extensor retinaculum, or where the tendons are contained in their dorsal compartments. In zone 4, tendons are sheathed in canals beneath the dorsal carpal retinaculum. The hand or orthopedic surgeon should leave some of the retinaculum intact to prevent extensor tendon bow-stringing during extension and hyperextension of the wrist. Zone V is the area proximal to the extensor retinaculum; in this zone the musculotendinous unit requires surgical repair.

de Quervain's Disease

Inflammation of the first dorsal tendon extensor compartment can cause pain, tenderness, and crepitus with movement of the wrist. Pain is aggravated by picking up objects and is not uncommon among new mothers who

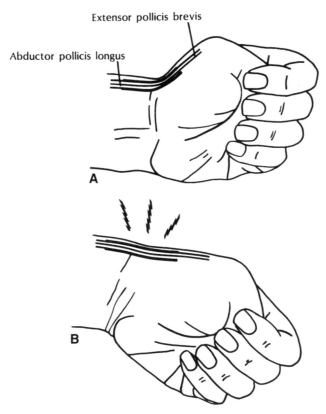

Extensor pollicis brevis

Abductor pollicis longus

A

B

Figure 4-46 Finkelstein's Test for de Quervain's Disease. A, With the wrist in neutral position the tendons of the first dorsal tendon compartment are free of pain. **B,** Ulnar deviation of the wrist stretches the first dorsal compartment tendons, causing exquisite pain. (From Noble J, editor: *Textbook of primary care medicine,* ed 3, St Louis, 2001, Mosby.)

flex the wrist and extend the thumb while holding their infants. Pain radiates along the radial aspect of the thumb and forearm.

History. Pain usually begins insidiously and worsens over time. It is often described as a burning or deep aching sensation. Carrying an infant, picking up a gallon jug of milk, or repetitive grasping movements may aggravate pain. Resting the thumb often decreases symptoms. Numbness and tingling are rare.

Physical Examination and Diagnosis. Visible thickening of the tendon sheath along the radiocarpal border of the thumb may be present with de Quervain's disease. Both active and passive movements tend to cause pain. Neurovascular status is usually normal.

The classic test for de Quervain's disease is Finkelstein's test (Figure 4-46). This test is performed by asking the patient to make a fist around the thumb and to relax the wrist. The practitioner then ulnarly deviates the wrist. A positive test is reproduction of the patient's pain and is usually sufficient for a diagnosis of de Quervain's disease.

Treatment. Conservative treatment with splinting, NSAIDs, application of moist heat, and activity modification often results in complete resolution of symptoms. An effective splint should support the thumb in a neutral, comfortable position. These splints are commercially available by prescription or can be fabricated out of fiberglass or plaster.

If symptoms persist beyond 2 weeks, corticosteroid injection into the tendon sheath may be useful. At this stage, it is appropriate to refer the patient to an orthopedic surgeon. Occasionally surgical release of the tendon sheath is necessary.

Flexor Tendons

In flexor tendon injuries, repair is also based on zones (Figure 4-47). As a general rule, all patients with flexor tendon injuries of the hand should be referred to a hand surgeon. As mentioned earlier, the A2 and A4 pulleys need to be preserved to maintain function of the flexor tendon. A basic understanding of the flexor zones of the hand can assist the practitioner in identifying and communicating the potential severity of the injury.

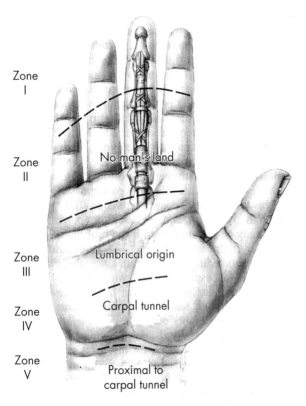

Zone
I

Zone
II

No man's land

Zone
III

Lumbrical origin

Zone
IV

Carpal tunnel

Zone
V

Proximal to carpal tunnel

Figure 4-47 Flexor tendon zones of the hand and wrist. (From Canale ST, editor: *Campbell's operative orthopedics*, ed 10, vol 1, St Louis, 2003, Mosby.)

Zone I is the area distal to the flexor digitorum superficialis insertion into the middle phalanx. The most common injury in zone I is an avulsion, typically sports-related, of the flexor digitorum profundus. An example is jersey finger, so named because this injury is often a result of a player attempting to tackle another by grabbing the sport jersey. The result can be forced extension of a flexed DIP joint, tearing the tendon. For reasons not completely understood, the ring finger is most commonly involved.

Typically the patient is unable to flex the DIP joint. Pain is variable, but sensation is usually intact. A zone I injury needs to be repaired, and repair is easy if recognized early. Commonly, however, a zone I injury is recognized late and often needs to be repaired with a graft or a DIP fusion. In older patients the latter treatment is favored. To reduce the incidence of complications, the patient should be referred to a hand surgeon.

Zone II is the area commonly known as "no man's land" and extends from the metacarpal neck to the insertion of the flexor digitorum superficialis at the midportion of the middle phalanx. It is the area where the two flexor tendons are found in the fibroosseous tunnel. Successful repairs in this area are quite difficult because of flexor sheath adhesions that occur during healing. Any patient with a tendon laceration in zone II requires immediate referral to a hand surgeon.

Zone III ranges from the transverse carpal ligament to the fibroosseous canal. Zone IV comprises the area of the transverse carpal ligament plus the area under the transverse carpal ligament. In both zones tendon repair is recommended.

Zone V extends from the musculotendinous junction to the transverse carpal ligament; accurate identification of the proximal and distal stumps can be difficult in this area. An injury in zone V is known as "a spaghetti wrist."

NONTRAUMATIC FLEXOR TENDON PROBLEMS

Trigger Finger

History. The formation of scar tissue around a flexor tendon often causes a catching of the tendon under the first annular (A1) pulley of the hand. When this occurs, the finger catches, or locks, in a flexed position. As the finger is extended, the nodule of scar tissue slides beneath the pulley and then releases, causing a sudden and painful "triggering" of the finger. A similar condition may sometimes be found in the newborn, commonly in the thumb, often requiring surgical release for extension of the thumb IP joint to be regained.

Physical Examination and Diagnosis. Pain with palpation over the MCP joint of the affected digit is common. (The A1 pulley lies in this area.) Sometimes there is a palpable nodule and the patient can trigger the finger for the practitioner. Diagnosis is based on history and physical examination.

Treatment. Initial treatment of trigger finger is a corticosteroid injection into the tendon sheath at the A1 pulley. This treatment will not usually eliminate the triggering, but it is successful in eliminating the pain associated with triggering. Definitive treatment requires surgical release; for such, the patient should be referred to a hand surgeon.

Ganglion Cyst

A ganglion cyst is an encapsulated, frequently mobile mass of tissue usually found near a joint or tendon sheath. A ganglion may be filled with a thick mucoid material. By itself the cyst generally causes no clinical problem unless it impinges on nearby tissue, such as a joint, blood vessel, or nerve. Ganglia are common on either the dorsum or palmar aspect of the wrist (Figure 4-48). Ganglion cysts are more common among people who engage in repetitive motion near the site of cyst formation, as well as in patients with underlying arthritic conditions.

History. Most cysts appear spontaneously, but some may occur after trauma to the affected area. The patient may note changes in the size of the cyst depending on activity. Typically the cyst will enlarge, causing pain after a period of repetitive use; it often decreases in size after a period of rest.

Physical Examination. A well-defined, usually mobile cyst over a tendon sheath is the most common presentation in the hand. Asking the patient to flex (for a palmar cyst) or extend (for a dorsal cyst) the fingers or wrist may accentuate the movement of the cyst. Pain can occur with compression of the mass.

Diagnosis. Diagnosis of a ganglion cyst is based primarily on history and clinical findings. No special tests are usually indicated. The determination of a fluid-filled cyst can often be aided by transillumination, or holding a small otoscope or opthalmoscope against the mass in a darkened room and noting a uniform glow throughout the mass.[30]

Treatment. Initial treatment of a ganglion cyst should be noninvasive. If the cyst can be manually reduced by applying finger or thumb pressure, a padded button or coin can be firmly secured to the area with an elastic bandage for a 3-week period to prevent reaccumulation of the cyst.[16] Ganglia that have been present for less than 3 months are most likely to fall into this category.

A ganglion that has a more well-defined capsule can be treated with aspiration using a large-bore needle followed by a corticosteroid injection. Extreme caution must be used if the ganglion is near a nerve or artery. Application of a compressive dressing follows aspiration and injection. Surgical excision is another option. Unfortunately, ganglia can recur after either of these treatments, and the patient should be so advised.

Dupuytren's Contracture

History. Another common hand problem is Dupuytren's disease, an inherited autosomal dominant fibrodysplasia of the palmar fascia that leads to flexion contractures from nodules and cords that develop progressively (Figure 4-49).[4] Typically, patients are men of age 40 or older, of northern European ancestry, and with a positive family history. Alcohol use and smoking, as

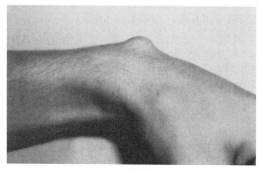

Figure 4-48   Appearance of ganglion cyst on the dorsum aspect of wrist. (From Hartley A: *Practical joint assessment: upper quadrant,* ed 2, St Louis, 1995, Mosby.)

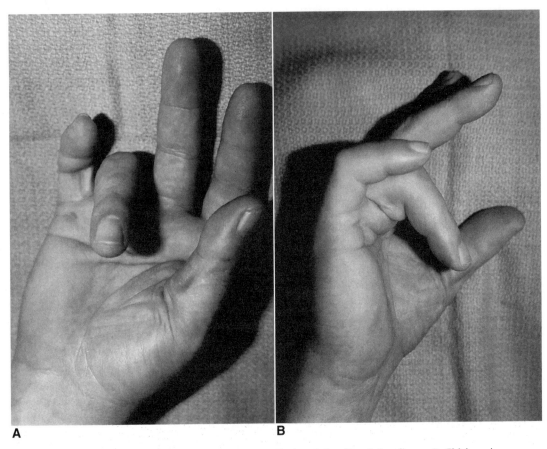

A   B

Figure 4-49   Dupuytren's Contracture. A, Flexion deformity of ring finger. **B,** Thickened palmar cord. (From Noble J, editor: *Textbook of primary care medicine*, ed 3, St Louis, 2001, Mosby.)

well as diabetes and seizure disorders, are found in association with this disease. Dupuytren's contracture can also be associated with a diathesis in which a similar fibrosis develops in the feet. This condition is called Lederhose's syndrome. Associated fibrosis of the penis is known as Peyronie's disease. Dupuytren's diathesis is generally understood to be a more aggressive form of the disease and tends to have a poorer surgical outcome. Patients often complain of the inability to place their hand within a pocket because of the flexion contracture.

Physical Examination. There are no symptoms of Dupuytren's contracture other than progressive deformity of the affected digit, often the small and ring fingers; it can be seen bilaterally. As the disease pro-

gresses, the palmar skin adheres to the fascia, forming a palpable band in the palm of the hand and causing a progressive flexion deformity of the PIP and MCP joints. Nodules are often palpable along with the cords. Multiple fingers can be affected.

Diagnosis. Diagnosis of Dupuytren's contracture is based on history and physical examination. No special tests are generally necessary.

Treatment. In general, as long as patients with Dupuytren's contracture pass the "flat hand" test, they do not need surgery. The flat hand test is simply the ability to flatten the fingers and palm of the hand against a hard surface. However, a patient with *any* PIP joint contractures that cannot be straightened should be immediately referred to a hand surgeon for correction. Contractures of the MCP joint of 30 degrees or greater that cannot be straightened also require referral to a hand surgeon.

COMPRESSIVE NEUROPATHIES

Compressive neuropathies commonly occur around the hand and wrist. They are the result of the mechanical entrapment of peripheral nerves, which cause localized ischemia. These neuropathies can be initiated by postural, developmental, inflammatory, metabolic, neoplastic, iatrogenic, and idiopathic causes, as well as anatomic ones.

Loss of sensation is usually the first manifestation. Treatment is initially nonoperative, using splinting, occupational therapy, and nonsteroidal medications.

Median Nerve

Carpal Tunnel Syndrome

The most common median nerve compression phenomenon is carpal tunnel syndrome (CTS), the result of compression of the median nerve in the carpal canal at the wrist. Its cause can be idiopathic or it can be associated with other diseases such as diabetes, hypothyroidism, alcoholism, rheumatoid arthritis, and amyloidosis.[31] Women are affected more often than men, at least in part because women have smaller wrists and therefore a smaller carpal tunnel through which the nerves can pass. Those who work in occupations requiring repetitive wrist motion often have complaints of CTS.

Although CTS is often a single entity, it can occur in combination with cervical radiculopathy or other compressive neuropathies. The symptoms of CTS may be quite atypical when present in combination with another neuropathy. The compression of a single nerve at two different sites is referred to as a "double crush" phenomenon, such as might occur if a nerve root at the C-spine level is compressed as well as axons of the same nerve at the carpal canal.[38]

History. Symptoms of CTS usually begin spontaneously, but recent trauma such as a wrist fracture can also be noted before the onset of symptoms. Patients classically report nighttime symptoms that include pain, numbness, and tingling, which wake them from a sound sleep. The patient often describes a "wake and shake" history of shaking his or her hand awake before being able to fall back to sleep. The most frequently affected digits are the long and index fingers, but the thumb and the radial half of the ring finger can also be involved. Patients may complain of burning pain in the arm or an inability to engage in activities requiring repetitive wrist movements (e.g., keyboarding, hammering, working with hand tools, crocheting, or, occasionally, even writing). A feeling of clumsiness or weakness is not uncommon when using the affected hand.

Pain and aching may progress proximally to the elbow or shoulder. Left untreated, symptoms become more constant, eventually occurring even at rest.

Physical Examination. On physical examination the patient usually has a positive Tinel's sign at the wrist, as well as the reproduction of symptoms in Phalen's wrist flexion test (Figure 4-50). Tinel's test is performed by percussing the median nerve at the carpal tunnel. Phalen's test is performed by asking the patient to flex the wrist to 90 degrees and hold it in that position. A reproduction of symptoms should occur within 60 seconds.

Diagnosis. The patient with CTS may also show weakness of the thenar musculature, the presence of which indicates more advanced nerve entrapment. A simple method to test for this condition is to ask the patient to pinch the thumb to the little finger while the practitioner taps the thenar muscles to see if they are firing. Normally the thenar eminence should feel tense to the practitioner's tap.

Treatment. Activity modification, use of a cock-up wrist splint, and administration of NSAIDs are usually the initial steps in treating CTS. Activity modification is aimed at removing or reducing possible causes of the symptoms. Proper ergonomics at work and home (e.g., maintaining proper computer keyboard placement) and avoiding extremes of wrist flexion may lessen symptoms.[31] To prevent wrist flexion while sleeping, splints such as a simple cock-up wrist splint can be worn at night. NSAIDs relieve inflammation and reduce pain. Vitamin B_6 in twice-daily doses of 100 mg has also been found to be helpful.

Steroid injections are often useful but are not recommended as an initial treatment. Failure to respond to conservative treatment after a period of at least 6 weeks should lead the practitioner to consider electromyography

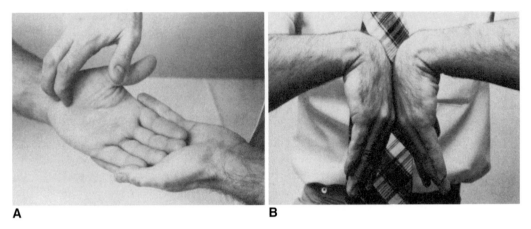

A   **B**

Figure 4-50   Tests for Carpal Tunnel Syndrome. A, Tinel's test is performed by percussing the median nerve at the carpal tunnel. **B,** Phalen's test, considered to be a more accurate test for carpal tunnel syndrome, is performed with the wrists flexed to 90 degrees; symptoms should be reproduced within 60 seconds. (From Mercier LR: Practical orthopedics, ed 5, St Louis, 2000, Mosby.)

(EMG) and nerve conduction studies (NCS). These tests can be helpful but are not always diagnostic.[33] Evidence of CTS from EMG or NCS is sufficient reason to refer the patient to a hand surgeon or an orthopedic surgeon who performs carpal tunnel surgery.

Surgery is indicated after failure of conservative measures and can be performed in several ways. The standard of care is the release of the transverse carpal ligament through an open carpal tunnel procedure with an incision in the palm. However, a procedure growing in popularity over the last few years is an endoscopic tunnel release, for which there are both one- and two-incision techniques. Many believe that the rehabilitation after endoscopic carpal tunnel release is shorter. However, studies have shown that in 6 months, recovery is the same after either open or endoscopic release.[35]

Pronator Syndrome

Pronator syndrome is an entrapment of the median nerve in the forearm at the pronator teres. This proximal entrapment is less common than CTS. Patients may have vague symptoms of forearm pain or hand numbness along the median nerve distribution. This syndrome tends to occur in individuals who have large forearm muscles and is associated with activity. Nighttime pain, numbness, and tingling is uncommon.

Numbness and tingling in the median nerve palmar cutaneous branch distribution suggests a problem with the median nerve more proximal than the wrist. This symptom usually involves the palm and wrist more than the digits. Tinel's and Phalen's tests are usually negative, as is evaluation with NCS.

Initial treatment for pronator syndrome is similar to that for CTS. Additionally, avoidance of repetitive forearm pronation and flexion may be helpful. If these measures fail, surgical release of the nerve is indicated, and the patient should be referred.

Anterior Interosseous Syndrome

Entrapment of the anterior interosseous nerve, a large motor nerve branch of the median nerve, can occur in the forearm. A result of this entrapment is the inability to flex the DIP joints of the index and long fingers and the IP joint of the thumb.[5] Clinically it causes a loss of a precise pinch or the ability to make the "OK" sign. There is no sensory deficit. Typically, patients report pain in the forearm that may precede development of weakness of the thumb and index and long fingers. Pain is aggravated by upper extremity exercise. The findings of EMG and NCS are often normal in this disorder.

Initial treatment of anterior interosseous syndrome consists of the use of NSAIDs and the avoidance of activities requiring resisted upper extremity strength. Surgery is indicated only if the patient fails to progress after 3 months of conservative treatment.

Ulnar Nerve

Cubital Tunnel Syndrome

The most common ulnar nerve neuropathy is cubital tunnel syndrome, the entrapment of the ulnar nerve at the elbow. Several factors play a role in this problem, including the narrowing and reduced capacity of the cubital tunnel during elbow flexion.[16] Because the nerve is quite superficial at the elbow, it may subluxate in and out of the groove.

Symptoms of cubital tunnel syndrome include numbness and tingling and sometimes pain along the distribution of the ulnar nerve. Patients experience pain radiating down from the elbow or up toward the elbow to the area of the medial epicondyle, under which the nerve runs.

Pain at night is rare. Symptoms of numbness and tingling may be present on the dorsum and palmar aspects of the hand. Complaints of muscle weakness and atrophy indicate more severe entrapment.

On physical examination, patients with cubital tunnel syndrome have a positive Tinel's sign over the ulnar nerve at the cubital tunnel of the elbow. They will also have a positive elbow flexion test. This test is performed by simply holding the elbow in a flexed position; symptoms should be reproduced within 3 minutes.

Treatment of cubital tunnel syndrome is conservative. If conservative treatment has not improved symptoms after 6 weeks, EMG can be helpful, but it is not always diagnostic. Surgical release of the ulnar nerve can be performed but is less predictable than that done in carpal tunnel surgery.

Ulnar Tunnel Syndrome

Ulnar tunnel syndrome, which is the compression of the ulnar nerve in Guyon's canal, is usually caused by repetitive trauma. It can also result from thickened ligaments, hypertrophied muscles, injury to or anatomic variations in the carpal bones, or an ulnar artery aneurysm at the base of the hypothenar eminence.[16]

Typically patients report aching, numbness, and tingling along the ulnar border of the hand. Like CTS, symptoms may be worse at night. If entrapment is severe the patient will experience severe intrinsic muscle weakness and atrophy, as well as sensory changes.

Although sensation on the palmar surface of the little finger and the ulnar half of the ring finger may be diminished, sensation on the dorsum of the hand and digits is usually intact in the patient with ulnar tunnel syndrome. This is because the ulnar nerve passes to the dorsum of the hand proximal to Guyon's tunnel.

Allen's test (see Figures 4-12 and 4-13) can be helpful to determine whether compression of the ulnar nerve is caused by arterial thrombosis or aneurysm.

Treatment for ulnar tunnel syndrome is similar to that for CTS. Surgical release of the ulnar nerve is frequently necessary.

Radial Nerve

Radial nerve entrapments are much less common. Radial tunnel syndrome is the compression of the radial nerve in the radial tunnel, which is bounded by the brachioradialis and brachialis muscles and extends distally to the distal border of the supinator muscles. There are several levels within this tunnel where the nerve can be compressed.

Because there are no motor deficits, radial tunnel syndrome is often confused with tennis elbow. The pain is localized to an area approximately 5 to 7 cm distal to the lateral epicondyle and is aggravated by resisted extension of the middle finger. Resisted forearm supination can also reproduce the patient's symptoms.[17]

Treatment of radial nerve entrapment includes activity modification that avoids pronation and supination, as well as splinting and use of NSAIDs. Surgical exploration or release may be necessary if 3 to 6 months of conservative treatment fails.

Cheiralgia Paresthetica

The dorsal sensory branch of the radial nerve may become trapped near the wrist, causing a mononeuritis along the path of the nerve. This entity has also been called "prisoner's palsy" or "handcuff disease."

Symptoms of cheiralgia paresthetica typically include pain, numbness, hyperesthesia, and burning over the dorsoradial wrist and forearm. Symptoms may begin after a blow to the wrist, or while wearing tight wrist bands.

Diagnosis is primarily clinical. Performing Tinel's test over the radial aspect of the forearm usually causes pain. Flexion of the thumb with ulnar deviation of the wrist can also cause pain. With cheiralgia paresthetica, there is no swelling over the first dorsal tendon compartment, unlike with de Quervain's disease. Grip strength may be weak secondary to pain.[17] EMG or NCS may be helpful in making a definitive diagnosis.

As with other compressive neuropathies, treatment of cheiralgia paresthetica begins with use of NSAIDs, activity modification, and splinting. Referral to an occupational therapist for fabrication of a thumb spica splint is appropriate. Once the compressive device is removed, most cases of cheiralgia paresthetica will resolve with further conservative treatment.

Other Compressive Neuropathic Anomalies

Other compressive neuropathies include thoracic outlet syndrome, either from cervical ribs, anterior scalene muscle constriction, abnormal fibrous bands, or compression by the head of the sternocleidomastoid muscle of the lateral cord of the brachial plexus. Anatomic anomalies of the peripheral nerves can also cause symptoms. Cervical radiculopathy from disk degeneration or spondylosis can also mimic compressive peripheral neuropathies.

DEGENERATIVE AND DEVELOPMENTAL PROBLEMS

Kienböck's Disease

Kienböck's disease is an osteonecrosis of the lunate. It is a problem that is more common in women. Chronic wrist pain that worsens over several months is often the presenting symptom. It is associated with ulnar negative variance where the distal ulna is shorter than the radius on a neutral PA x-ray film. Several stages have been described for Kienböck's disease.

History. Pain after an injury to the wrist is a common history for Kienböck's disease. Sometimes no specific incident can be recalled by the patient, but those in occupations requiring repetitive wrist flexion and extension may be at greater risk. Pain is worse with hyperextension of the wrist, and motion may be limited.

Physical Examination. Swelling without discoloration may be present. Usually there is exquisite ten-

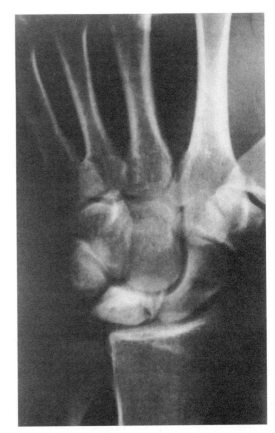

Figure 4-51   Kienböck's Disease. Sclerosis and the collapse of the lunate that occurs in later stages is shown. Chronic wrist pain is the result of osteonecrosis of the bone. (From Mackin EJ et al, editors: *Rehabilitation of the hand and upper extremity*, ed 5, vol 1, St Louis, 2002, Mosby.)

derness to palpation of the lunate bone. Pain with passive extension of the middle finger is often present.

Diagnosis and Treatment. Diagnosis of Kienböck's disease is made by history, examination, and x-ray evaluation. On an AP view of the wrist, the presence of sclerotic bone causes the lunate to appear white (Figure 4-51). In its later stages the lunate may collapse. MRI is an important tool for staging the disease, since early changes are not visualized on x-ray films (Figure 4-52). The patient with Kienböck's disease should be treated by a hand surgeon, since surgical excision or stabilization may be necessary.

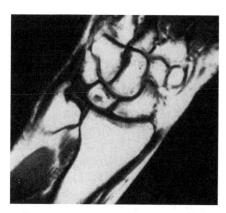

Figure 4-52   Stage III Kienböck's Disease. MRI appearance of the area of decreased signal (*dark spot*) on the lunate that corresponds with changes of osteonecrosis. (From Firooznia H et al, editors: *MRI and CT of the musculoskeletal system*, St Louis, 1992, Mosby.)

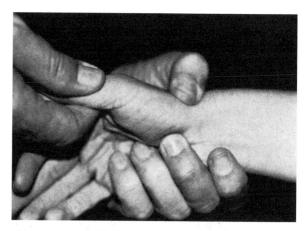

Figure 4-53   Grind Test for Carpometacarpal Arthritis of the Thumb. Pushing the metacarpal against the trapezium will cause pain in the presence of osteoarthritis of the joint. (From Mackin EJ et al, editors: *Rehabilitation of the hand and upper extremity*, ed 5, vol 1, St Louis, 2002, Mosby.)

Arthritis

Arthritis around the hand and wrist area is very common. As previously mentioned the CMC joint of the thumb is one of the joints of the hand most commonly involved in osteoarthritis. The incidence of arthritis at the CMC joint is believed to be the result of the large amount of flexibility at this saddle joint combined with the substantial forces placed upon it.[3] Typically women are affected more than men. Pain and weakness with pinch types of thumb motion are common complaints, as is a constant aching at the base of the thumb.

On physical examination, generally there is tenderness at the CMC joint of the thumb, and crepitus may be palpable with the movement of the thumb. The grind test, a type of joint loading, is performed by stabilizing the wrist and then holding the metacarpal and applying force directly to the trapezium; this test will reproduce or aggravate pain (Figure 4-53). Bony hypertrophy may be palpable at the joint.

Diagnosis of arthritis is confirmed with x-ray evaluation. Treatment includes a trial of nonnarcotic analgesics, followed by administration of NSAIDs. Intraarticular injection of a corticosteroid may significantly improve symptoms. If these treatments are unsuccessful it is appropriate to refer the patient to an orthopedic hand surgeon. Although synthetic implants

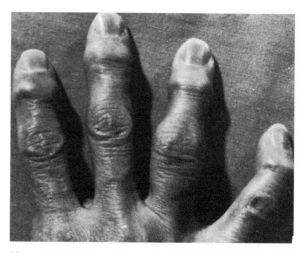

Figure 4-54   Osteoarthritis of the hand. Heberden's nodes are shown at the DIP joints. (From Mackin EJ et al, editors: *Rehabilitation of the hand and upper extremity*, ed 5, vol 2, St Louis, 2002, Mosby.)

are still used, optimal treatment is probably an excisional arthroplasty with ligament reconstruction.[25]

The DIP joints of the digits are also commonly involved in osteoarthritis and display Heberden's nodes (Figure 4-54) and mucous cysts. Less commonly the PIP joints will be involved.

Treatment of arthritis can include splinting, occupational and physical therapy, corticosteroid injections, glucosamine, and the use of medications such as analgesics and NSAIDs. There are also surgical options, which should be left to the discretion of a competent hand surgeon.

Rheumatoid Disease

Hand involvement in rheumatoid disease is common. In fact, as a rule the small joints of the hands are the first seen to be affected with rheumatoid arthritis (RA) and often the most severely affected (Figure 4-55). Tenosynovitis is also a common finding in the wrist and hand.

History. Aching pain that is worse in the morning is a classic finding in RA. Stiffness and limited ROM are also common. The patient usually complains of joint pain and may or may not have associated swelling. Generalized complaints of fatigue and weakness, as well as weakness in the fingers or wrist, are frequently encountered.

Physical Examination. In established RA, deformity is usually the most obvious sign. Ulnar deviation of the fingers occurs in combination with bony hypertrophy of the joints, joint subluxation, and ankylosis; multiple finger deformities are seen (Figures 4-56 and 4-57).

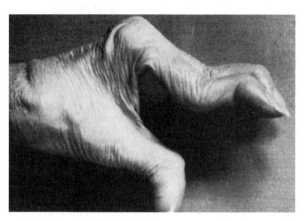

Figure 4-56 Swan-neck Deformity of the Fingers. The metacarpophalangeal and distal interphalangeal joints are fixed in flexion while the proximal interphalangeal joint is hyperextended. (From Mackin EJ et al, editors: *Rehabilitation of the hand and upper extremity*, ed 5, vol 1, St Louis, 2002, Mosby.)

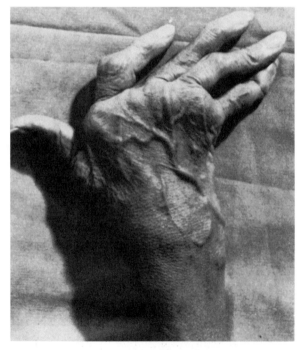

Figure 4-55 Late Rheumatoid Arthritis. Typical hand appearance of both boutonnière and swan-neck deformities. (From Mackin EJ et al, editors: *Rehabilitation of the hand and upper extremity*, ed 5, vol 2, St Louis, 2002, Mosby.)

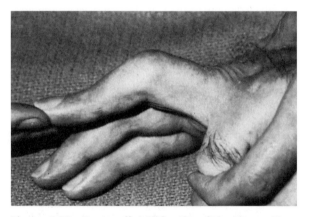

Figure 4-57 Boutonnière Deformity of the Finger. There is fixed flexion of the proximal interphalangeal joint and hyperextension of the distal interphalangeal joint. (From Mackin EJ et al, editors: *Rehabilitation of the hand and upper extremity*, ed 5, vol 1, St Louis, 2002, Mosby.)

Joint instability is seen when connective and supportive tissues are involved.

Palpation of the radial and ulnar aspects of the joints may reveal an obscured joint line caused by synovial thickening.[23] Manual compression of the metacarpal heads tends to increase pain.

Diagnosis. The American College of Rheumatology has established clear guidelines for the diagnosis of RA. The reader is referred to a general rheumatologic text for these criteria.

Treatment. Consultation with or referral to a rheumatologist should be made, especially if this is the patient's first work-up for the disease. If the patient is being treated for RA but joint symptoms are progressing to the point of incapacitation, the patient should be referred to an orthopedic hand surgeon.

INFECTIONS

Because the hand receives a good supply of blood, infections are uncommon. However, hand injuries in the presence of diseases such as diabetes or peripheral vascular disease, trauma such as human and animal bites, farm injuries, intravenous (IV) drug use, or chronic immunosuppressed states should cause the practitioner to reach a high index of suspicion for polymicrobial infection.

The most common organism identified in hand infections is *Staphylococcus aureus*. Other common pathogens include *Streptococcus* and gram-negative organisms. Treatment of hand infections is based on patient history, an idea of which organisms are likely to have caused them, and their course.

Many times, initial treatment with IV antibiotics helps resolve or localize the infection. If at all possible, cultures should be obtained before starting antibiotics; not, however, if obtaining cultures incurs a delay in beginning antibiotic therapy that places the patient or the limb at risk.

Examination of an individual with a hand infection should include palpation of the lymph nodes. It should be kept in mind that the epitrochlear nodes drain the ring and small fingers; the axillary nodes drain the radial digits.

Cellulitis

Most practitioners have seen cellulitis in their clinical practice. Classically it appears as an erythematous, warm, diffusely tender, edematous area. Lymphangitis is also frequently present. In the hand, cellulitis may be attributable to local penetration of or other trauma to the skin, or dermatitis; its cause may be idiopathic. The primary concern in cellulitis is to rule out an underlying, more serious infection, such as a septic joint or a deep space infection.

Group A β-hemolytic streptococcus is the most common causative organism, but *Staphylococcus aureus* is also often involved. In the absence of constitutional symptoms such as fever, chills, nausea, vomiting, or headache, oral antibiotics are appropriate initial therapy. Cephalexin or erythromycin generally provides adequate coverage. If no improvement is noted within 24 to 48 hours after instituting antibiotic therapy, a deeper or more serious infection should be considered. At that point, the patient should be referred to an infectious disease specialist or a hospital.

Paronychia

Hand infections that are encountered in a typical primary care practice include paronychia, which involves infections of the nail bed (Figure 4-58). Typically the term paronychia refers to an abscess. Paronychia is more

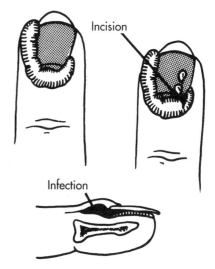

Figure 4-58 Typical appearance of paronychia and the location for incision for drainage. (From Noble J, editor: *Textbook of primary care medicine*, ed 3, St Louis, 2001, Mosby.)

common in persons who bite their nails, wear artificial nails, or have hangnails.

Antibiotics are generally of little use without drainage of the abscess. As a result patients with paronychia should be treated by a hand surgeon, especially if a trial of antibiotics has failed to reduce the infection.

Felon

Another common infection is felon, a subcutaneous abscess of the distal pulp on the volar side of the distal phalanx. The distal pulp contains a network of septa, effectively making the area a closed compartment. Early in the course of felon, the distal phalanx is cellulitic. At this point, warm soaks, elevation, and oral antistaphylococcal antibiotics may resolve the symptoms.

If felon progresses to abscess formation, incision and drainage are necessary. An incision over the area of greatest tenderness and the disruption of the septa are usually the treatments of choice. Because of the problems associated with skin and the closeness of nerves, vessels, and flexor tendon sheaths, these procedures should be performed by a qualified hand surgeon.

Human Bites

Human bite wounds can be severe, especially if they involve bone or joints. Human bite wounds should always be considered infected and usually require incision and drainage. When a human bite wound is inflicted during an altercation, lacerations to the hand most commonly involve the ring and little finger MCP joints.

Although the most common infecting organism is *S. aureus*, up to 42 bacterial strains have been isolated from human bite wounds.[1] Fortunately, coverage for group A *Streptococcus* and *Eikenella corrodens* (a gram-negative organism) in addition to *S. aureus* is usually sufficient. Clindamycin, penicillin, or amoxicillin/clavulanate is recommended for prophylaxis.

Dog and Cat Bites

Dog and cat bites can also be serious. Cat bites are more likely to become infected than dog bites. Vigorous wound irrigation and cleansing with soap and water are the initial treatment steps. Antibiotics used must cover *Pasteurella multocida* (also a gram-negative coccobacillus); these include amoxicillin/clavulanate or penicillin.

Rabies is another consideration in animal bites, especially those of a wild animal (e.g., raccoon, fox, or skunk).

Suppurative Flexor Tenosynovitis

One hand infection that is an urgent surgical emergency is suppurative flexor tenosynovitis (infection of the flexor tendon sheath). This infection is usually the result of penetrating trauma, but hematogenous spread is typical for gonococcal infection.[1] If untreated, suppurative flexor tenosynovitis leads to tendon adhesions, decreased ROM, and necrosis.

The classic presenting symptoms are Kanavel's four cardinal signs: (1) severe pain on passive extension; (2) affected finger held in a flexed position; (3) severe tenderness along the flexor tendon sheath; and (4) symmetric swelling or "sausage digit." Any patient who exhibits these signs should be urgently referred to an orthopedic hand surgeon or an emergency department.

Treatment begins with IV administration of antibiotics, elevation, and splinting. Surgical treatment is indicated if significant improvement is not noted within 24 hours.[11] This infection can spread to the adjoining deep spaces of the hand. These deep spaces lie internal to the flexor tendons and include the thenar space, which is deep to the thumb and index finger. The middle and ring fingers border the midpalmar space and the small finger, which has the ulnar bursa. These deep spaces also require treatment through surgical procedures.

Another deep infection that can occur around the web space is the "collar button" abscess. This infection usually needs to be treated with incision and drainage, with incisions on both the dorsal and volar aspects of the web space.

Septic Joint

Infection of a hand or finger joint is another surgical emergency. In the hand, *S. aureus*, *Streptococcus*, and gonococcus are the most common offending organisms. As with other joint infections, the more rapid the treatment, the better the outcome.

Any patient who has a red, swollen, and exquisitely tender immobile joint should be evaluated for a possible intraarticular infection.

Pain with motion and guarding of the joint (hence its relative immobility) are typical symptoms of joint infection. The joint should be aspirated as soon as possible; this treatment may necessitate a referral to an emergency department or orthopedic surgeon.

Aspiration and laboratory analysis of joint fluid will identify the causative organism and can rule out gout, which can closely mimic a septic joint. Fluid should be sent for white blood cell count, Gram's stain, culture, and crystal examination.

Treatment consists of IV administration of antibiotics and irrigation and débridement of the joint. Often the wound is left open to prevent abscess formation.

Herpetic Whitlow

Herpetic whitlow is a fairly common infection in medical and dental personnel. This is a herpes virus infection that typically involves the distal phalanx of a digit, often the thumb or index finger. Symptoms may begin after a viral illness. The patient experiences pain, swelling, and tenderness of the involved digit. The presence of a vesicular rash is typical.

The disease is self-limited, usually resolving in 7 to 10 days. Unfortunately it is quite contagious as long as vesicles are present. The practitioner should not treat this infection with incision and drainage but rather with splinting and elevation.

Miscellaneous Infections

Another rare but interesting infection that needs to be discussed is sporotrichosis, a fungal infection usually caused by handling roses. Lymphatic spreading causes discoloration and small bumps on the skin. Sporotrichosis is treated with potassium iodide supersaturated solution.

Mycobacterial infections, especially with the marinum strain, are commonly seen in fishermen or pool workers. This infection can initially cause swelling and a nonhealing ulcer that often becomes chronic. Treatment with oral medications, such as rifampin and ethambutol, is often successful, but incision and débridement may be required.

Insect bites, such as that of the brown recluse spider, can cause areas of focal necrosis and require early wide local excision.

With hand infections the probability of hand surgery is high, and early consultation with a hand specialist is recommended for these problems.

MISCELLANEOUS CONDITIONS

Complex Regional Pain Syndrome

The phrase complex regional pain syndrome (CRPS) has been introduced to replace the term reflex sympathetic dystrophy. The disorder, which is characterized by a large, localized area of pain following an inciting event, is divided into two types: CRPS I and CRPS II. Type I CRPS occurs without an identifiable nerve injury; whereas type II is associated with a specific nerve injury. The hallmark sign for this syndrome is pain out of proportion to that expected from a given injury or event. Other characteristic clinical findings include stiffness, atrophic skin changes, underlying bone osteopenia, and vasomotor and autonomic nervous system disturbances. These will manifest as a decrease in function, changes in skin color, cold intolerance, and dry skin. Sympathetic blocks are useful in that they can be both diagnostic and therapeutic. The most important features of successful treatment of CRPS are early diagnosis, prompt initiation of physical therapy, and treatments that diminish sympathetic activity, such as a stellate ganglion block.[18]

Hypothenar Hammer Syndrome

Hypothenar hammer syndrome is ulnar artery spasm or thrombosis. Symptoms include pain, cold intolerance, numbness, and often, in smokers and heavy users of alcohol, ulceration. It can also occur in persons who use their hands as substitutes for tools (e.g., hammers).

The syndrome can be verified with Doppler studies. Angiography is also used to diagnose this condition. Microvascular surgery, which requires resection and grafting of the ulnar artery, is the treatment of choice for hypothenar hammer syndrome.

Raynaud's Disorders

Another common vascular ailment is Raynaud's phenomenon, syndrome, or disease. All three disorders are related to problems with vascular spasms. Young adult women are most frequently affected.

Usually the patient has pallor of the digits, especially with exposure to the cold or with emotional stress. Once pallor resolves, the digits become cyanotic, then hyperemic. These characteristics explain the "red, white, and blue" of the disease.

Treatment is symptomatic and should include avoidance of cold exposure, cessation of tobacco use, and stress management. Referral to an orthopedic surgeon is not necessary.

Raynaud's phenomenon has identical symptoms to Raynaud's disease. The phenomenon, however, occurs in the course of other diseases, most often scleroderma and systemic lupus erythematosus.

Compartment Syndrome

Another occlusive problem that is seen relatively rarely in office practice is compartment syndrome. Compartment syndrome occurs when increased tissue pressure in a limited space leads to decreased blood flow and function. This disorder can be caused by fractures, soft-tissue injury, arterial injury, IV drug infusion, burns, or crush injuries.

EVALUATION MODALITIES

Plain Radiographic Films

Plain x-ray films are probably the quickest and most cost-effective diagnostic imaging modality to assess bony anatomy. Standard AP, lateral, and oblique x-ray projections will provide information about bones, articular surfaces, and soft-tissue shadows. Fractures, dislocations, and degenerative conditions can be visualized. Dislocated or displaced bony structures of the wrist and hand provide preliminary evidence of associated soft-tissue damage.

Special views may be necessary to visualize the thumb. A Robert's view is used to evaluate the MCP joint. This view requires the patient to rotate internally the shoulder, pronate the forearm, and extend the fingers, placing the thumb on the film cassette.

A carpal tunnel view is used to evaluate osseous obstructions in the carpal canal and fractures of the hook of the hamate and pisiform bones. This view requires a degree of hyperextension of the wrist, with the x-ray beam directed horizontally between the thenar and hypothenar eminences.[37] Other specialized views can provide improved visualization of other carpal bones, but these projections are best left to the discretion of the orthopedic or hand surgeon.

Computed Tomography

The large number of bones and their overlying shadows, as well as the types of fractures found in the wrist, render x-ray evaluation insufficient in some instances. CT is considered the imaging modality of choice for evaluating the position of dislocated or displaced bony structures. Carpal bone fractures, including occult or suggested scaphoid fractures, can be evaluated in greater detail with CT than with plain x-ray studies. CT is also preferred in evaluating joint congruity in intraarticular fractures, as well as in distal radioulnar joint subluxation and dislocation.[6] Assessment of fracture nonunion (as in a scaphoid fracture) is best visualized with CT.

Arthrography

Arthrography is one of the least expensive types of imaging study available, but it is invasive and uncomfortable for the patient. It remains, however, an excellent way to detect tears of the TFCC. It is also quite useful in evaluating scapholunate tears. In some instances, arthrography can be combined with CT to evaluate joint or ligamentous disruption.

Magnetic Resonance Imaging

MRI has a utility in certain wrist and hand injuries that cannot be matched by other imaging modalities. In addition to visualizing early changes in bone associated with osteonecrosis (e.g., Kienböck's disease), soft-tissue abnormalities are easily seen.

Tendonitis, synovitis, fibrous tissue masses, ligamentous injuries, and ganglion cysts can all be evaluated by MRI. Evaluation of infection, particularly in the deep spaces of the hand, is another use for MRI.

INDICATIONS FOR REFERRAL

See the following Red Flags box for referral information.

Red Flags *for Wrist and Hand Disorders*

Patients with these findings may need to be referred for more extensive work-up.

Signs and Symptoms	Response
Phalangeal fracture caused by rotational force results in rotated digit	Usually unstable injury; refer to orthopedic hand surgeon. (It is appropriate to refer any phalangeal fracture to an orthopedic surgeon.)
Rotated metacarpal fracture; ROM may reveal inability to fully extend metacarpal joint of affected digit; pain and palpable deformity over fracture site	Rotated fractures should be referred to orthopedic surgeon.
Comminuted, intraarticular fracture of base of fifth metacarpal	Possible Rolando fracture. Splint fracture and immediately refer to orthopedic surgeon. Rolando fracture is difficult to stabilize even with surgery.
Intraarticular fracture of base of first metacarpal; injury displaced as abductor pollicis longus pulls shaft more radially; remaining piece of bone rotated by pulling capsular attachment	Possible Bennett's fracture. Confirm with plain x-ray film. Splint entire thumb, and refer to orthopedic surgeon. Fracture may require operative stabilization.
Anatomic snuff-box tenderness	Possible scaphoid fracture. Refer to orthopedic or preferably hand surgeon because of high complication rate with treatment, including high rate of nonunion.
Displaced or nondisplaced isolated ulnar shaft fracture	
Colles' fracture—dorsal angulation and often some radial deviation of distal fragment; may involve articular surface	Generally, all wrist fractures should be treated by orthopedic surgeon, especially if displaced.
Smith's fracture—occurs in opposite direction of Colles' fracture	Diagnose fracture, immobilize it, and refer to orthopedic surgeon.
Barton's fracture—through articular surface of dorsal aspect of distal radius; distal fracture fragment displaced dorsally and proximally	
Chauffeur's fracture—intraarticular fracture of radial styloid; distal fragment displaces distally and may be rotated	
Pain from wrist "sprain" continues beyond 6 to 8 weeks	Possible radiocarpal joint dislocation. Refer to hand surgeon.

Continued

Signs and Symptoms	Response
Lunate dislocated away from distal radius, usually from fall on outstretched hand with resultant hyperextension of wrist	Possible carpal dislocation. Injury is usually significant and requires attention of hand surgeon.
Dislocation of CMC joint, most frequently occurring at ring and little fingers and often with associated fracture	Splint hand and reduce dislocation (if possible). Refer to orthopedic hand surgeon. Unstable nature of this injury may require surgical treatment.
Digit (usually thumb) forced into hyperextension; on x-ray film, sesamoid bone may be interposed between metacarpal and proximal phalanx; tenting of skin often present at joint	Possible complex MCP joint dislocation. Injury needs to be treated surgically. Refer to hand surgeon.
Disruption of volar plate and usually of radial or ulnar collateral ligament; no associated fracture	Possible PIP dislocation. Splint PIP joint at approximately 45 degrees of flexion. Refer to orthopedic hand surgeon.
Swelling and dislocation over dorsal aspect of hand; palpation may elicit tenderness just ulnar to anatomic snuff-box; movement of fingers usually normal; making tight fist causes increased pain as does hyperextension of wrist; Watson's test elicits symptomatic clicking and sometimes palpable clunk over scaphoid; x-ray films show increased space between scaphoid and lunate bones on AP projection	Possible scapholunate injury. Ligament reconstruction may be required. Refer to orthopedic hand surgeon.
Twisting injury to wrist; exquisite tenderness between ECU and FCU tendons; may be localized swelling over ulnocarpal area	Possible TFCC tear. Refer to hand surgeon.
Thumb abruptly radially deviated because of fall; pain and swelling after injury; unstable thumb and weakness when twisting bottle cap; weakness when pinching thumb and forefinger; swelling on ulnar side of metacarpal joint of thumb	Possible ulnar collateral ligament injury (also known as gamekeeper's thumb or skier's thumb). Operative repair may be necessary if there is complete rupture of ligament. Refer to orthopedic hand surgeon.
Complete disruption of ligament from finger sprain; no end point when ligament is stressed; joint painful and feels unstable to patient	Possible grade III collateral ligament injury. Buddy tape injured finger. Refer to orthopedic surgeon for definitive treatment.
Digits rotate away from side of torn collateral ligament after wrist is flexed and extended	Possible disruption of radial or ulnar collateral ligament of metacarpal joint. Refer to orthopedic hand surgeon.
Symptoms of de Quervain's disease persist after corticosteroid injection into tendon sheath	Surgical release of tendon sheath may be necessary. Refer to orthopedic surgeon.

Signs and Symptoms	Response
Injury to any flexor tendon from zone I to zone V	Refer to hand surgeon for repair to reduce incidence of complications.
Formation of scar around flexor tendon resulting in catching of tendon under A1 pulley of hand; as finger extends, nodule of scar tissue slides beneath pulley and releases, causing sudden and painful "triggering" of finger	Possible trigger finger. Definitive treatment requires surgical release. Refer to hand surgeon.
Progressive deformity of affected digit, often ring finger; seen bilaterally; palmar skin may adhere to fascia, forming palpable band in palm of hand; nodules often palpable with cords; multiple fingers affected	Possible Dupuytren's contracture. If patient has PIP or MCP contracture of >30 degrees, refer to orthopedic hand surgeon.
Failure of response to conservative treatment for CTS after 6 weeks; EMG and NCS reveal evidence of CTS	Carpal tunnel surgery may be indicated. Refer to hand surgeon or orthopedic surgeon.
Failure of response to conservative treatment for pronator syndrome	Surgical release of nerve may be indicated. Refer to orthopedic surgeon.
Failure to progress after 3 months of conservative treatment for anterior interosseous syndrome	Refer to orthopedic surgeon.
Aching, numbness, and tingling along ulnar border of hand; symptoms worse at night; severe intrinsic muscle weakness and atrophy, as well as sensory changes; Allen's test negative for arterial thrombosis or aneurysm	Possible ulnar tunnel syndrome. Surgical release of the ulnar nerve is frequently necessary. Refer to orthopedic surgeon.
Failure of response to 3 to 6 months of conservative treatment for radial nerve entrapment	Refer to orthopedic surgeon. Surgical exploration or release may be necessary.
Exquisite tenderness of lunate bone; may be painful with passive extension of middle finger; may be swelling of wrist without discoloration; pain worsens with hyperextension of wrist; motion may be limited	Possible Kienböck's disease. Refer to hand surgeon. Surgical excision or stabilization may be necessary.
Treatment for arthritis (nonnarcotic analgesics and NSAIDs and intraarticular injections of corticosteroids) unsuccessful	Refer to orthopedic hand surgeon. Patient may need synthetic implants or arthroplasty with ligament reconstruction.

Continued

Signs and Symptoms	Response
Ulnar deviation of fingers occurs in combination with bony hypertrophy of joints, joint subluxation, and ankylosis; may be multiple finger deformities; joint instability seen when connective and supportive tissue involved; palpation of radial and ulnar aspects of joints may reveal obscured joint line attributable to synovial thickening; manual compression of metacarpal heads increases pain	Consult with or refer to rheumatologist, especially if this is patient's first work-up for RA.
RA joint symptoms progressing to point of incapacitation	Refer to orthopedic hand surgeon for possible surgical intervention.
No improvement of hand infection in 24 to 48 hours after antibiotic treatment	Refer to infectious disease specialist or to hospital.
Infection at fold between nail plate and fold	Possible paronychia. Refer to hand surgeon for drainage of abscess, especially if antibiotics have failed to reduce symptoms.
Felon progresses to abscess formation	Incision and drainage are necessary. Because of problems with skin and closeness of nerves, vessels, and flexor tendon sheaths, refer to qualified hand surgeon.
Severe pain on passive extension; affected finger held in flexed position; severe tenderness along flexor tendon sheath; symmetric swelling, or sausage digit	Possibly suppurative flexor tenosynovitis. Immediately refer to orthopedic hand surgeon or emergency department.
Red, swollen, exquisitely tender immobile joint; pain with motion and guarding of joint	Possible septic joint. Refer to an emergency department or orthopedic surgeon to aspirate joint as soon as possible.
Ulnar artery spasm or thrombosis; pain, cold intolerance, numbness, and often ulceration in smoker, heavy alcohol user, and those who use hands as substitutes for tools	Possible hypothenar hammer syndrome. Refer to orthopedic hand surgeon for treatment with microvascular surgery that requires resection and grafting of ulnar artery.

AP, Anteroposterior; *CMC,* carpometacarpal; *CTS,* carpal tunnel syndrome; *ECU,* extensor carpi ulnaris; *EMG,* electromyography; *FCU,* flexor carpi ulnaris; *MCP,* metacarpophalangeal; *NCS,* nerve conduction studies; *NSAIDs,* nonsteroidal antiinflammatory drugs; *PIP,* proximal interphalangeal; *ROM,* range of motion; TFCC, triangular fibrocartilage complex.

REFERENCES

1. Abrams RA, Botte MJ: Hand infections: treatment recommendations for specific types, *J Am Acad Orthop Surg* 4:219, 1996.

2. Amadio PC et al: Anatomy and pathomechanics of the flexor pulley system, *J Hand Ther* 2:138, 1989.

3. Ateshian GA et al: Contact areas in the thumb carpometacarpal joint, *J Ortho Res* 13:450, 1995.

4. Benson LS, Williams CS, Kahle M: Dupuytren's contracture, *J Am Acad Orthop Surg* 6:1, 1998.

5. Brown DE, Neumann RD: *Orthopedic secrets*, St Louis, 1995, Mosby.

6. Chidgey LK: The distal radioulnar joint: problems and solutions, *J Am Acad Orthop Surg* 3(2):95, 1995.

7. Reference deleted in Proofs.

8. Gan BS, Richards RS, Roth JH: Arthroscopic treatment of triangular fibrocartilage tears, *Orthop Clin North Am* 26:721, 1995.

9. Gellman H et al: Comparison of short and long arm thumb spica casts for non-displaced fractures of the carpal scaphoid. *J Bone Joint Surg Am* 71:353, 1989.

10. Gutierrez G: Office management of scaphoid fractures, *Physician Sportsmedicine* 24(8):60, 1996.

11. Gutowski KA et al: Closed catheter irrigation is as effective as open drainage for treatment of pyogenic flexor tenosynovitis, *Ann Plastic Surgery* 49(4):350, 2002.

12. Harris C et al: The functional anatomy of the extensor mechanism of the finger, *J Bone Joint Surg Am* 54:713, 1972.

13. Helms A, Brodell RT: Surgical pearl: prompt treatment of subungual hematomas, *J Am Acad Dermatol* 42(3):508, 2000.

14. Inoue G, Sakuma M: The natural history of scaphoid nonunion. Radiographical and clinical analysis of 102 cases, *Arch Orthop Trauma Surg* 115:1, 1996.

15. Kaplan SJ, Springfield VA: The Stener lesion revisited: a case report, *J Hand Surg (Am)* 23:833, 1998.

16. Khoo D, Carmichael SW, Spinner RJ: Ulnar nerve anatomy and compression, *Orthop Clin North Am* 27(2):317, 1996.

17. Kleinert JM, Mehta S: Radial nerve entrapment, *Orthop Clin North Am* 27(2):305, 1996.

18. Koman LA, Poehling GG, Smith TL: Complex regional pain syndrome: Reflex sympathetic dystrophy and causalgia. In Green DP, Hotchkiss RN, Pederson WC, editors:

Operative hand surgery, ed 4. New York, 1999, Churchill Livingstone.

19. Kozin SH, Bishop AT: Gamekeeper's thumb: early diagnosis and treatment, *Orthop Rev* 23:797, 1994.

20. Kuschner SH et al: Scaphoid fractures and scaphoid nonunion, *Orthop Rev* 23:861, 1994.

21. Lewis HG, et al: A 10 year review of high pressure injection injuries to the hand: *J Hand Surg (Br)* 23(4):479, 1998.

22. Mayfield JK et al: Carpal dislocations: pathomechanics and prospective perilunar instability *J Hand Surg Am* 35:226, 1980.

23. Moder KG: A working guide to joint examination in rheumatoid arthritis, *J Musculoskel Med* 12(11):17, 1995.

24. Perron AD, Miller MD, Brady WJ: *Orthopaedic pitfalls in the ED: fight bite. Am J Emerg Med* 20(2):114, 2002.

25. Pomerance JF: Painful basal joint arthritis of the thumb, part II: treatment, *Am J Orthop* 24(6):466, 1995.

26. Rayan GM: Scaphoid fractures and nonunions, *Am J Orthop* 24:227, 1995.

27. Rockwell WB et al: Extensor tendon: anatomy, injury and reconstruction, *Plast Reconstr Surg* 106:1592; 2000.

28. Ruby LK: Carpal instability, *J Bone Joint Surg Am* 77:476, 1995.

29. Reference deleted in Proofs.

30. Soren A: Clinical and pathologic characteristics and treatment of ganglia, *Contemp Orthop* 31(1):34, 1995.

31. Steyers CM, Schelkun PH: Practical management of carpal tunnel syndrome, *Physician Sportsmedicine* 23(1):83, 1995.

32. Tiel-van Buul MMC et al: Choosing a strategy for the diagnostic management of scaphoid fracture: a cost effective analysis, *J Nucl Med* 36:45, 1995.

33. Terrono AL, Millender LH: Management of work-related upper-extremity nerve entrapments, *Orthop Clin North Am* 27(4):783, 1996.

34. Totterman SM, Miller RJ: MR Imaging of the triangular fibrocartilage complex: *Magn Reson Imaging Clin North Am* 3:213-228; 1995.

35. Trumble TE, Diao E, Abrams RA, Gilbert-Anderson MM: Single-portal endoscopic carpal tunnel release compared with open release: a prospective, randomized trial, *J Bone Joint Surgery Am* 84(7):1107; 2002.

36. Wehbe MA: Tendon graft donor sites, *J Hand Surg (Am)* 17:1130, 1992.

37. Weisman TL, Donahue BJ, Fletcher DJ: Radiology of the wrist and hand, *Orthopedics* 19:957, 1996.

38. Wilbourn AJ, Gilliat RN: Double-crush syndrome: a critical analysis, *Neurology* 49:21, 1997.

Chapter 5

Lumbar Spine

Approximately 60% of the adults in the United States have had an episode of back pain during the past year. At any time, 2.6 million people are temporarily disabled because of back pain. Although estimations are difficult, it is believed that between $38 and $50 million dollars are spent annually for back disorders in the United States.[1,13] Estimated total annual costs for health care related to low back pain may exceed $5 to $20 billion.[26] Approximately 15 million people seek advice each year from a health care professional for low back complaints, more than for any other problem. Because of the frequency with which these complaints are discussed, it is necessary for the primary care practitioner to have a good understanding of the problems associated with the lumbosacral spine.

ANATOMY AND PHYSIOLOGY

The lumbar spine cannot be studied without discussing its relationship to the sacrum. The lumbar spine normally consists of five lumbar vertebrae, with L1 the most proximal. However, it is not uncommon for L6 to be present, an additional normal vertebra. The lumbar spine consists of the vertebral body, posterior elements, intervertebral disks, and ligaments. This complex provides protection for the neural structures (Figure 5-1).

The sacrum is the most distal of all segments and is the base of the spine. At birth it consists of multiple vertebrae, which by adulthood fuse to form the sacrum; the coccyx is the most distal segment. The lumbosacral spine

provides the lordosis to the spinal column that completes its sagittal contour. Both the cervical and lumbar areas of the spine are lordotic, and the thoracic spine is kyphotic. Lumbar lordosis is measured in degrees of arc and is usually between 30 and 60 degrees, depending on where the measurements are taken. Exaggerated lumbar lordosis may be an anomaly and related to an underlying bony, muscular, or neurologic problem.

The way in which the lumbar vertebral bodies and joint complex interact allows motion between the segments. Interruption of or injury to those relationships can cause decreased range of motion (ROM) and pain.

The lumbar vertebrae are the largest of the spinal column and, by nature of their location, bear the weight of the torso and head. The vertebral body is made up of a strong cancellous bone that is connected to the posterior elements by pedicles; these elements are called the lamina, transverse process, and spinous process (Figure 5-2). The association of two vertebrae creates a joint between vertebral bodies; this articulation is called a *facet joint*. Multiple ligaments connect the vertebral bodies to one another; these include the posterior longitudinal ligament, anterior longitudinal ligament, intertransverse ligaments, interspinous ligaments, and supraspinous ligaments.

An intervertebral disk is located between each two vertebrae and is connected to the vertebral body. This disk is made up of a strong outer layer, the annulus fibrosis, and the nucleus pulposus, which is a jellylike material that moves in the center of the annulus and

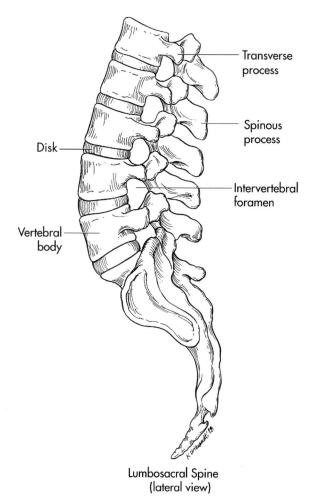

- Transverse process
- Spinous process
- Intervertebral foramen
- Disk
- Vertebral body

Lumbosacral Spine
(lateral view)

Figure 5-1 Lateral drawing of the lumbar spine.

redistributes as different stresses are placed on the disk. A third component, consisting of intertwined annular bands, helps strengthen the disk and dissipate forces placed on the spine. The disk acts like a shock absorber between the vertebrae.

The spinal canal is the round opening at the center of the vertebral column. This canal provides the necessary room for the spinal neurologic structures to function and to be protected. The size of the spinal canal varies along its length; in the cervical spine it is at its largest, and in the thoracic spine at its smallest. In the lumbar spine the normal anterior-posterior dimension is

15 mm, and the transverse measurement is 23 mm. When the canal is smaller, the condition is called *congenital spinal stenosis*. The neural structures are thus confined to a smaller area.

Integral to the discussion of lumbar spine abnormalities are numerous muscle groups across the lower back that receive innervation from the lumbar nerve roots. The low back musculature is divided into the superficial, the intermediate, and the deep muscle layers. This complex system provides support of the torso and facilitates the motion of the lumbar spine.

Most of the muscles of the lumbar spine are located posteriorly, with the exception of the psoas and quadratus lumborum muscles. The spinal musculature extends over multiple segments; no muscle extends the entire length of the spine. To understand lumbar muscle complaints it is important to note the interconnection of muscle groups (Figures 5-3 and 5-4). In addition, the interspinous musculature between the vertebrae facilitates lateral bending and extension of the spine (Figure 5-5).

The cauda equina, which is the continuation of the spinal cord below the first lumbar level in the adult, literally means "horse's tail" (Figure 5-6). It consists of an array of nerves that exit the conus and continue down the lumbar spine, then exiting through the foramen at different lumbar and sacral levels. These nerves are responsible for specific sensory and motor functions. Therefore a problem can be pinpointed by the symptoms, and the specific anatomic level or levels can be determined.

Physical Examination

History

The examination of the spine begins with the identification of the chief complaint and is followed by a focused history related to the problem. How long has the patient had the problem? What was the precipitating incident? If no incident is recalled, in what types of activity did the patient participate before the onset of symptoms? What is the exact mechanism of the spinal injury—flexion, extension, or rotation? If there are no symptoms, but a deformity exists, how long has this condition been noticed?

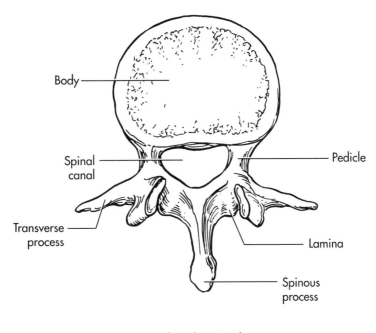

Body

Spinal
canal

Pedicle

Transverse
process

Lamina

Spinous
process

2nd Lumbar Vertebra
(superior view)

Figure 5-2   Coronal drawing of the spinal canal showing the L2 vertebra.

The history of the patient with a low back anomaly is extremely important.[29] Other medical factors such as a recent febrile illness, gynecologic complaints, urinary symptoms, or cardiovascular problems may be related to the low back problem. A thorough family history is also necessary to identify any familial orthopedic or neurologic problem.

Observation

Much information can be gained during the interview process. The examiner should observe the patient as he or she sits in the chair. Does the patient sit comfortably or often shift positions? Is the patient unable to sit because of pain? Does the sitting-to-standing maneuver cause discomfort, or is it accomplished without difficulty? The patient should be asked to walk around the examination room and be observed for his or her ability to move freely. Once the patient is standing, the practitioner should note the stance. Listing to one side may indicate scoliosis or a herni-

ated disk. Exaggerated lordosis of the lumbar spine can be a sign of poor abdominal muscle tone. The patient who is able to move quickly and easily with no outward signs of pain and yet complains of severe pain should be approached cautiously, and concern should be raised over the possibility of symptom enhancement or fabrication.[31,39]

If the patient appears to be stable when walking, the examiner should ask him or her to walk on toes and on heels and to squat down. These three maneuvers offer a quick assessment of gross muscle strength in the lower extremities. If there is concern regarding strength, the examiner should protect the patient from falling or test lower extremity muscle groups while the patient is sitting.

Inspection

The entire spine should be inspected for any signs of deformity, unusual skin markings or clefts, and hairy patches, all of which may indicate underlying congenital

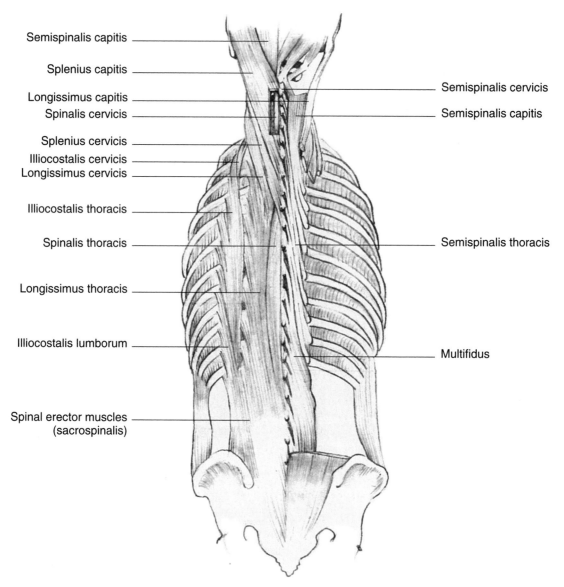

Figure 5-3   Posterior view of intermediate layer of the spinal muscles. (From Reckling FW et al: *Orthopedic anatomy and surgical approach*, St Louis, 1990, Mosby.)

abnormalities. Signs of previous surgical procedures should also be noted, and surgical scars investigated and included in the history. In addition to inspecting the spine, the practitioner should note any leg-length discrepancy and pelvic obliquity, because either may play a role in spine abnormality.

Range of Motion

With the patient in the standing position the ROM can be easily measured. The examiner should ask the patient to flex forward as if touching the toes with knees straight. The patient should then extend backward with the examiner close to prevent falling. Normal flexion of

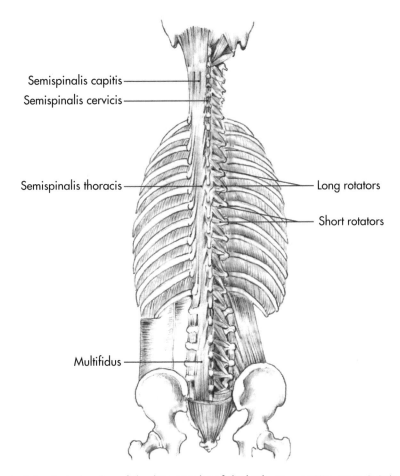

Figure 5-4   Posterior view of the deep muscles of the back. (From Reckling FW et al: *Orthopedic anatomy and surgical approach*, St Louis, 1990, Mosby.)

the lumbar spine should be 90 degrees, and normal extension should be 30 degrees. With the patient standing in the erect position with the examiner's hands on the iliac crests for stabilization, the patient rotates from one side to another. The patient should then laterally flex on each side. Normal rotation is 15 degrees, and normal lateral flexion is 40 degrees. Measurement of costovertebral joint ROM is also important in the patient who complains of generalized back or sacroiliac pain. The examiner should place a tape measure around the chest at the level of the nipples on a man or under the breasts on a woman. The patient should be instructed to completely exhale and then fully inhale. In most adults the measurement between inhaling and exhaling should differ a minimum of 2 inches. Extreme reduction in this measurement may suggest a pathologic condition.

Muscle Strength and Reflexes

Muscle strength and reflexes are often approached together, moving from the upper extremities to the lower. The upper extremities of the patient with a suggested problem of the lumbar spine should be examined to confirm that there is no upper motor neuron abnormality. With the patient in the seated position, the

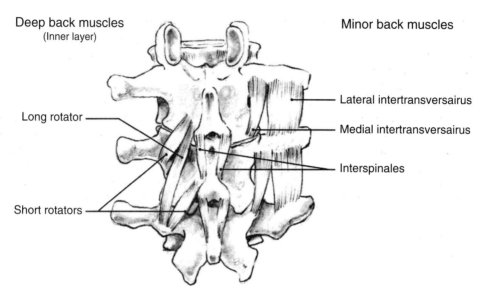

Figure 5-5   Interspinous muscles of the lumbar spine. (From Reckling FW et al: *Orthopedic anatomy and surgical approach*, St Louis, 1990, Mosby.)

examination begins with the upper extremities and progresses to the lower. All muscle groups and reflexes should be evaluated in all extremities. Any pathologic reflexes or weaknesses should be reevaluated later in the examination to confirm that the reflexes and weaknesses are consistent.

While still seated, the patient looks at the bottom of the feet. By examining the sole of his or her foot in this manner, the sciatic nerve is stretched. By performing this test in this manner the examiner has the opportunity to accomplish a straight leg examination out of the usual context. The findings may become important later when conducting a lying down straight leg examination. Inconsistencies in the results of the sitting and lying straight leg raise examinations should be noted.

Lumbar Spine Algorithms

In the last decade the use of algorithms, critical pathways, and care maps has been encouraged to help provide a standardized way to approach similar patients. Algorithms provide a specific time frame into which health care providers incorporate the treatment plan.

The Agency for Health Care Policy and Research (AHCPR), in conjunction with clinical practitioners, developed the algorithms for low back pain (Figures 5-7 through 5-11). These algorithms focus on an organized, methodic approach to lumbar spine evaluation. Seasoned practitioners who have tried to implement them in the clinical setting have criticized algorithms as cumbersome and impractical. However, for the new practitioner, algorithms are a valuable tool for understanding the complexity of the lumbar spine. Although not all patients will fit an algorithm, the AHCPR algorithms help the practitioner who has limited experience with complaints of the lumbar spine and their management.

TRAUMATIC PATHOLOGIC CONDITIONS AND TREATMENTS

Lumbosacral Sprain and Strain

A sprain refers to damage to a ligament, whereas a strain refers to damage to a muscle by either injury or overuse. It is difficult to differentiate between ligament and muscle when examining the patient with low back pain. Often the words strain and sprain are interchanged when diagnosing conditions of the lumbar spine. The Quebec system, a recognized system used to delineate

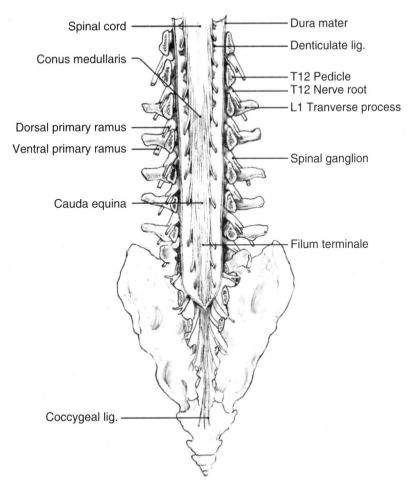

Spinal cord

Conus medullaris

Dorsal primary ramus

Ventral primary ramus

Cauda equina

Coccygeal lig.

Dura mater

Denticulate lig.

T12 Pedicle

T12 Nerve root

L1 Tranverse process

Spinal ganglion

Filum terminale

Figure 5-6   Drawing showing the end of the spinal cord (conus medullaris) and the cauda equina. (From Reckling FW et al: *Orthopedic anatomy and surgical approach*, St Louis, 1990, Mosby.)

diagnoses, actually classifies the pain rather than the tissue from which it arises.

The patient often relates a change in activity level or a change of participation in a normal activity (e.g., lifting) that has lead to the onset of back pain. The pain can be located in any segment of the spine, but most commonly pain arises from the lumbar area. Typically the patient describes the pain as lateral to the spine in the flank area. The practitioner can often manually identify muscle tightness by palpating the affected side.

The initial phase of treatment for a lumbar sprain or strain includes modalities such as cold, massage, and ultra-

sound; heat therapy is started 48 to 72 hours after injury. Mild analgesics and muscle relaxants should be prescribed for the patient who continues to complain of pain. Mild restriction of activity should be encouraged for the first few days after injury. However, researchers have shown that prolonged bed rest is less effective than a gradual return to normal activities. Patients who return to their usual activities have more rapid resolution of pain.

Acute Cauda Equina Syndrome

Although many diagnoses related to the lumbar spine are discussed, acute cauda equina compression is an

Text continued on p. 141

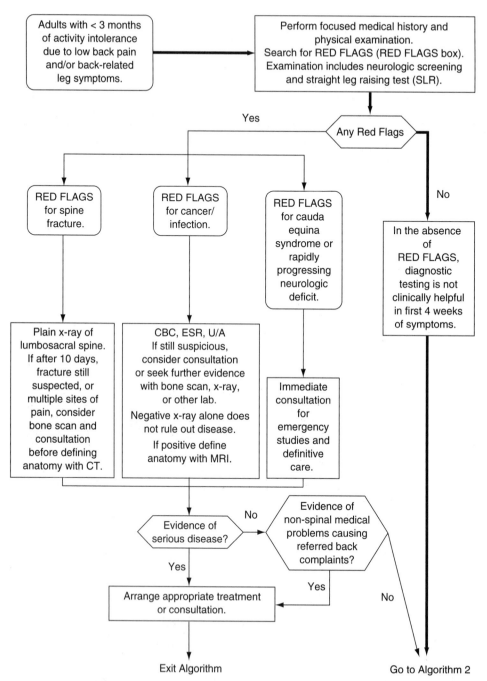

Figure 5-7   Algorithm 1. Initial evaluation of acute low back problem. (From Agency for Health Care Policy and Research: Algorithms for the management of acute low back pain in adults, *Clinical Practice Guideline 14, Attachment A,* Publication No. 95-0642, 1994, AHCPR.)

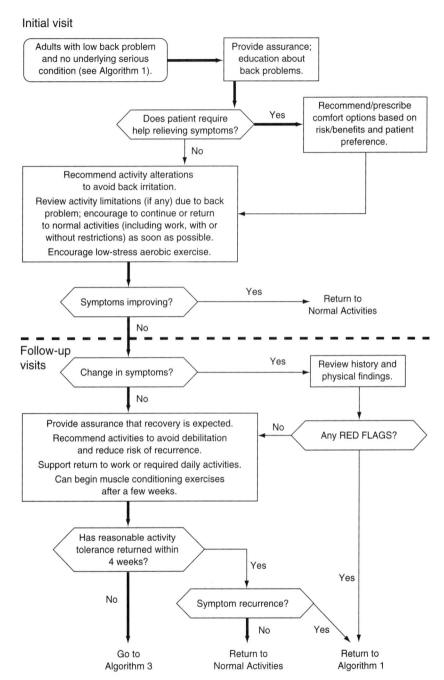

Initial visit

```
┌─────────────────────────┐        ┌─────────────────────┐
│ Adults with low back    │        │ Provide assurance;  │
│ problem and no underlying│───────▶│ education about      │
│ serious condition        │        │ back problems.       │
│ (see Algorithm 1).       │        └─────────────────────┘
└─────────────────────────┘
```

Does patient require help relieving symptoms? — Yes → Recommend/prescribe comfort options based on risk/benefits and patient preference.

No

Recommend activity alterations to avoid back irritation.
Review activity limitations (if any) due to back problem; encourage to continue or return to normal activities (including work, with or without restrictions) as soon as possible.
Encourage low-stress aerobic exercise.

Symptoms improving? — Yes → Return to Normal Activities

No

Follow-up visits

Change in symptoms? — Yes → Review history and physical findings.

No

Provide assurance that recovery is expected.
Recommend activities to avoid debilitation and reduce risk of recurrence.
Support return to work or required daily activities.
Can begin muscle conditioning exercises after a few weeks.

No ← Any RED FLAGS?

Has reasonable activity tolerance returned within 4 weeks?

No → Go to Algorithm 3

Yes → Symptom recurrence?

No → Return to Normal Activities

Yes → Return to Algorithm 1

Yes (RED FLAGS) → Return to Algorithm 1

Figure 5-8   Algorithm 2. Treatment of acute low back problem on initial and follow-up visits. (From Agency for Health Care Policy and Research: Algorithms for the management of acute low back pain in adults, *Clinical Practice Guideline 14, Attachment A,* Publication No. 95-0642, 1994, AHCPR.)

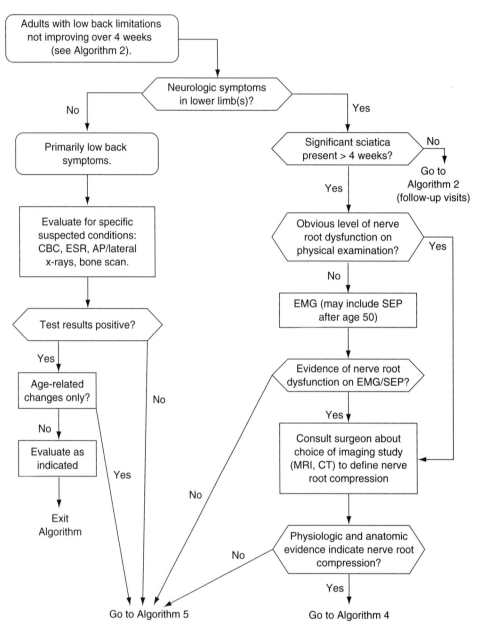

Figure 5-9   Algorithm 3. Evaluation of the slow-to-recover patient with low back problems (symptoms >4 weeks). (From Agency for Health Care Policy and Research: Algorithms for the management of acute low back pain in adults, *Clinical Practice Guideline 14, Attachment A*, Publication No. 95-0642, 1994, AHCPR.)

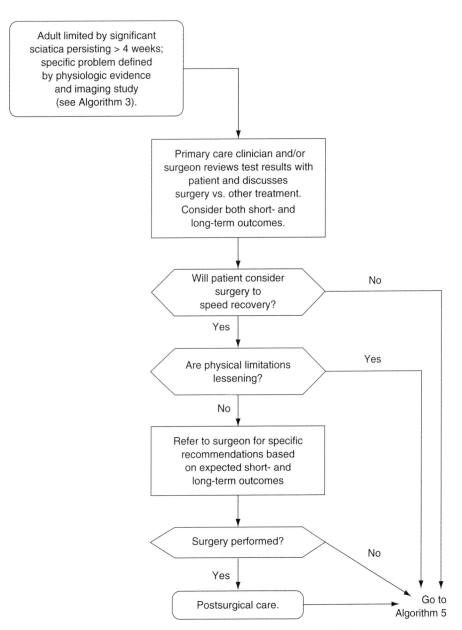

Figure 5-10   Algorithm 4. Surgical considerations for patients with persistent sciatica. (From Agency for Health Care Policy and Research: Algorithms for the management of acute low back pain in adults, *Clinical Practice Guideline 14, Attachment A,* Publication No. 95-0642, 1994, AHCPR.)

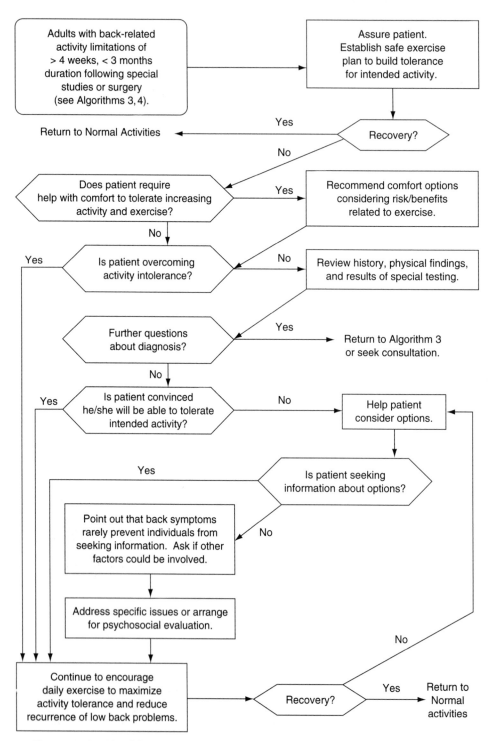

Figure 5-11 **Algorithm 5.** Further management of acute low back problem. (From Agency for Health Care Policy and Research: Algorithms for the management of acute low back pain in adults, *Clinical Practice Guideline 14, Attachment A*, Publication No. 95-0642, 1994, AHCPR.)

orthopedic emergency and must be foremost in the practitioner's mind when evaluating the patient with low back pain. Although the incidence is low, a misdiagnosis of acute cauda equina compression is devastating. Cauda equina syndrome results from compression of the nerve roots distal to S1. Whether acute or chronic, the presenting symptoms of this syndrome are typically the onset of low back pain, weakness and sciatica of the bilateral lower extremities, sensory deficit in the perineal and rectal area ("saddle anesthesia"), and possible bowel and bladder incontinence.[12,28] Often the pathologic condition is an acute herniation of a large disk. The patient with these symptoms should be urgently referred to the care of the surgeon with expertise in spinal surgery. Emergent diagnostic testing is necessary, including myelography or magnetic resonance imaging (MRI). If cauda equina compression is confirmed, surgical lumbar decompression within 48 hours is the treatment of choice to halt neurologic deterioration,[7] unless contraindicated because of other medical problems.

Intervertebral Disk Disease

Many terms are used to describe disk pathologic disease, often confusing health care providers. The most commonly used terms to describe disk abnormalities are a bulging or a slipped, herniated, ruptured, or extruded disk. The size of the individual's spinal canal becomes an important consideration when diagnosing a disk problem. A small canal will tolerate less disk material that is bulging or is herniated, ruptured, or extruded. A small, herniated disk in one patient will not be a problem; in another, the same-sized herniation may cause significant compression to the neural structures.

Disk anomalies begin when there is injury or degeneration to the annulus fibrosis, the outer portion of the disk. The nucleus pulposus begins to bulge in the area of weakness or tear. Bulging is an initial indication that the disk is showing signs of wear and tear. In most patients a bulging disk will cause no symptoms. In patients who have a small spinal canal and neural compression, symptoms may be seen.

A herniated or ruptured disk describes the nucleus pulposus pushing through a tear in the annulus fibrosis (Figure 5-12). The location and amount of disk material in the canal will determine the symptoms. A small

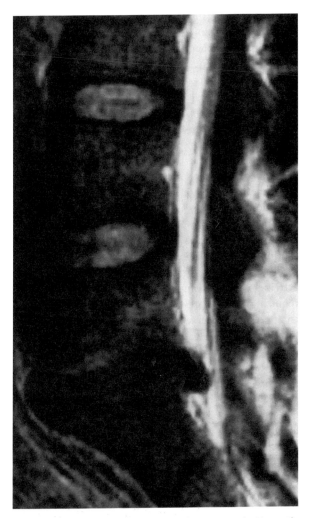

Figure 5-12 Herniated Disk at the L5 Level. Magnetic resonance image visualizing the indentation of the disk material into the spinal canal, compressing the cauda equina.

amount of nucleus pulposus in a congenitally small canal can cause significant symptoms. Not all bulging or herniated disks result in clinical symptoms, so it is imperative to correlate clinical and any imaged abnormalities.[8] Most disks will herniate more to one side than the other, compressing the nerve roots on the affected side. Symptoms include ipsilateral buttock and leg pain. In a large, centrally herniated disk, bilateral symptoms may be present. Bowel and bladder incontinence can also occur with significant compression.

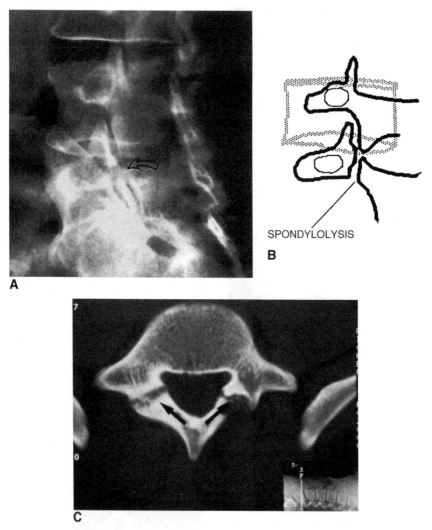

Figure 5-15   Lumbar Spondylolysis. A, An oblique radiograph demonstrating spondylolysis or "a collar on the Scotty dog;" **B,** schematic drawing of the defect; **C,** computerized axial tomographic scan showing a pars defect. (**A,B** from Wimberly RL, Lauerman WC: Spondylolisthesis in the athlete, *Clin Sports Med* 21(1): 137, 2002)

occur because of a developmental weakness of the pars interarticularis, repetitive stress over time, or an acute extension injury to the lumbar spine. Instability at this level may result. Many patients with spondylolysis may not be aware of a problem and have relatively few symptoms except for occasional backache.[35] Often spondylolysis is discovered on a preemployment physical examination for an occupation that requires

manual labor. However, the patient with acute spondylolysis can usually report a specific incident (e.g., a gymnast performing a routine) at the onset of severe low back pain.

There has been some success in placing the patient whose spondylolysis is believed to be acute in a custom-made orthosis with the lumbar spine in extension to achieve healing of the fracture. This regimen is often sufficient to relieve symptoms. It can be difficult for every patient to maintain this position because of body habitus. Whether actual bony healing occurs or whether a fibrous union is present is debatable.

Conservative management for the patient who has symptoms related to an existing spondylolysis includes a short course of rest, mild analgesics, and muscle relaxants as indicated. Most patients respond to this type of treatment within 1 week of the onset of symptoms. For the patient who has frequent and significant episodes of disability related to the spondylolysis, spinal surgery to fuse the pars fracture may be indicated.

Spondylolisthesis

Spondylolisthesis is a forward subluxation or slip of one vertebra on another, which can occur at any level of the spinal column. It can involve one or more levels of the spine.[17] However, spondylolisthesis is most commonly seen in the lumbar spine. Spondylolisthesis is classified into two categories, developed or acquired. Although other categories are used, these two classifications are the most logical and easiest to understand. Developed spondylolisthesis occurs when there is congenital dysplasia of the lumbar vertebrae. If the normal architecture of the vertebral structures is absent, the vertebra is at more risk for instability. Depending on the degree of dysplasia and which elements are involved, the risk of further slippage of the vertebra is either likely or unlikely. For the most part, this is the type of spondylolisthesis seen in children.

Acquired spondylolisthesis occurs after a significant injury to the lumbar spine and more often occurs in adults. Most adult spondylolisthesis is secondary to spondylolysis. Adults may also have developmental spondylolisthesis that is first identified in adulthood. Patient complaints typically include low back pain that sometimes radiates into the buttocks. Pain is worse with activity and relieved by rest.

The degree to which a vertebra slips forward onto the next is graded in a I through IV classification system. This system, developed by Meyerding, helps practitioners communicate the severity of the spondylolisthesis. Grade I is the lowest degree of forward slippage; grade IV represents the highest degree of slippage (Figure 5-16, *A* and *B*). Spondyloptosis is the term used to

describe a vertebra that has completely slipped off and over the edge of the lower vertebra (Figure 5-16, *C*). A standing lateral plain radiograph can often provide the diagnosis. A standing radiograph is important because some low-grade slippages can reduce if the patient is lying on an x-ray table.[5] Forward flexion may accentuate the slippage.

Treatment for spondylolisthesis ranges from observation to surgical intervention.[22] Approximately 5% of the population is believed to have a spondylolisthesis, many of whom have few or no symptoms. Identifying which grade of spondylolisthesis will cause neurologic symptoms or persistent back and leg pain is essential when determining treatment.

The child who has a grade I or II spondylolisthesis with low dysplasia and minimal symptoms should be closely observed and involved in a physical therapy program that teaches the child and family abdominal and low back strengthening exercises. This child should be restricted from activities, such as gymnastics or football, which cause significant stress to the lumbar spine. Any episode of acute back pain with leg pain, weakness, or bowel and bladder symptoms should be evaluated immediately.

Children who have significant dysplasia and a grade II or higher degree of slippage require surgical intervention to prevent further slippage and neurologic deficits. These children should be under advisement regarding physical activity and restricted from any that causes stress to the lumbar spine until successful surgical treatment is complete.

In adults, conservative treatment is often successful. Rest, weight loss, and nonsteroidal antiinflammatory drugs (NSAIDS) help relive symptoms. A lumbosacral corset will provide some stabilization. Abdominal strengthening exercises are beneficial. If symptoms progress in spite of conservative therapy, surgical intervention may be indicated.

The surgical management of spondylolisthesis varies among surgeons.[3,25] Although all agree that spinal fusion is necessary in a patient with a progressive spondylolisthesis or a spondylolisthesis that is accompanied by pain or neurologic symptoms, there is still debate over the approach. Many surgeons believe that the child or adult with a more significant slip will require fusion with segmental instrumentation (Figure 5-17, *A-D*). Because the

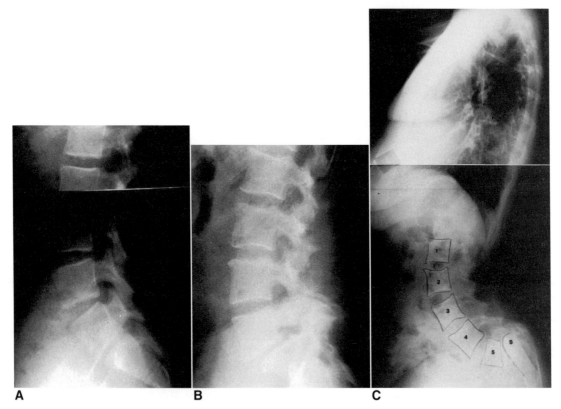

Figure 5-16 Lateral radiographs demonstrating Grade I spondylolisthesis **(A)**, grade IV spondylolisthesis **(B)**, spondyloptosis **(C)**.

determination is based on many complex issues, an orthopedic surgeon with an expertise in spinal surgery should provide care for this patient.

Scoliosis

Scoliosis is a lateral curvature of the spine that may be structural or functional in nature. Structural scoliosis has vertebral body rotation. It may be caused by congenital malformation of the vertebral structures, by neuromuscular, degenerative, or metabolic conditions, or by an unknown cause called *idiopathic scoliosis*. Idiopathic scoliosis (Figure 5-18) is the most common type seen and is often first diagnosed in adolescence. Although scoliosis can also be seen in infants or children under age 10, it is far less common.

A standing anteroposterior (AP) radiograph confirms the diagnosis of scoliosis. Once the film is taken, the degree of curvature can be objectively measured. The Cobb method is the most common means of assessing curvature. An extended line is drawn along the upper edge of the most tilted superior vertebra in the curve. Another line is drawn along the bottom of the most tilted inferior vertebra. The angle at the intersection of these two lines is then measured to obtain the degree of curvature.

Functional scoliosis is characterized by a lateral curvature of the spine with no structural changes, such as vertebral rotation. Functional scoliosis is found secondary to leg length inequality, local inflammation, nerve root irritation, or, in rare cases, hysteria. Treatment of

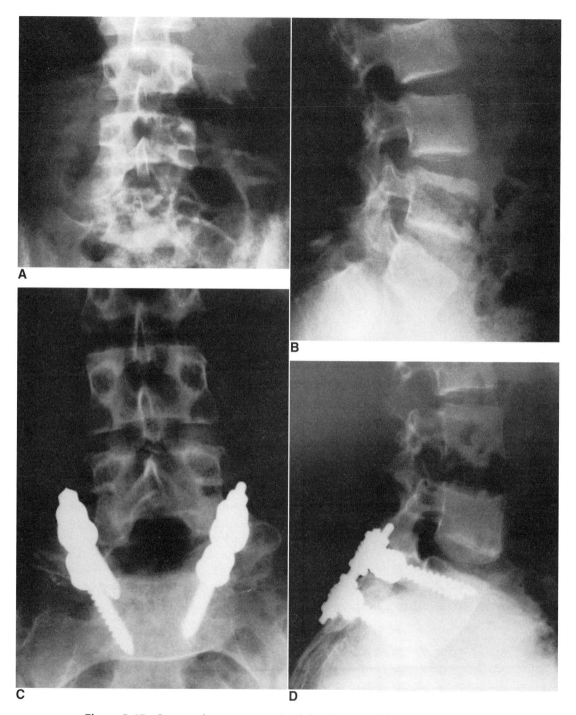

Figure 5-17 Preoperative anteroposterior **(A)** and lateral **(B)** radiographs of a grade II spondylolisthesis. Postoperative anteroposterior **(C)** and lateral **(D)** radiographs showing segmental fixation and partial reduction of the forward slip of L5 on the sacrum.

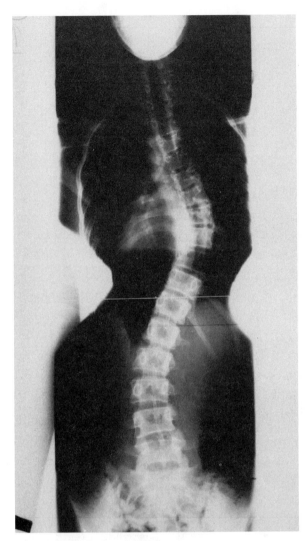

Figure 5-18 Standing posteroanterior radiograph of the spine showing an idiopathic scoliosis. Note the vertebral rotation indicative of a structural scoliosis.

the underlying condition generally results in resolution of functional scoliosis.

Treatment of scoliosis will range from observation of curves less than 20 degrees to surgical intervention in curves greater than 40 degrees. Prompt referral to a specialist should be made if the curvature reaches or exceeds 20 degrees. Children with minimal asymmetry should be assessed every 3 to 4 months with clinical evaluation. If

progression is suggested, a radiographic study should be ordered. Baseline radiographs should be obtained in the child who has asymmetry of the waist, shoulders that are not level, or rib or paravertebral prominence. Although it is recognized that radiographs of children should be done only when necessary, the early identification of a true scoliosis is appropriate reason to obtain standing anteroposterior and lateral films. Realizing that these children will be under observation for a long period, x-ray studies should be ordered only when a clinical change has occurred or at 1-year intervals.

Curves between 20 and 40 degrees in a growing child should be placed in a bracing program, with a custom-made orthosis that addresses the child's curve pattern. In most instances a full-time bracing program, consisting of 20 to 24 hours per day, is initially recommended until skeletal maturation has occurred. A hand film for bone age will help determine skeletal maturity and when a brace-weaning program can begin.

Many different types of braces are used for the management of scoliosis. The Boston brace (Figure 5-19) is the most common appliance used for a lumbar or thoracolumbar curve with an apex below the T9 level. The Lyon brace (Figure 5-20) is one example of an underarm brace that is used for curves in the thoracic or thoracolumbar areas. The Milwaukee brace (Figure 5-21) is used for sagittal plane deformities such as kyphosis. It is not routinely used for idiopathic scoliosis unless there is a kyphotic component to the deformity.

Adolescence is a difficult time for most children; as a result, a modified program that allows an adolescent to continue to participate in some routine activities may be necessary. Programs should be modified only when parents and patient understand the possible ramifications of less brace time, including progression of the curvature.

Surgical intervention is recommended for the child or adult patient with scoliosis greater than 40 degrees. Surgical stabilization with instrumentation, partial correction, and spinal fusion is necessary to avoid progression. Although correction of the scoliosis is important to restore normal coronal alignment and reduce deformity, the sagittal contour of the spine is equally important. Maintaining or restoring normal lumbar lordosis is necessary to place the lumbar segments that lie distal to the

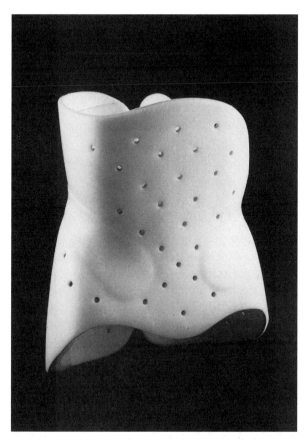

Figure 5-19   A Boston brace used for nonoperative lumbar scoliosis management.

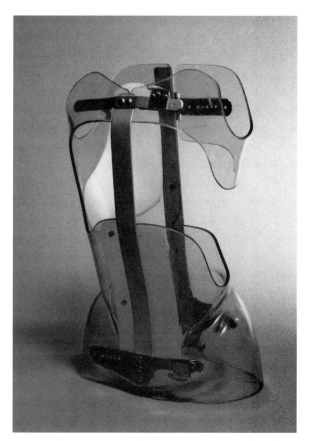

Figure 5-20   A Lyon brace used for nonoperative treatment of thoracic and lumbar scoliosis.

spinal fusion at the best possible advantage in order to avoid long-term deterioration below the fusion.

The common procedure has been posterior spinal fusion with segmental instrumentation using one of the many systems available (e.g., Cotrel-Dubousset, Texas Scottish Rite Hospital) (Figure 5-22, *A-D*). With the newer, anterior instrumentation systems (Figure 5-23, *A-D*) that are being developed, many surgeons prefer the anterior approach to the lumbar spine. Often fewer segments need to be included in the anterior fusion, thus leaving more segments mobile in the lumbar spine. Both anterior and posterior fusion may be necessary for larger lumbar curves or in the adult patient where posterior fusion alone is more difficult to achieve.

Postoperative immobilization using a thoracolumbosacral orthosis (TLSO) may be prescribed (Figure 5-24). Although instrumentation is often adequate, postoperative discomfort and anxiety are often improved with immobilization. The decision is based on the age of the patient, original deformity, bone strength, internal fixation, patient characteristics, and surgeon preference. The length of time in the TLSO ranges from 8 weeks to 6 months and is determined by the surgeon.

DEGENERATIVE DISK CONDITIONS AND TREATMENTS

The normal aging process can cause degeneration to occur between *any* joints, including those in the spine.

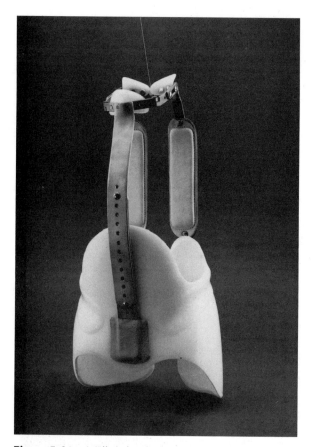

Figure 5-21 A Milwaukee brace is most commonly used for the treatment of kyphotic conditions.

The intervertebral disk dehydrates and begins to flatten. Disk degeneration is thought to have a biochemical basis caused by various chemical mediators, including prostaglandins, nitric oxide, and interleukins.[34] The degree to which the disk deteriorates differs with each person, and in fact there may be a genetic predisposition.[34] However, it has been documented that disks in men begin to degenerate before those in women, most showing early signs of degeneration by age 20. By the time of the sixth decade, more than 90% of all disks in both men and women show some signs of degeneration. However, it appears that the person who has engaged in a more rigorous lifestyle, whether recreational or work-related, will show signs of disk degeneration earlier. With disk degeneration and a reduction in height, the

relationships of the posterior elements are disturbed. Degeneration occurs at the motion segment of the spine. (A motion segment consists of two adjacent vertebral bodies, their shared disk, facet joints, and ligamentous supports.) The facet joints will degenerate, the foraminal openings will become smaller, and the nerve roots that exit through these openings will be encroached on.

Spinal Stenosis

In spinal stenosis the spinal canal is smaller than normal. Spinal stenosis can be congenital, acquired (e.g., a bulging disk or due to degenerative changes), iatrogenic (e.g., postsurgical), or due to miscellaneous causes such as Paget's disease or acromegaly.[34] In any case there is less room for the cauda equina, causing compression of the nerve roots. The term spinal stenosis is also used when describing the effect a herniated disk has on the neural structures, but this type of stenosis is related to disk material rather than being attributable to bony or cartilaginous changes. Spinal stenosis is also a term used to describe compression secondary to fracture, abscess, tumor, or instability.

Symptoms often begin insidiously and progress slowly with vague complaints of low back pain and stiffness. Examination may reveal a decrease in normal lumbar lordosis. Unilateral or bilateral leg pain or paresthesias may be present when walking. Prolonged standing is uncomfortable. Sitting or walking while hunched forward may help decrease discomfort. Lumbar extension may exacerbate any lower extremity symptoms.

The treatment for spinal stenosis is based on several considerations: (1) the degree of the stenosis; (2) the length of time the nerves have been compressed and the chances for significant recovery with decompression; (3) the presenting complaints; and (4) the health of the patient. After appropriate assessment with x-ray studies, computed tomography (CT), magnetic resonance imaging (MRI), or myelography, the treatment plan is developed. In the past, myelography was considered the best diagnostic tool available to demonstrate spinal stenosis; however, the combination of CT and MRI can provide excellent preoperative information (Figure 5-25, *A* and *B*).[34]

Initial treatment consists of NSAIDs, activity modification, and physical therapy. Williams' flexion exercises,

Text continued on p. 155

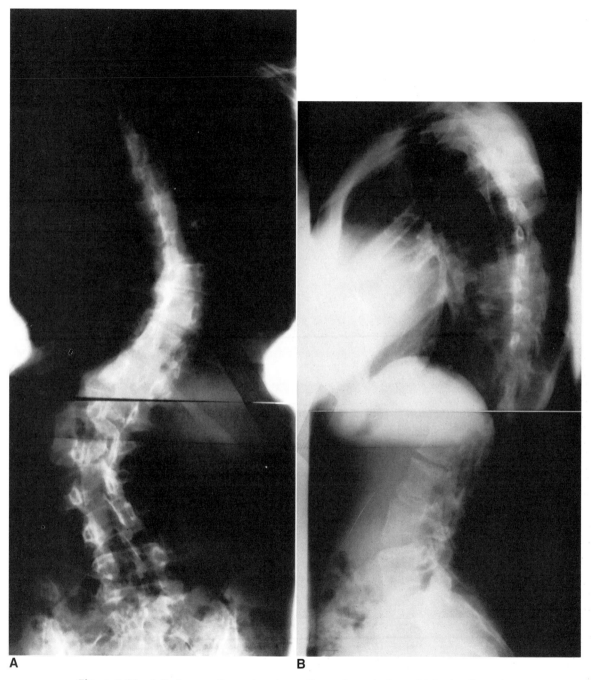

Figure 5-22   A-D, Preoperative and postoperative posteroanterior and lateral radiographs of a patient with posterior stabilization and partial correction of idiopathic scoliosis.

Continued

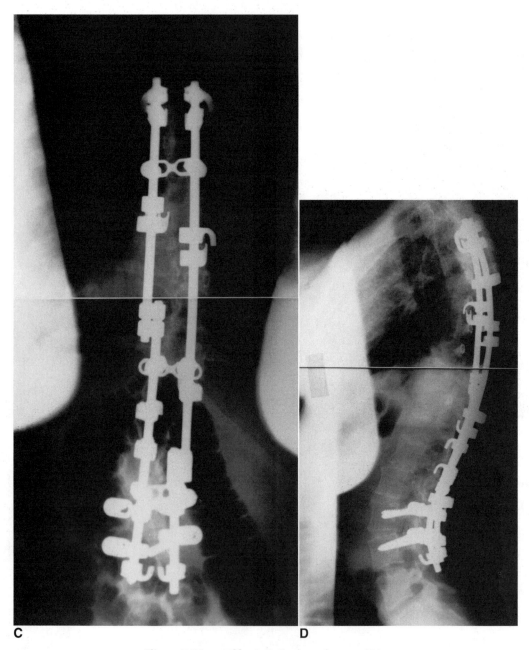

Figure 5-22, cont'd   A-D, For legend, see p.151.

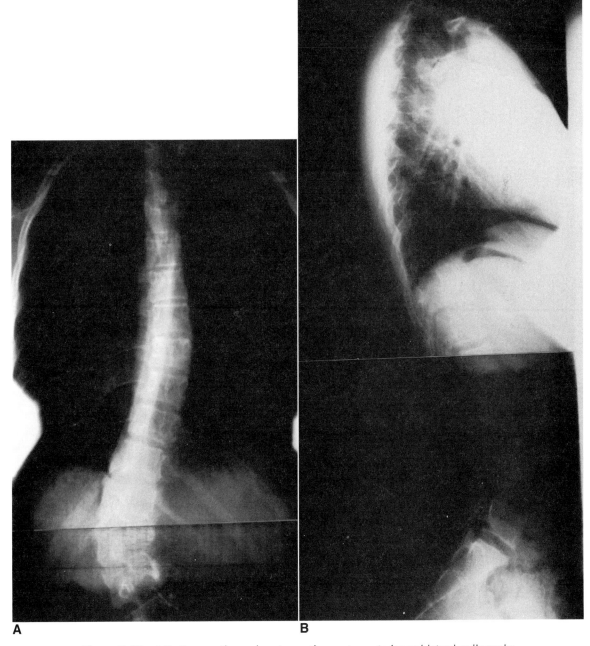

Figure 5-23 A-D, Preoperative and postoperative posteroanterior and lateral radiographs of a patient with lumbar scoliosis, anterior stabilization, and partial correction of idiopathic scoliosis. Note that only five vertebrae are fused.

Continued

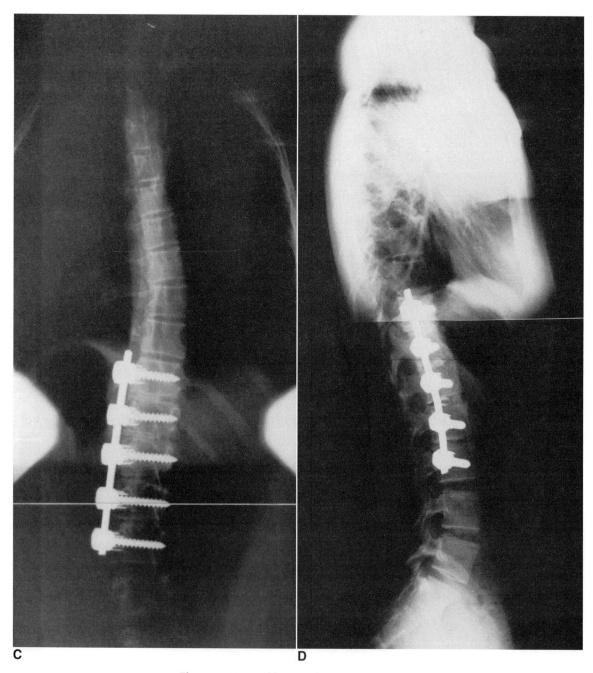

C   D

Figure 5-23, cont'd   A-D, for legend see p.153.

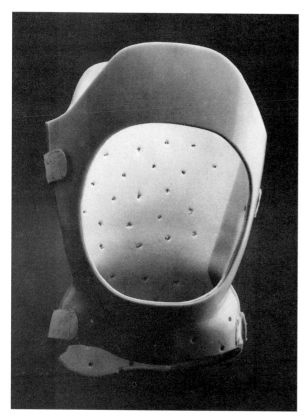

Figure 5-24 Thoracolumbosacral orthoses used for postoperative immobilization in select patients.

abdominal muscle strengthening, and aquatic therapy are often beneficial. Epidural steroid injections are useful in selected patients.

For the patient who does not respond to conservative management, surgical decompression may be indicated. Spinal surgery for spinal stenosis must be thoroughly considered, or the patient's postoperative status may be worse than it was before the surgical procedure. Surgery can range from simple, one-level decompression to multiple levels of decompression with or without instrumentation.[32]

Because many patients with spinal stenosis are older than ages 40 to 50, their bone density status is an important consideration. If the patient's bone is too soft to accept spinal instrumentation and if the spine would be rendered unstable after the decompression, surgery is of

no benefit to the patient. The better approach is a well-managed pain management program that allows the patient to function. Assuming that the neurologic status of the patient is not severely compromised, this nonsurgical approach is the better treatment option.

Arthritic Conditions

Ankylosing Spondylitis

Ankylosing spondylitis (AS) is a systemic, seronegative spondyloarthropathy that primarily affects the sacroiliac joints, spine, and hip; it is more commonly seen in men. There is a direct relationship between AS and the histocompatibility human leukocyte antigen (HLA)-B27, but not all individuals who are HLA-B27 positive will develop AS.[9] Sacroiliac (SI) joint involvement is necessary to establish the diagnosis of AS. Early symptoms are nonspecific and may only consist of morning stiffness. Initially the patient describes generalized back pain but has no objective findings on diagnostic radiographs, CT, MRI, or myelography. Early radiographs reveal a straight spine with no abnormalities. As the disease progresses, subchondral granulation tissue erodes the joint and is later replaced by fibrocartilage, eventually ossifying. In the spine this process initially affects the junction of the vertebrae and disks, finally progressing to the characteristic "bamboo spine" appearance seen on x-ray films.

Because patients' only complaint in the early stages is pain, often these individuals are thought to be malingering and may soon be labeled as such. Symptoms may be affected by weather and temperature conditions.[10] Patients often become depressed because of the inability of health care practitioners to make a diagnosis and because of the persistence of significant pain.

As the disease progresses, many of these patients may describe a feeling of stiffness and there is progressive loss of spinal ROM. Comfort is obtained by bending forward. At this time, radiographs may show signs of fusion of the intervertebral joints. Radiographs begin to show the characteristics of a "bamboo" spine (Figure 5-26). Spinal fragility is increased in AS, and relatively minor spinal trauma can result in significant neurologic deficit.[15]

Any young adult with generalized back pain should be assessed for decreased motion of the thoracic spine.

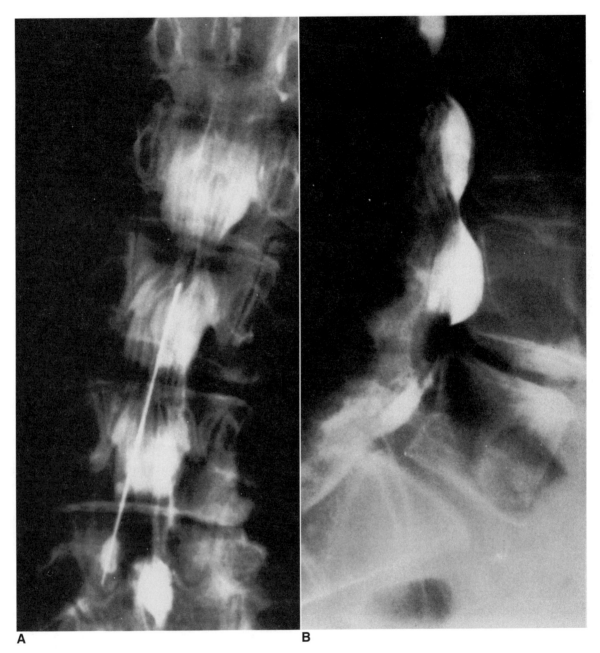

A   B

Figure 5-25 Lumbar **(A)** and lateral **(B)** myelographic images demonstrating spinal stenosis. Note the indentation into the dye column.

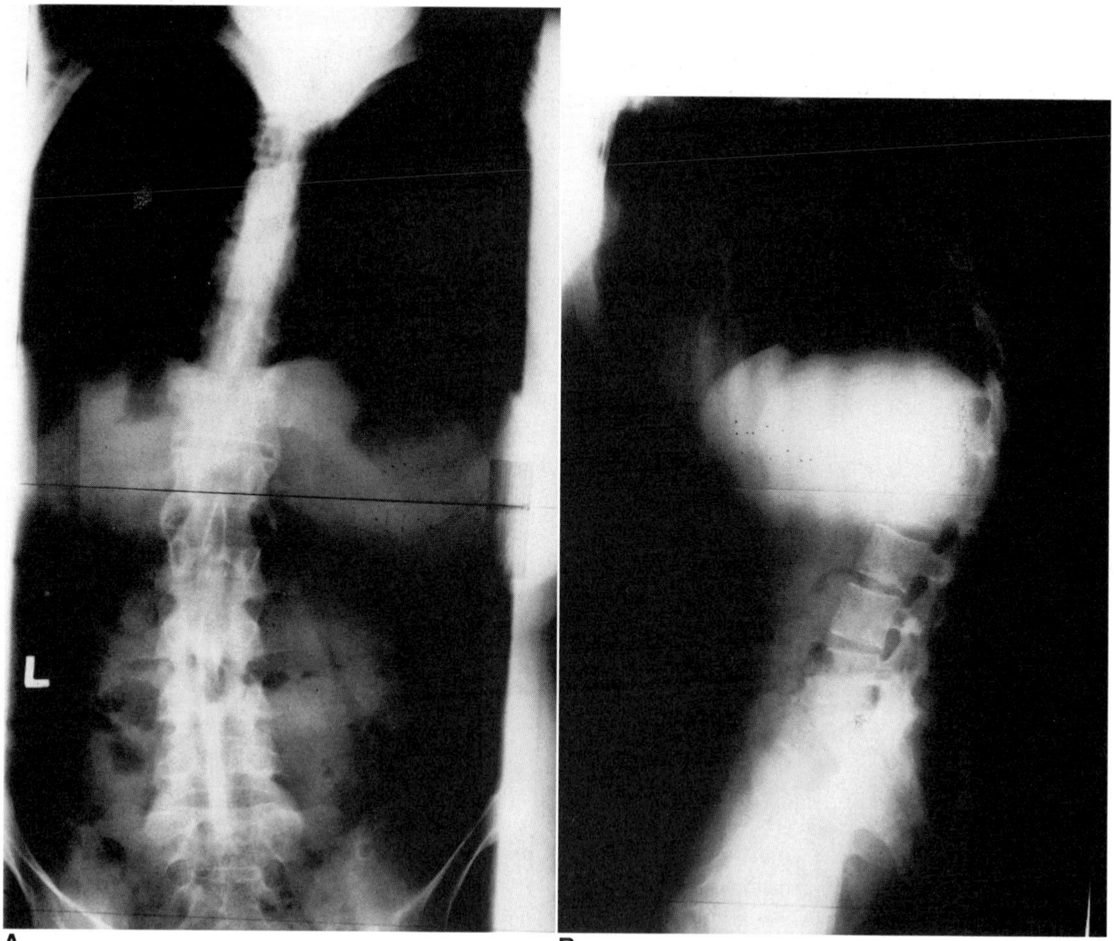

Figure 5-26　Posteroanterior **(A)** and lateral **(B)** radiographs showing a "bamboo spine" in a patient with ankylosing spondylitis. Note the fusion of the spine.

By simply measuring the chest expansion, a probable diagnosis can be made. The costovertebral joints will become stiff, and a loss of motion in this area will cause an inability to expand the rib cage. A chest expansion of less than 2 inches should be evaluated further. Because decreased expansion of the rib cage can also be seen in other conditions (e.g., emphysema), additional laboratory studies should be performed, including an HLA-B27 test. This antigen is almost universally present in the serum of Caucasian men with AS. A mild hypochromic anemia, elevated erythrocyte sedimenta-

tion rate (ESR), the presence of immunoglobulin-G antiglobulins, or an elevated creatine phosphokinase may also be present.

Referral to a rheumatologist may be needed to rule out any other seronegative spondyloarthropathies. Treatment for AS includes the use of antiinflammatory medication for pain relief and a physical therapy program that maintains extension of the thoracic spine, prevents the formation of a severe kyphotic condition, and maintains ROM of the hip joints. Disease-modifying antirheumatic drugs (DMARDs) and monoclonal antibodies such as infliximab show promise in controlling pain and symptoms.[6,23]

Osteotomy and realignment of the spine can be considered for the patient who has developed severe kyphosis. This treatment is a major undertaking and requires precise planning to achieve a good outcome. With the entire spine fused from occiput to pelvis, it is critically important to perfectly realign the spine, or the result will be poor. If the sagittal deformity is overcorrected, the patient may be left looking upward; this makes walking difficult and dangerous. Only those spinal surgeons with knowledge of AS and sagittal plane deformity should evaluate the patient with severe kyphosis.

Reactive Arthritis

Reactive arthritis includes AS, psoriatic arthritis, and arthritis that follows an enteric, urogenital, or pharyngeal infection. Chronic bacterial infection or the body's antigenic response to infection may play a role in the development of reactive arthritis.[33] A synovitis develops most commonly in the joints of the lower extremities, but it is occasionally seen in the sacroiliac joints as well. The presenting symptom is often an inflamed joint, and during the interview any history of recent infection should be noted. Many patients will be afebrile. The estimated sedimentation rate (ESR) is generally elevated.

Diagnosis is based on history, examination, and lack of positive serum markers for other arthritides. MRI examination of the axial skeleton can show early changes of synovium, subchondral bone, and articular cartilage.[21]

The treatment for reactive arthritis is treatment of the bacterial infection as normally indicated in urogenital and pharyngeal cases. Antiinflammatory medications are generally required for several weeks; most patients show improvement within 2 weeks.

Sacroiliitis

Sacroiliitis is an inflammation of the SI joints. It can be found in association with AS, rheumatoid or psoriatic arthritis, Reiter's syndrome, infection (tuberculosis, brucellosis), and enteropathology such as Crohn's disease or ulcerative colitis. Often thought to be referred pain from the lumbar spine, sacroiliitis sometimes goes undiagnosed for a time. The patient complains of posterior thigh pain and medial buttock pain that is often worsened with weight bearing on the affected side. Young, multiparous women may have bilateral SI joint pain thought to be due to laxity and stress on the joint during pregnancy and delivery. This condition is called *osteitis condensans ilii.*

Normally the SI joint is of uniform width. One of the earliest signs of sacroiliitis is a widening of the joint seen on a plain AP x-ray of the pelvis. A bone scan, CT, or MRI will demonstrate inflammation of the SI joint. Deep palpation of the sacroiliac joint will often exacerbate the symptoms.

The treatment of sacroiliitis is use of oral antiinflammatory drugs to help decrease the inflammation of the sacroiliac joint. In severe cases the use of crutches or a walker may be indicated. Injection of steroids into the sacroiliac joint is performed if oral agents do not reduce symptoms. Fusion of the sacroiliac joint is recommended only after all other treatment modalities fail.

Metabolic Conditions

Osteopenia

Osteopenia is a description of the bone as visualized on radiographs. To say that a patient has osteopenia means that the films show less bone density than normal. Osteopenia is therefore not a diagnosis but rather a descriptive term. By the time osteopenia is visualized on x-ray studies, the patient is experiencing at least a 20% decrease in bone mass. Further bone-density testing should be ordered to corroborate the findings of the films. If bone-mass loss is confirmed, the cause must be found; it may arise from either metabolic or neoplastic conditions.

Osteoporosis

Osteoporosis is a metabolic bone disease that primarily affects bone remodeling and is characterized by compromised bone strength. Osteoporosis is the most common metabolic bone disease in the United States and accounts for over 1.5 million fractures each year. The National Osteoporosis Foundation estimates that nearly 44 million adults in the United States over age 50 have low bone mass or osteoporosis.[27] Normally a balance of bone resorption and formation is maintained by the function of osteoclasts and osteoblasts. Trabecular bone, found in the spine, is more metabolically active than cortical bone; as a result, changes of bone mineral density are often evident there before they are seen in other sites. Bone remodeling is affected by a number of local and systemic factors, including cytokines, estrogen and androgen levels, parathyroid hormone, vitamin D levels, scoliosis, and the patient's level of physical activity. Low body weight, a small body frame, heavy alcohol intake, cigarette smoking, and high caffeine intake are also associated with low bone mass. Other risk factors for osteoporosis include eating disorders and radiation or chemotherapy. Postmenopausal women, particularly those of northern European or Asian descent, are at greatest risk for developing osteoporosis. A family history of osteoporosis may be predictive of low bone density. Women who sustain a fracture before menopause are also at increased risk for postmenopausal fracture.[16]

Secondary osteoporosis can result from other diseases or conditions such as multiple myeloma, insulin-dependent diabetes, Addison's disease, hyperparathyroidism, long-term use of glucocorticoids or anticonvulsants, and malabsorption syndromes. Osteoporotic hip fractures are commonly associated with significant morbidity and mortality; however, neither are osteoporotic spine fractures to be considered benign. In addition to causing pain, they can result in loss of height, spinal deformity (particularly kyphosis), reduced pulmonary function, and increased mortality.[18]

In an effort to identify those at risk for fracture, the World Health Organization (WHO) has defined four diagnostic categories of bone mineral density applicable to postmenopausal women.[40] These guidelines are summarized in Table 5-1.

Diagnosis of osteoporosis is generally made by evaluation of specified central (hip and spine) or peripheral (calcaneus, forearm, or finger phalanx) sites. Peripheral testing is not as accurate for predicting fracture risk as central testing, but peripheral tests are inexpensive and portable, and they provide a relatively fast screening method. Quantitative CT is currently the only available method to obtain true bone mineral density values, but its expense and relatively high ionizing radiation exposure prevent it from being widely used. Today, central dual-energy x-ray absorptiometry (DXA) scanning is the preferred method for determining bone mineral density.

Treatment of osteoporosis is a multifaceted process that includes lifestyle changes such as smoking cessation, adequate calcium and vitamin D intake, adequate weight-bearing exercise, and use of medications. Bisphosphonates such as alendronate and risedronate are preferentially directed to bone and cause apoptosis of the osteoclasts, thus reducing bone turnover. Bisphosphonates have been approved for the prevention and treatment of osteoporosis in postmenopausal women as well as for treatment of glucocorticoid-induced osteoporosis. Selective estrogen response modifiers such as raloxifene have estrogenic effects on bone, but without effect on breast or endometrial tissue. Calcitonin has been used for treatment but not prevention of osteoporosis. Anabolic agents such as parathyroid hormone and teriparatide are also being investigated. Hormone replacement therapy for the prevention of postmenopausal osteoporosis has become more controversial because of associated breast cancer risk.[11]

Newer treatments of osteoporotic spine fractures include vertebroplasty and kyphoplasty. Vertebroplasty is a minimally invasive technique of injecting low-viscosity

TABLE 5-1   WHO classification criteria for postmenopausal bone mineral density

Diagnostic Classification	Bone Mineral Density
Normal	<−1 standard deviation (SD) below the mean of BMD in young, healthy woman
Osteopenia	BMD>−1 but <−2.5 SD below the mean BMD in young, healthy women
Osteoporosis	BMD>−2.5 SD below the mean BMD in young, healthy women
Severe osteoporosis	Presence of a fracture and BMD >−2.5 SD below mean BMD in young, healthy women

BMD, Bone mineral density.

cement in to an osteoporotic vertebral body to prevent further fracture. The procedure is performed using a catheter under fluoroscopic guidance. Kyphoplasty is a more invasive procedure. It involves placing an inflatable bone tamp into the fractured vertebral body, inflating the tamp, and then injecting a more viscous bone cement into the void created by the balloon. This method has the advantage of decreasing pain as well as restoring vertebral body height, thus reducing spinal deformity.[20]

Osteomalacia

Osteomalacia, often called rickets when seen in children, is the inability of the body to mineralize osteoid. The most common cause is a vitamin D deficiency. Laboratory studies reveal decreased calcium levels. Low-fat and vegetarian diets provide little vitamin D, and vitamin supplements should be encouraged for patients who follow them. The older population is also at risk for low serum vitamin D levels, often because of lack of sun exposure, poor dietary habits and loss of appetite.

The treatment of both osteoporosis and osteomalacia in its earliest stages centers around the identification of the problem's cause. Dietary supplements are essential for patients who do not receive adequate calcium or vitamin D. Although there are differing opinions on the correct amount of calcium, it is generally believed that between 1200 and 1500 mg of calcium should be consumed each day. Consumption is best achieved by diet. For patients who cannot or will not eat dairy products, calcium supplements should be encouraged. A calcium diary should be kept for a time to determine the actual amounts of calcium that are normally consumed. Whatever is lacking should be supplied by means of supplements.

INFECTIONS

Infections of the spine can be divided into disk space infections and vertebral osteomyelitis. Disk space infections in the pediatric patient are usually bacterial and result from hematogenous transmission to the disk space. Disk space infections in adults are the result of a hematogenous seeding of the disk space or are secondary to complication of lumbar diskectomy or diskogram.

The treatment for a disk space infection is normally bed rest for comfort; biopsy for culture and sensitivity is followed by appropriate antibiotic therapy. Most patients respond well to this therapy and will be ambulatory when comfortable.

Vertebral osteomyelitis can be bacterial, fungal, granulomatous, or parasitic. Bacterial infections tend to be acute whereas fungal or tuberculous infections are often chronic.[2] Often diagnosis is delayed because the onset is insidious in nature and the white blood cell count may be normal or only slightly elevated; the ESR will be elevated. An infection should be considered when the patient with back pain has had recent spinal surgery, urinary tract surgery (e.g., cystoscopy), tooth abscess, or any other type of skin sore or infection or has a compromised immune system. Spinal epidural abscess is a serious infection of the epidural space that may begin as a skin abscess or furuncle that leads to back pain, radicular irritation, and finally neurologic deficit.[30]

Blood cultures may be helpful in determining the organism causing the infection. However, if no organism is identified, direct biopsy must be obtained before instituting therapy, since there are tremendous differences in which agent should be used. In injection drug users, antibiotic therapy should not wait until culture results are returned. While awaiting culture reports, the practitioner should begin empiric antibiotics that include coverage for Staphylococcus and aerobic gram-negative bacilli.[38] In tuberculosis cases, a multidrug approach is certainly necessary. Consultation with infectious disease specialists should be obtained to identify appropriate drug therapy.

Early diagnosis of the patient with a spine infection is imperative. Spinal infection must be considered when persistent back pain of unknown causes is the presenting system of a patient who has contributing medical factors or history. It is not uncommon for the spinal surgical practice to see several patients each year who have become paraplegic while a diagnosis eluded the primary care practitioner (Figure 5-27, A-C). An early bone scan or MRI is indicated for these patients.[14]

When spinal column stability has been eroded because of an infectious process or the neural structures are compressed causing neurologic deficit, surgical management may be necessary to decompress and stabilize

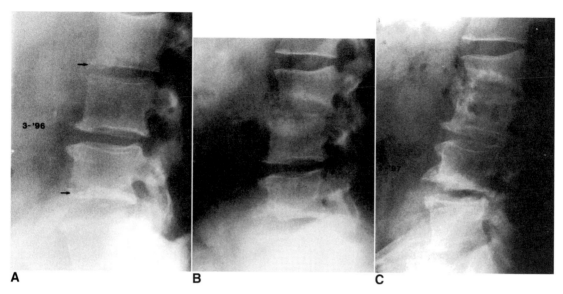

Figure 5-27 A-C, Serial radiographs demonstrating the progression of vertebral osteomyelitis. **(A)** Initial areas of infection indicated by arrows; **(B)** destruction of superior vertebral endplate; **(C)** erosion of vertebral body and collapse of initially affected vertebra.

the spine. Stabilization and reconstruction may be necessary, even with infection, to protect or improve neurologic function. This type of major spinal reconstruction should be undertaken in close collaboration with infectious disease specialists. The patient must maintain adequate antibiotic therapy for many months or until the ESR has returned to normal. Discontinuing antibiotic therapy too early allows reemergence of the infection.

TUMORS

Spinal tumors can be divided into benign and malignant; malignant tumors are further divided into primary and metastatic. By far the most common spine tumor is metastatic; primary spinal bone tumors are very rare. Pain is usually the presenting symptom. For the patient with a diagnosis of cancer, spine pain elicits instant concern and workup. However, for the patient with no known cancer history, such back pain may remain undiagnosed for some time. Back pain secondary to tumor is generally well located, is exacerbated with percussion, does not go away when the patient lies down, and is pro-

gressive. Pain may be secondary to microfracture or macrofracture of the tumorous bone or caused by enlargement of the tumor itself.

Radiographs are obtained and reviewed with a degree of concern about the presence of a tumor. In the event films are negative with the history of symptoms as previously stated, a bone scan or MRI should be obtained. MRI better evaluates early metastases since bone medullary changes often occur before cortical involvement becomes apparent on bone scan images.[36] After correlating imaging studies and the physical examination, a CT scan of the appropriate vertebral level should be obtained.

Benign tumors of the spine include osteoid osteoma, osteoblastoma, hemangioma, aneurysmal bone cyst, giant cell tumor, and eosinophilic granuloma. Each of these tumors is treated on the basis of vertebral column stability, aggressiveness of the tumor, and symptomatology.

Primary malignant tumors include plasmacytoma, multiple myeloma, osteosarcoma, Ewing's sarcoma, chordoma, chondrosarcoma, and lymphoma. Over 50% of metastatic tumors to the spine result from primary sites of the breast, lung, prostate, thyroid, or kidney.[19]

The diagnosis of the spinal tumor should be confirmed even with a known cancer elsewhere in the body. Certain tumors such as renal cell carcinoma are known to be highly vascular. If renal cell carcinoma is known or suspected, embolization of the vertebrae is necessary before biopsy and surgery. Once a biopsy has been obtained and the tissue type confirmed, the appropriate treatment course can be planned. Some tumors respond well to chemotherapeutic agents and/or radiation. If the spine is not unstable, this course may be followed. If the spine is unstable from vertebral tumor invasion, surgical intervention may be necessary.

Staging of the disease is necessary before proceeding with major reconstructive spinal surgery. It is generally accepted that surgery should be considered if it can be accomplished quickly and safely and if the patient (1) has a minimum of 6 weeks of life remaining, (2) can achieve ambulatory status from stabilization of the spine, (3) can avoid paraplegia or quadriplegia, or (4) is more comfortable during the final days. Only the patient with a competent immune system should be taken to the operating room unless neurologic deficits are present. Even with neurologic deficits, the patient with a severely compromised immune system will require more time to heal large surgical wounds and may develop devastating infection. The surgeon must make surgical decisions based on the patient's general medical status and prognosis.

If only a few weeks of life are expected, a less aggressive procedure may be performed to stabilize the spine. For the patient who has months of life or longer, a procedure designed to offer long-term stability is recommended (Figure 5-28, A to C).

DIFFERENTIAL DIAGNOSIS

Many of the differential diagnoses of lumbar spine problems have been discussed. In addition to those stated, other nonmusculoskeletal conditions that can cause lumbar spine pain should be considered when interviewing and examining the patient. These conditions include abdominal aortic aneurysm; genitourinary abnormalities such as urinary tract infection, kidney stones, and endometriosis; and neoplastic conditions, including infrapelvic tumors, pancreas, and liver. Each of these medical conditions can cause primary back pain. The patient often seeks orthopedic consultation rather than a general medical assessment. However, the practitioner should ask questions regarding these medical diagnoses of any patient with low back pain, as well as auscultating and examining the abdomen as indicated.

EVALUATION MODALITIES

Radiographic Studies

After the history and physical examination are complete, radiographs are obtained to assess the spine for vertebral irregularities, loss of disk height, and deformity. An x-ray study is not routinely ordered for the patient with lumbar spine complaints but rather follows a detailed assessment. If the symptoms of pain have been present for a short time and there are no neurologic findings, a short course of observation is recommended with a follow-up evaluation to confirm resolution of the problem. If symptoms are severe or persist, standard AP, lateral, and oblique x-ray views of the lumbar spine should be obtained. Standing flexion and extension views should be obtained if instability is suspected.

Bone Density Tests

Bone density tests are important to help identify at an early stage those who have osteomalacia or osteoporosis and who require medical management to increase bone strength. For the patient undergoing spinal surgery, bone density is important if reconstructive surgery and instrumentation are needed.

Computed Tomography

The CT scan is recommended when the bony architecture needs to be evaluated. The CT scan provides multiple axial and sagittal images at every vertebral level. This test uses radiation. The CT scan is the test of choice when evaluating a spondylolysis or spondylolisthesis or when there is concern regarding fracture, infection, or tumor. The patient is placed on the CT scanning table, which moves slowly through a machine. Movement by the patient causes distortion of the images and will result in a poor test.

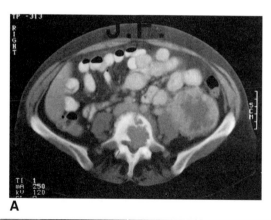

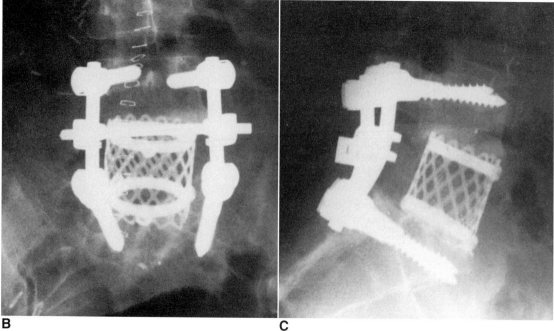

Figure 5-28 **A,** Computed tomographic scan demonstrating tumor invasion into L5. Anteroposterior **(B)** and lateral **(C)** radiographs of a lumbar spine reconstruction after metastatic breast carcinoma rendered the spine unstable.

Magnetic Resonance Imaging

MRI provides better visualization of soft-tissue structures, such as vertebral disks, and it is more useful for evaluating infections or tumors of the spine. There is no radiation exposure for this test. MRI is very helpful when examining the soft-tissue material and its relationship to the spinal cord or cauda equina. Diffusion-weighted MRI is a new technique that allows greater differentiation of edema, tumor, and fracture.[4] The MRI scan should be explained to the patient and a pretest checklist should be reviewed to determine whether the patient should be a candidate for the procedure. Before proceeding with an MRI test, any patient who has a cardiac pacemaker, intracranial aneurysm clips, neurostimulators, or a history of employment that includes grinding metal or being in close proximity to it, should be evaluated by a neuroradiologist. Any patient whose plain radiographs show the presence of metallic fragments is excluded from MRI. The patient who has spinal surgical implants will not have good imaging in the same area of the spine, unless the implants are titanium.

The patient should be told that the test will require a period of lying flat on a table in a cylindrical tube that encircles the body. The patient will hear loud knocking during part of the examination. Any patient who has a history of claustrophobia should be scheduled in an open MRI scanner or sedated to obtain the best scanning result and decrease patient concerns.

Electromyography

Electromyography (EMG) consists of the placement of electrodes into the various muscles to stimulate them under different circumstances: during insertion of the needle, after the needle is placed, with slight muscle contraction, and with maximal muscle contraction. This test helps identify peripheral motor nerve or root injury.

EMG is an uncomfortable test, and the patient should be advised of this before beginning. Many patients say, "It is the worst test I have ever had." With this in mind, EMG should be explained to the patient and ordered only when no other diagnostic test can fully explain the pathologic condition.

Myelography

The myelogram is used less frequently today because of the capabilities of the CT and MRI scanning methods. A water-soluble contrast material is introduced under sterile conditions into the subarachnoid space in the cervical or lumbar area. The patient is then manipulated by the use of a specialized table so that the contrast material can be visualized as it moves up and down the spinal canal. A compromise of the spinal canal can be readily seen, and routine radiographs are taken to document the procedure. The patient should understand the procedure, including the placement of a needle in the subarachnoid space and the introduction of contrast material. A thorough review of any allergy history is imperative. The patient is observed in the outpatient area for several hours after the test and before returning home. The most common complication after a myelogram is a spinal headache that, in some cases, does not resolve after bed rest but requires a blood patch to seal a dural leak.

Diskography

A diskogram is a study that consists of placing a needle into the nucleus of the disk with the introduction of contrast material to visualize whether the annulus is intact (Figure 5-29). This test helps further identify a problematic disk. Pain symptoms are often reproduced with the injection of the fluid into the disk space, confirming disk disease.

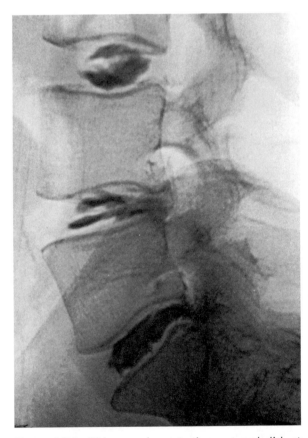

Figure 5-29 Diskogram demonstrating a normal disk at L3-L4 and abnormal disks at L4-L5 and L5-S1. Note the extravasation of dye out of the nucleus at this level.

Selective Nerve Root Block

Based on a physical examination and diagnostic tests, a particular nerve root may be considered for selective nerve root block. Under fluoroscopy the nerve root sleeve is injected with an anesthetic agent to determine if pain relief can be achieved. A small amount of contrast material may be placed; an x-ray is taken to document the nerve root that is injected. This test can pinpoint a particular nerve root problem, but it must be performed and assessed by a knowledgeable person.

CONCLUSION

The study of the lumbar spine is imperative for any health care practitioner. Each year, millions of people seek evaluation for low back complaints. The majority of these people will resolve their problems with little or no intervention. However, because of the relationship of abnormalities of the lumbar spine and neurologic deficits, a timely diagnosis is beneficial.

INDICATIONS FOR REFERRAL

See the following Red Flags box for referral information.

Red Flags *for Lumbar Spine Disorders*

Patients with these findings may need to be referred for more extensive workup.

Signs and Symptoms	Response
Acute onset of low back pain; bilateral lower extremity weakness and sciatica; sensory deficit in perineal and rectal areas; possible bowel and bladder incontinence	Possible acute cauda equina syndrome; urgently transfer to orthopedic spine surgeon for myelogram or MRI and lumbar decompression
Patient with intervertebral disk disease does not respond to conservative management of herniated disk or has significant neurologic symptoms that include lower extremity weakness and bowel and bladder incontinence	Refer to orthopedic surgeon for possible decompression of lumbar neural structures—laminectomy, hemilaminectomy, microscopic disk excision, or percutaneous disk excision
Neurologic injury associated with lumbar spine fracture	Refer to orthopedic spine surgeon, preferably in spinal trauma facility for best possible surgical, rehabilitative, and emotional care
Patient with spondylolysis has frequent episodes of disability after conservative management of symptoms	Refer to orthopedic spine surgeon; surgery to fuse pars fracture may be indicated
Patient with significant dysplasia and grade II or higher slip of one vertebra onto another	Refer to orthopedic spine surgeon; may require surgical intervention to prevent further slippage and neurologic defects
Patient with scoliosis of greater than 40 degrees	Refer to orthopedic spine surgeon; surgical stabilization with instrumentation, partial correction, and spinal fusion are necessary to avoid progression
Patient does not respond to conservative management of degenerative disk disease	Surgical decompression may be indicated; refer to orthopedic spine surgeon
Patient with unexplained generalized pain in lower back; ankylosing spondylitis ruled out	Refer to rheumatologist to rule out pathologic condition
Patient with ankylosing spondylitis has developed severe kyphosis	Realignment of spine should be considered; refer to spinal surgeon with knowledge of ankylosing spondylitis and sagittal plane deformity
All treatment modalities for sacroiliitis (antiinflammatory drugs, crutches or walker, corticosteroid injection) have failed	Fusion of sacroiliac joint may be necessary; refer to orthopedic spinal surgeon
Spinal column stability eroded or neural structures compressed resulting in neurologic deficit in patient with late-diagnosed spine infection	Refer to orthopedic spinal surgeon; surgical management may be necessary to decompress and stabilize spine; reconstruction of spine may also be necessary; also refer to infectious disease specialist
Spine is unstable from vertebral tumor invasion	Refer to orthopedic spinal surgeon for surgical intervention

REFERENCES

1. Andersson GB: Epidemiological features of chronic low back pain, *Lancet* 354:581, 1999.

2. Arce D et al: Recognizing spinal cord emergencies, *Am Fam Physician* 64:631, 2001.

3. Bassowitz H, Herkowitz H: Lumbar stenosis with spondylolisthesis: current concepts of surgical treatment, *Clin Orthop* 384:54, 2001.

4. Baur A et al: Diffusion-weighted imaging of the spinal column, *Neuroimaging Clin N Amer* 12:147, 2002.

5. Bendo JA, Ong B: Importance of correlating static and dynamic imaging studies in diagnosing degenerative lumbar spondylolisthesis, *Amer J Orthop* 30:247, 2001.

6. Brandt J et al: Infliximab treatment of severe ankylosing spondylitis: one-year follow-up, *Arthritis Rheum* 44:2936, 2002.

7. Borenstein DG: Epidemiology, etiology, diagnostic evaluation and treatment of low back pain, *Curr Opin Rheumatol* 13:128, 2001.

8. Borenstein DG et al: The value of magnetic resonance imaging of the lumbar spine to predict low-back pain in asymptomatic subjects: a seven-year follow-up study, *J Bone Joint Surg Am* 83A:1306, 2001.

9. Bowness P: HLA-B27 in health and disease: a double-edged sword? *Rheumatology* 412:857, 2002.

10. Challier B et al: Is quality of life affected by season and weather conditions in ankylosing spondylitis? *Clin Exp Rheumatol* 19:277, 2001.

11. Clemons M, Goss P: Estrogen and the risk of breast cancer, *N Engl J Med* 344:276, 2001.

12. Della-Giustina D, Kilcline BA: Acute low back pain: recognizing the "red flags" in the workup, *Consultant* 42:1277, 2002.

13. Deyo R, Weinstein J: Low back pain, *N Engl J Med* 344:363, 2001.

14. Hetem SF, Schils JP: Imaging of infections and inflammatory conditions of the spine, *Semin Musculoskelet Radiol* 4:329, 2000.

15. Hitchon PW et al: Fractures of the thoracolumbar spine complicating ankylosing spondylitis, *J Neurosurg* 97(suppl 2):218, 2002.

16. Hosmer WD et al: Fractures before menopause: a red flag for physicians, *Osteoporos Int* 13:337, 2002.

17. Iguchi T et al: Lumbar multilevel degenerative spondylolisthesis: radiological evaluation and factors related to anterolisthesis and retrolisthesis, *J Spinal Disorders Techniques* 15:93, 2002.

18. Kado DM et al: Vertebral fractures and mortality in older women: a prospective study. Study of Osteoporotic Fractures Research Group, *Arch Intern Med* 159:1215, 1999.

19. Kostuik J: Metastatic spine tumors. In Frymoyer JW, editor: *The adult spine*, Philadelphia, 1997, Lippincott-Raven.

20. Linville DA II: Vertebroplasty and kyphoplasty, *South Med J* 95:583, 2002.

21. Luong AA, Salonen DC: Imaging of the seronegative spondyloarthropathies, *Curr Rheumatol Rep* 2:288, 2000.

22. Marchetti PG, Bartolozzi P: Classification of spondylolisthesis as a guideline for treatment. In Bridwell K, DeWald R, editors: *The textbook of spinal surgery*, Philadelphia, 1998, Lippincott-Raven.

23. Marzo-Ortega H et al: Efficacy of etanercept in the treatment of the entheseal pathology in resistant spondyloarthropathy: a clinical and magnetic resonance imaging study, *Arthritis Rheum* 44:2112, 2001.

24. McGraw JK, Silber JS: Intradiscal electrothermal therapy for the treatment of discogenic back pain, *Appl Radiol* 30:11, 2001.

25. Molineri RW et al: Anterior column support in surgery for high-grade, isthmic spondylolisthesis, *Clin Orthop* (394):109, 2002.

26. Chronic pain: Hope through research. National Institute of Neurological Disorders and Stroke, Bethesda, Md, Sept. 1997, National Institutes of Health. website: www.thebody.com/nih/pain/triad.html.

27. National Osteoporosis Foundation: *America's bone health: the state of osteoporosis and low bone mass*, Washington, DC, 2001, National Osteoporosis Foundation.

28. Orendacova J et al: Cauda equina syndrome, *Prog Neurobiol* 64:613, 2001.

29. Patel AT, Ogle AA: Diagnosis and management of acute low back pain, *Am Fam Physician* 61:1779, 2000.

30. Reihsaus E et al: Spinal epidural abscess: a meta-analysis of 915 patients, *Neurosurg Rev* 23:175, 2000.

31. Rodts MF: Disorders of the spine. In Maher A, Salmond S, Pellino T, editors: *Orthopaedic nursing*, Philadelphia, 1998, WB Saunders.

32. Sheehan JM et al: Degenerative lumbar stenosis: the neurosurgical perspective, *Clin Orthop* 384:61, 2001.

33. Sieper J: Pathogenesis of reactive arthritis, *Curr Rheumatol Rep* 3:412, 2001.

34. Spivak JM, Bendo JA: Lumbar degenerative disorders. In Koval KJ, editor: *Orthopaedic Knowledge Update 7: Home Study Syllabus*, Rosemont, Ill, 2002, American Academy of Orthopaedic Surgeons.

35. Standaert CJ et al: Spondylolysis, *Phys Med Rehabil Clin North Am* 11:785, 2000.

36. Taoka T et al: Factors influencing visualization of vertebral metastases on MR imaging versus bone scintigraphy, *Am J Roentgenol* 176:1525, 2001.

37. Teasell RW: Compensation and chronic pain, *Clin J Pain* 17(suppl 4):546, 2001.

38. Tunkell AR, Pradhan SK: Central nervous system infections in injection drug users, *Infect Dis Clin North Am* 16:589, 2002.

39. Waddell G et al: Objective clinical evaluation of physical impairment in chronic low back pain, *Spine* 17:617, 1992.

40. World Health Organization: *Assessment of fracture risk and its application to screening for postmenopausal osteoporosis,* Geneva, Switzerland, 1994, World Health Organization (Technical report series).

Chapter 6

Hip and Thigh

Hip complaints in primary care are often the result of degenerative or traumatic processes; they may also be attributable to congenital problems or be the result of referred pain from the back, pelvis, or leg. Because the hip joint is one of the largest in the body and is a major weight-bearing joint, disorders of the hip are often noticeable during walking. Weight-bearing stresses on the hip during walking can be greater than five times an individual's body weight.

ANATOMY

Similar to the shoulder, the hip is a ball-and-socket joint, but it has far greater stability. Hip stabilization begins with a deep socket—the acetabulum. A strong joint capsule and its surrounding muscles and ligaments provide additional stabilization. This high degree of stabilization causes some limitation of movement.

Bony Structures

Composed of the cup-shaped acetabulum and ball of the femoral head, the hip joint is responsible for joining the lower extremity to the pelvis and trunk (Figure 6-1). Similar to the shoulder, the depth of the acetabulum is increased by a fibrocartilagenous labrum.[40] Compared with the shoulder, the socket of the hip encompasses a greater area of the ball.

Portions of three pelvic bones—the ilium, the ischium, and the pubis, form the acetabulum. These bones fuse into a Y in the acetabular depression. The shape of the acetabulum is half of a sphere; the femoral head is about two thirds of a sphere and is somewhat globular. The acetabulum-femoral head complex does not articulate very congruently; however, as load increases on the joint, the congruency is enhanced to increase surface contact area and joint stability.

When standing, the body's center of gravity passes through the midpoint of the pelvis and the center of the acetabulae. Acetabular injury can disrupt this normal weight distribution.

The femoral neck extends from the femoral head downward, outward, and a little posteriorly. The neck connects the femoral head with the shaft of the femur. The angle of the femoral neck relative to the femoral shaft is known as the "angle of inclination." The degree of this angle is not as great in women as in men because the female pelvis tends to be wider. The angle of inclination varies during an individual's lifetime. Normally the angle of the femoral neck is about 140 degrees in children and 125 to 130 degrees in adults; this angle can decrease even more in the older adult (Figure 6-2). It is important to understand that, as the angle of inclination approaches 90 degrees (i.e., a smaller angle), the weight-bearing stresses on the femoral neck increase, thereby raising the risk of a femoral neck fracture occurring. The posterior portion of the femoral neck serves as the attachment for the posterior part of the capsular ligament of the hip joint. The neck ends distally at the greater and lesser femoral trochanters (Figure 6-3).

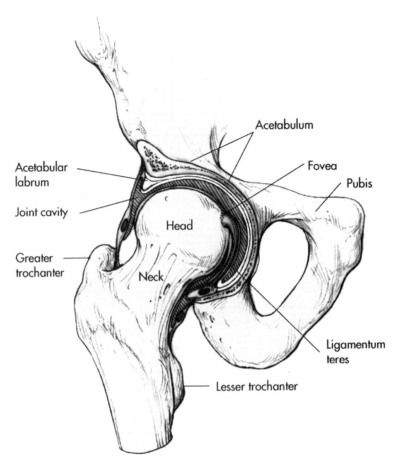

Figure 6-1   Anatomy of the Hip Joint and Proximal Femur. The acetabulum encompasses slightly more than one-half of the femoral head. (From C.L.A.S.S.: *Clinical anatomy principles*, St Louis, 1996, Mosby.)

The greater trochanter abuts the femoral neck and shaft; it is fairly prominent and relatively easy to palpate on the lateral thigh. It is the widest portion of the lower extremities and serves as an attachment for the tendons of several muscles, including the gluteus medius, gluteus maximus, obturator externus, obturator internus, gemelli, and piriformis (Figure 6-4).

The lesser trochanter extends out from the lower back part of the base of the femoral neck. Both the iliopsoas and iliacus muscle tendons insert at the lesser trochanter. A fairly prominent ridge of bone extending between the greater and lesser tuberosities roughly marks the intertrochanteric line.

Soft-Tissue Structures

Muscles

The four basic movements of the hip are flexion, extension, abduction, and adduction. Muscles that encompass the hip joint accomplish each motion.

The muscles of the hip can be divided into three basic groups based on their location: anterior, posterior, and medial. The muscles of the anterior thigh—the vastus medialis, the vastus intermedius, the vastus lateralis, and the rectus femoris—make up the quadriceps muscles (Figure 6-5). The quadriceps account for approximately 70% of the muscle mass of the thigh. Their primary

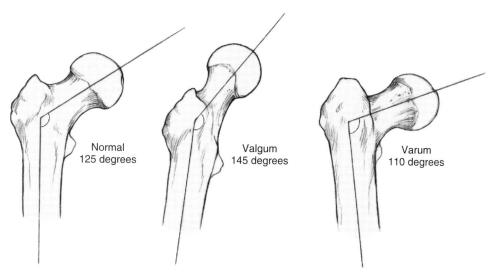

Figure 6-2 Variations in the Angle of the Femoral Neck. Also known as the "angle of inclination," this angle is measured from the center of the femoral head to the center of the femur. In children the angle may be as great as 145 degrees. The normal angle in adults is 125 degrees. As the angle decreases, the femoral neck becomes more prone to fracture. (From C.L.A.S.S.: *Clinical anatomy principles*, St Louis, 1996, Mosby.)

function is flexion of the hip and extension of the knee. The rectus femoris is the only muscle of the group that crosses the hip joint; the other three cross the knee joint. When there is injury to the rectus femoris muscle, hip flexion when the knee is flexed causes greater pain than it does when the knee is extended.

Posteriorly, the gluteal, hamstring, and piriformis muscles are all located in the buttock area. The gluteus maximus is the predominant hip extensor. In concert with the tensor fascia lata, the gluteus maximus helps maintain normal tone of the iliotibial band. The gluteal muscles also abduct the hip. Lying almost parallel to and near the posterior border of the gluteus medius, the piriformis muscle assists in lateral rotation of the hip. The muscles of the hip insert farther from the joint than the comparable rotator cuff muscles of the shoulder; this arrangement further stabilizes the hip joint.

The gluteus maximus and hamstring muscles extend the hip joint. The hamstrings extend from the hip to the knee and aid with both flexion of the knee and extension of the hip. In normal walking the hamstrings provide sufficient hip extension, but the more powerful gluteus maximus is necessary for walking up stairs or climbing. Extension is more limited than flexion, because the iliofemoral ligament generally restricts the extension to 15 degrees or less (Figure 6-6). Flexion of the hip is primarily the result of contraction of the anterior muscles—the iliopsoas, iliacus, rectus femoris, and sartorius.

Abduction, necessary for walking sideways, is primarily attributable to contraction of the gluteus medius, gluteus minimus, and gluteus maximus muscles. Adduction is enabled by the medial thigh muscles, primarily the pectineus and gracilis, as well as the adductor magnus, the adductor longus, and the adductor brevis (Figure 6-7). The commonly used term to describe this muscle group is the hip adductors.

The hip also has the capability to rotate both internally (medially) and externally (laterally). Table 6-1 summarizes the basic movements of the hip. Medial rotation is necessary for squatting; the muscles of the internal femoral area are responsible for this motion. Lateral rotation of the hip is made possible by the piriformis, obturator externus, gemellus, and other

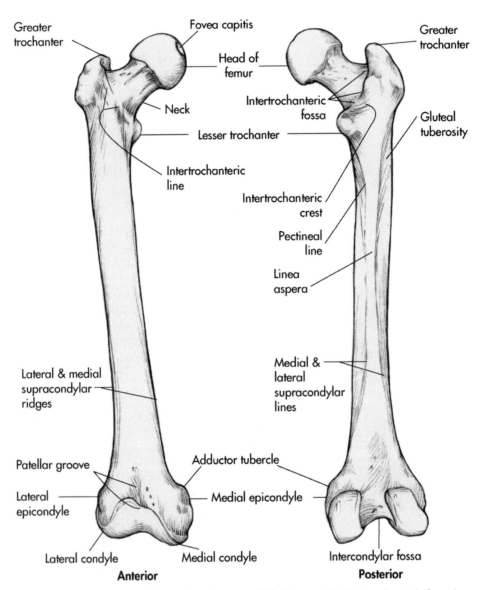

Figure 6-3 Anterior and Posterior Anatomy of the Femur. The intertrochanteric fossa is the line between the lesser and greater trochanters that defines the distal border of the femoral neck. The greater trochanter serves as the attachment for several posterior hip muscles. (From C.L.A.S.S.: *Clinical anatomy principles*, St Louis, 1996, Mosby.)

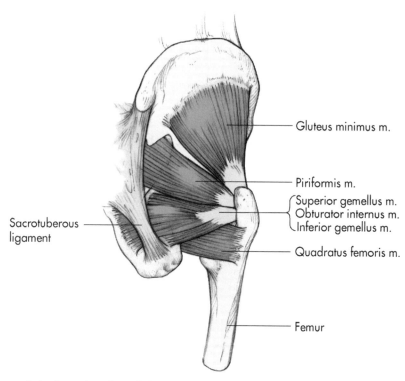

Figure 6-4 Deep Muscles of the Posterior Hip. Primarily, these muscles function to rotate the hip laterally. Note that the piriformis muscle passes through the sciatic notch. (From C.L.A.S.S.: *Clinical anatomy principles*, St Louis, 1996, Mosby.)

posteriorly lying muscles of the hip (see Figure 6-4). Lateral rotation occurs when one leg is crossed over the other.

Neurovascular Structures

Innervation of the hip and thigh originates from the lumbar plexus (i.e., portions of the upper four lumbar nerves). Unlike the brachial plexus, the nerves of the lumbar plexus tend to be less interwoven and branch more into each lower level.

The largest branch of the lumbar plexus, the femoral nerve, originates from L2, L3, and L4. It supplies the psoas major and iliac muscles. Branches of the nerve supply the pectineal, sartorius, and quadriceps femoris muscles. Standing from a squatting position will test the strength of the quadriceps and rectus femoris muscles. Hip flexion is mainly attributable to the integrity of the iliopsoas muscle, which is supplied by the branches of L1, L2, and L3.

The lateral femoral cutaneous nerve arises from L2 and L3; its terminal branches supply the anterolateral thigh from the greater trochanter to the knee. Injury to the superficial branches can cause persistent numbness of the anterolateral thigh, a condition known as *meralgia paresthetica*.

Hip adduction depends on an intact obturator nerve that arises from L2, L3, and L4. Sensation over the medial thigh is also partly a function of this nerve, but the distribution of the nerve varies. Table 6-2 summarizes the action, range of motion (ROM), and area of nerve root innervation of the major hip muscles.

The sciatic nerve is the most well-known nerve in the hip and thigh. Originating from L4, L5, S1, S2, and S3, the sciatic nerve is large, measuring 16 to 20 mm in

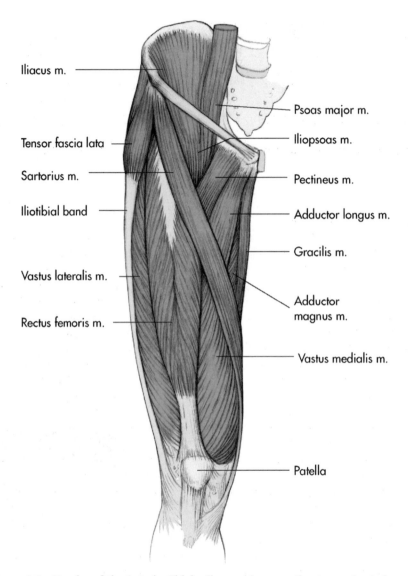

Figure 6-5 Muscles of the Anterior Thigh. The quadriceps are the strongest anterior muscles. The fourth muscle of the quadriceps, the vastus intermedius, lies beneath the rectus femoris muscle. (From C.L.A.S.S.: *Clinical anatomy principles*, St Louis, 1996, Mosby.)

diameter. It travels beneath the gluteus maximus muscle and lies on the posterior surface of the ischium (Figure 6-8). The sciatic nerve begins its course down the posterior thigh about halfway between the ischial tuberosity and the greater trochanter. The nerve has several branches, including the tibial and common peroneal nerves; it eventually terminates in the medial and lateral calcaneal branches and the lateral dorsal cutaneous nerve of the foot. Hip trauma, particularly dislocations, can cause sciatic nerve injury. Differentiating sciatic pain

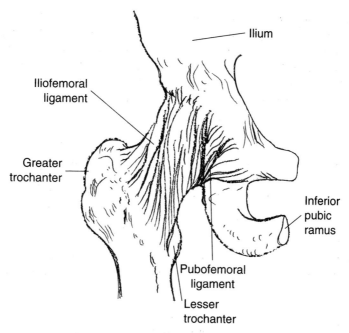

Figure 6-6   Anterior View of the Right Hip Showing the Iliofemoral Ligament. As the hip extends, the ligament tightens and restricts hip extension. (From C.L.A.S.S.: *Clinical anatomy principles*, St Louis, 1996, Mosby.)

from lumbar radiculopathy can present a diagnostic challenge. Table 6-3 summarizes the features of each entity.

The internal and external iliac, femoral, obturator, and superior and inferior gluteal arteries provide the primary blood supply to the hip and thigh. These vessels continue to branch off into smaller vessels throughout the thigh. The veins of the area generally correspond with their associated arteries.

There are no major lateral muscles, since the gluteus minimus and medius do not extend below the level of the greater trochanter. The tensor fascia lata extends from the iliac crest down and over the gluteus medius and maximus muscles, courses laterally, and inserts into the superior portion of the iliotibial band. In the hip area the function of the iliotibial band is to prevent lateral dislocation of the hip. Muscles of the hip are involved in many normal activities other than walking and running. However, injury to these muscles most frequently occurs with running or sports-related activities.

Ligaments

Strong ligaments encircle the hip joint and increase its stability. The hip joint itself has been described as a capsular ligament because the iliofemoral, pubofemoral, and ischiofemoral ligaments almost continuously encompass the joint. These three ligaments extend spirally from the pelvis to the anterior intertrochanteric line of the femur (Figure 6-9). Posteriorly they attach to the middle of the femoral neck. The majority of ligamentous joint reinforcement is anterior, superior, and posterior.

Anteriorly the iliofemoral ligament, the strongest in the body,[16] can be used by the surgeon as a fulcrum to a lever when manually reducing a hip dislocation. With normal hip extension the ligament becomes tight, aiding

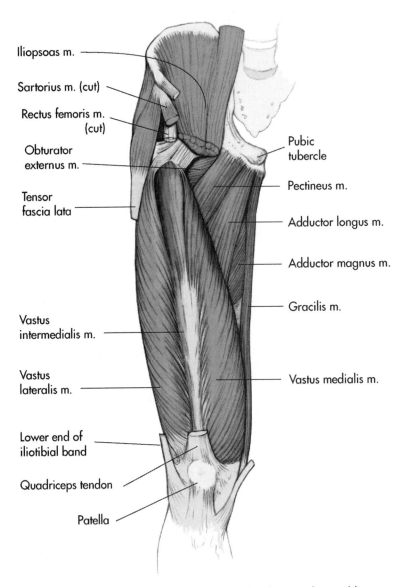

Iliopsoas m.

Sartorius m. (cut)

Rectus femoris m.
(cut)

Obturator
externus m.

Tensor
fascia lata

Vastus
intermedialis m.

Vastus
lateralis m.

Lower end of
iliotibial band

Quadriceps tendon

Patella

Pubic
tubercle

Pectineus m.

Adductor longus m.

Adductor magnus m.

Gracilis m.

Vastus medialis m.

Figure 6-7 Hip Adductor Muscles. These muscles lie deep to the quadriceps muscles.
Their primary function is adduction and flexion of the hip. The adductor magnus and gracilis
also medially rotate the knee. (From C.L.A.S.S.: *Clinical anatomy principles,* St Louis, 1996, Mosby.)

in the maintenance of upright posture by assisting in
rolling the pelvis backward onto the femoral heads. The
pubofemoral ligament helps limit abduction of the hip.
The ischiofemoral ligament makes up the posterior margin of the joint capsule and allows flexion of the hip; it
has no role in hip extension.

The ligamentum teres emerges from a small depression (the fovea capitus) in the femoral head (Figure 6-10).
This ligament may be congenitally absent in as much as
20% of the population. Even when the ligament is present, the blood vessels that emerge with it are more important, particularly the posterior branch of the obturator

| TABLE 6-1 | Selected Hip Muscles and Their Primary Actions |

Muscle	Location	Primary Action(s)
Psoas major	Lumbar vertebrae to lesser trochanter	Hip flexion, internal rotation of thigh
Sartorius	Anterior superior iliac spine to proximal medial tibia	Flexion, abduction, lateral rotation of hip
Quadriceps	Anterior inferior iliac spine or proximal femur to tibial tuberosity	Hip flexion
Gluteus maximus	Posterior iliac fossa and sacrum to iliotibial band and gluteal tuberosity	Hip extension, abduction
Gluteus medius and minimus	Middle iliac crest to greater trochanter	Abduction of hip
Gemellus superior and inferior	Sciatic notch to greater trochanter	Lateral rotation of hip
Tensor fascia lata	Superior iliac crest to iliotibial band	Flexion or extension of knee
Piriformis	Inner sacrum and sacroiliac joint to greater trochanter	Lateral rotation of hip

| TABLE 6-2 | Hip Range of Motion and Primary Muscles and Nerve Roots |

Motion	Range (degrees)	Muscle	Range of Nerve Root Innervation
Flexion	110-120	Iliopsoas Rectus femoris Sartorius Iliacus	L1-L3
Extension	10-20	Hamstrings Gluteus maximus Semimembranosus	L5-S2
Abduction	30-50	Gluteals Sartorius	L2-S1
Adduction	30	Adductors Gracilis Pectineus	L2-4
Medial rotation	30-40	Adductors Gluteus medius and minimus Tensor fascia lata	L2-S1
Lateral	40-60	Gluteus maximus Obturator internus Externus gemellus	L2-S2

artery. This vessel supplies a significant portion of blood to the femoral head. When these structures are present, injury to the ligament can also damage the artery and result in osteonecrosis (ON) of the femoral head.

Bursae

Usually found near a joint, a bursa is a fluid-filled sac lined with a synovial membrane. The function of a bursa is to decrease friction between tendon and bone, between ligament and bone, and between muscles. Typically there are three to four bursae around the greater trochanter, although as many as twenty have been described in the hip region.

Hip Examination

The hip and its surrounding structures play an important role in ambulation, but many other daily

TABLE 6-3   Potentially Differentiating Features of Sciatica and Lumbar Disk Disease

Sciatica	Lumbar Disk Disease
Describes leg pain along distribution of lumbosacral dermatome	Often a mechanical process aggravated by prolonged sitting or standing
Pain in buttock and posterior thigh into lateral ankle and sole of feet	Painless when spine is "balanced" by activities that unload compressive forces (e.g., walking, bending forward)
May involve neurologic deficit from disk disease	May result in sciatic pain

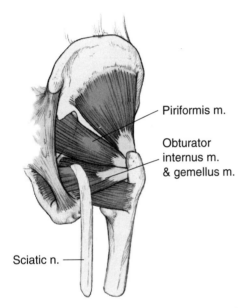

Piriformis m.

Obturator
internus m.
& gemellus m.

Sciatic n.

Figure 6-8 Typical anatomy of the sciatic nerve as it exits from the posterior hip and travels down the posterior thigh. (From C.L.A.S.S.: *Clinical anatomy principles*, St Louis, 1996, Mosby.)

activities also depend on normal hip function. Standing and sitting, crossing one leg over the other, standing from a squatting position, and ascending and descending stairs all require normal hip function. Observing these movements can provide clues to evaluate hip function.

In spite of the strong stabilization of the hip, it still has a fairly extensive ROM. Although circumduction is possible, generally the greatest plane of motion of the hip is flexion. Normal flexion ranges from 120 to 150 degrees. Extension of the hip is limited to 15 degrees or less by the tightening of the iliofemoral ligament. Abduction up to 50 degrees allows walking sideways. Adduction of 20 to 30 degrees is normal; this motion is limited because of the compression of the muscle and soft tissue of the thighs. Table 6-4 shows normal ROM for the hip.

Flexion of the hip is easily assessed by asking the patient to stand or lie supine (Figure 6-11) and then to draw the ipsilateral knee toward the chest. Initial assessment of hip extension can be made by asking the patient to get up from a sitting position without using the arms. More specific evaluation is made by asking the patient to lie prone on the examining table and slightly bend the knee (to relax the hamstrings). The practitioner stabilizes the pelvis with one arm while placing his or her other hand under the thigh and lifting the patient's leg upward off the table.

Abduction is measured by asking the patient to lie supine on the examining table while the practitioner stabilizes the pelvis by both placing his or her forearm across the patient's lower abdomen (between the iliac crests) and holding the contralateral anterior iliac spine. With a free hand, the examiner grasps the patient's ankle and abducts the leg. The degree of abduction is measured from an imaginary line running down the patient's midline.

Adduction is measured in a manner similar to abduction, but the patient's leg is brought across the midline (Figure 6-12). At the end point of adduction, some motion of the pelvis is palpable. Patients with large thighs may have limited adduction.

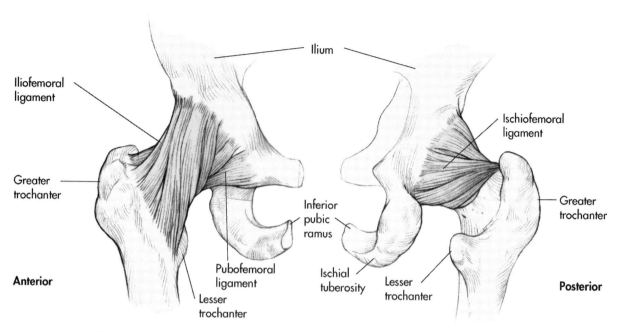

Figure 6-9 Anterior and posterior views of the three primary ligaments that stabilize the hip. The iliofemoral ligament is the strongest ligament in the body. (From C.L.A.S.S.: *Clinical anatomy principles*, St Louis, 1996, Mosby.)

Pathologic Abnormalities

Hip Fracture

Hip fractures in the United States occur at the rate of over 300,000 per year and have a substantial socioeconomic impact.[23,33] The incidence of hip fracture doubles for each decade of life after 50 years. Women are afflicted more than twice as often as men. One-year mortality for hip fractures in the elderly ranges from 14% to 36%.[8] Deep vein thrombosis is a serious complication that occurs in 40% to 83% of hip fracture patients. Secondary fatal pulmonary embolus occurs in 14% to 36% of patients who don't receive thromboprophylaxis.[31]

Risk factors for hip fracture are well documented. They include advancing age, muscle weakness, cognitive impairment, use of psychoactive medications, a history of stroke, tripping hazards in the house, physical inactivity, low body weight, previous hip fracture, tall stature, visual impairment, dementia, institutionalization, and osteoporosis.[39]

Pain in the hip area after trauma such as a fall or a motor vehicle accident, especially in patients over age 50, should give rise to the suggestion of fracture. Most hip fractures occur in the proximal femur. Fractures of the femoral head are considered intracapsular; extracapsular fractures are those that occur in the femoral neck. However, fractures of the sacrum, pubic ramus, acetabulum, or greater trochanter can also cause acute hip pain. Neither a lack of trauma nor the presence of a long-standing history of hip pain rules out a fracture.

Femoral Neck Fracture

Femoral neck fractures often occur in the older person. The costs of these fractures are significant. One study found the average total hospital charges per patient with a femoral neck fracture to be higher than $16,000.[33] Osteoporosis and a diminished angle of inclination of the femoral neck predispose a person to fracture in this area. Injury may range from a nondisplaced, impacted

Hip joint opened

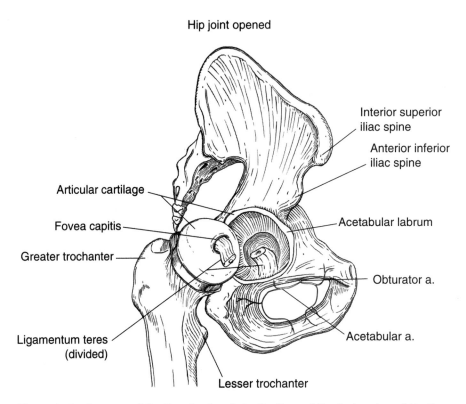

Figure 6-10   Anatomy of the Vascular Supply to the Femoral Head. An artery of the ligamentum teres is present in about 80% of the population. This artery arises from a posterior branch of the obturator artery.

TABLE 6-4	Normal Range of Motion for the Hip
Movement	Normal Range (degrees)
Flexion	120-150
Extension	10-15 (occasionally up to 30)
Abduction	45-50
Adduction	20-30
Internal rotation	35
External rotation	45

fracture of the neck into the femoral head to a complete displacement of the femoral head from the femoral neck (Figure 6-13). In the younger person these fractures are usually the result of significant trauma such as motor vehicle accidents and are considered an orthopedic emergency.

Pain is typically the cardinal symptom of any femoral neck fracture. However, in those younger than age 50, in osteoporotic patients, or even in some older persons, an inability to bear weight may be the presenting complaint. The affected leg appears shortened and is externally rotated from the contraction of the iliopsoas and gluteus maximus muscles.

ON of the femoral head is a serious complication of femoral neck fractures and corresponds with the degree of displacement of the fracture. Up to 50% of femoral neck fractures are complicated by osteonecrosis.[22] If the femoral head is completely displaced from the femoral neck, there is a greatly increased risk of damage to the

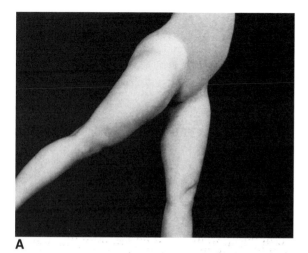

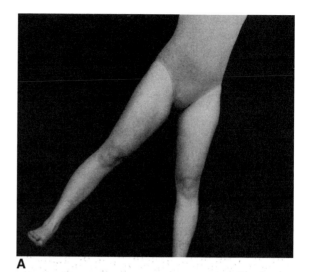

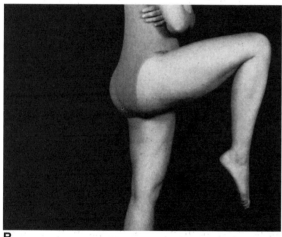

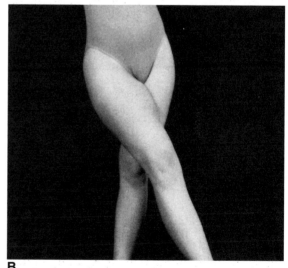

Figure 6-11 Extension (**A**) and flexion (**B**) of the hip can be measured with the patient either standing or supine, but hip extension is more accurately measured with the patient supine. (From Evans RC: *Illustrated orthopedic in physical assessment,* ed 2, St Louis, 2001, Mosby.)

Figure 6-12   Active Abduction and Adduction of the Hip. To accurately measure both motions, the patient's pelvis should be stabilized by the practitioner's forearm. Normal abduction ranges from 45 to 50 degrees; adduction ranges from 20 to 30 degrees. (From Evans RC: *Illustrated orthopedic physical assessment,* ed 2, St Louis, 2001, Mosby.)

nutrient vessels that emerge from the fovea capitis and supply the femoral head. ON may not manifest itself for months to years after injury. The anterolateral femoral head is most likely to be affected.

Most femoral neck fractures, especially in patients under age 50, are seen and managed as emergencies by orthopedic surgeons. Patients with chronic hip pain,

especially in the presence of osteoporosis, may have far more subtle symptoms indicating a fracture. Regardless of presentation, femoral neck fracture

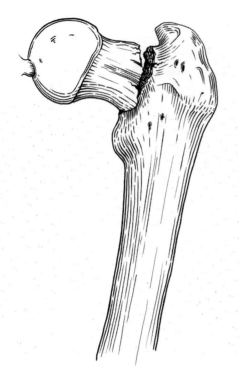

Figure 6-13 A displaced femoral neck fracture.

requires reduction and surgical fixation by an orthopedic surgeon.

Intertrochanteric Femur Fracture

It is fairly uncommon in the primary care setting to see fractures along the line connecting the greater and lesser tuberosities of the trochanter. These types of fractures are the result of forces and conditions similar to those responsible for femoral neck fractures. The causes include trauma, osteoporosis, rheumatoid arthritis, or metabolic diseases that affect the organs, as well as being older than age 50. Patients with short femoral necks may be at greater risk for intertrochanteric fracture than for femoral neck fracture. Unlike fractures of the femoral neck, those of the intertrochanteric femur involve the shaft (metaphysis) in a well-vascularized area of bone. As a result, the incidence of complications is generally less than that of femoral neck fractures.

The primary concern regarding intertrochanteric fractures is stability. An unstable fracture can result in malunion and a shortening of the femur. The angle of the imaginary line connecting the greater and lesser trochanters is oblique, thus predisposing the fracture to compressing down if any weight is placed on the affected limb. Intertrochanteric fracture lines that extend beyond the subtrochanteric region are among those classified as unstable.

Diagnosis. Physical examination, history, and plain radiographic films usually provide enough information to diagnose an intertrochanteric fracture. It is important to remember that not all fractures are easily visible on x-ray films and may be missed. If there is any suggestion of fracture, the patient should be referred to an orthopedic surgeon for further evaluation, including a possible bone scan or magnetic resonance imaging (MRI), and definitive treatment.

Treatment. Patients, especially young people, require urgent referral to an orthopedic surgeon. Treatment is surgical fixation, typically with a sliding hip screw or intramedullary nail. In some cases a total joint replacement may be necessary. Surgery within 24 to 48 hours of injury tends to produce a better outcome.

Subtrochanteric Femur Fracture

A fracture of the subtrochanteric femur occurs in the proximal third of the femur and may begin at or just distal to the lesser trochanter. When seen in young patients, subtrochanteric fractures are typically associated with high-energy injuries, such as vehicular trauma, falls from heights, or a direct blow. It is not unusual for a subtrochanteric fracture to be comminuted. The presence of multiple bone fragments requires greater hardware stabilization. In the older patient, a simple fall may cause such a fracture. Pathologic fractures from metastatic disease are not uncommon in this area.

On examination, the hip is abducted (because of contraction of the gluteus medius muscle), and the femur is externally rotated (due to contraction of the iliopsoas and gluteus maximus muscles). Weight bearing is difficult and may be impossible. Patients with a subtrochanteric fracture require immediate referral to an emergency department or orthopedic surgeon. Surgical fixation is the treatment of choice.

Similar to intertrochanteric fractures, the stability of subtrochanteric fractures is critically important. Unstable subtrochanteric fractures have the highest risk for surgical failure and healing complications. The high incidence of complications is at least partly due to the tremendous biomechanical stresses in this area.

Stress Fractures

Femoral neck stress fractures are not commonly seen in primary care. One of the primary risk factors for a stress fracture is repetitive stress to the femoral neck. Athletes, older person, and military personnel may be at greater risk for a stress fracture. These fractures are classified as either tension- or compression-type injuries. Tension fractures affect the superior portion of the femoral neck and are unstable. Compression fractures occur on the inferior portion of the femoral neck. Although compression-type stress fractures can be treated nonsurgically, both types of fracture should be referred to an orthopedic surgeon.

Recurrent groin or hip pain, especially with weight bearing, is the most frequent symptom of a stress fracture. There is usually no history of significant trauma. Percussing the femur distal to the suspected fracture may cause pain at the area of interest. Having the patient stand or hop on the affected leg will usually exacerbate pain. ROM may be uncomfortable, especially with internal rotation and joint compression, but there is no real limitation. Plain x-ray films are almost universally negative unless the process has persisted for several weeks. Diagnosis is made from a bone scan or MRI. MRI is the preferred diagnostic test because bone scan may not be positive until 2 to 3 days after the fracture (Figure 6-14 *A* and *B).* Left unrecognized or untreated, a stress frac-

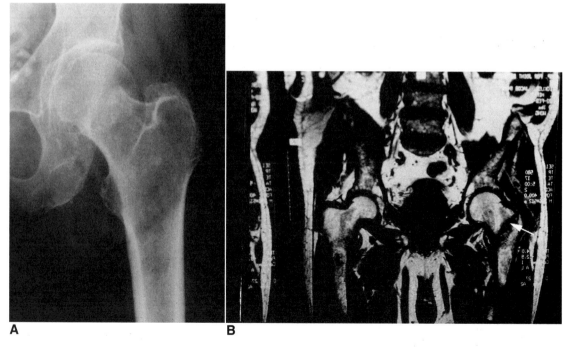

A   **B**

Figure 6-14 A patient with a suggested femoral neck fracture. A, Anteroposterior radiographic film does not show any obvious abnormality. **B**, Magnetic resonance image within 24 hours of injury clearly shows an intertrochanteric fracture. (From Loth TS: *Orthopaedic boards review II: a case study approach,* St Louis, 1996, Mosby.)

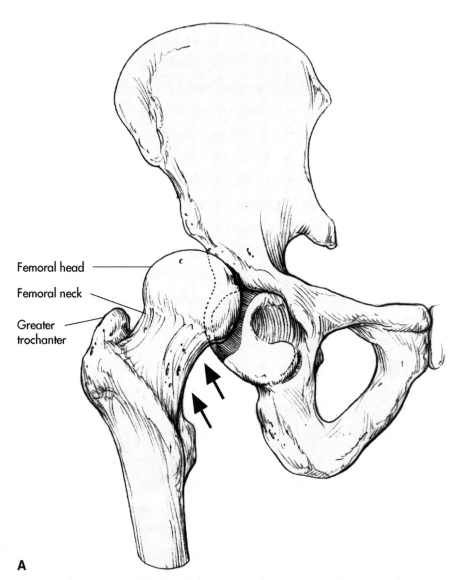

Femoral head
Femoral neck
Greater
trochanter

A

Figure 6-15   A Simple Posterior Dislocation of the Right Hip. A, The direction of force applied to create this dislocation is indicated by arrows. (From C.L.A.S.S.: Clinical anatomy principles, St Louis, 1996, Mosby.)

Continued

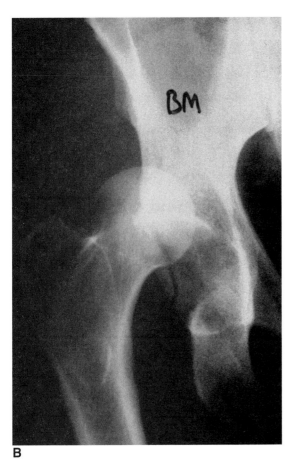

Figure 6-15, cont'd   B, A posterior fracture-dislocation of the hip. Note the fracture of the acetabulum on this x-ray projection. This type of injury carries a high risk of developing osteonecrosis of the femoral head. (From Loth TS: *Orthopaedic boards review II: a case study approach,* St Louis, 1996, Mosby.)

ture can progress to an unstable fracture that may predispose the injury to nonunion or osteonecrosis.

Initial treatment is directed at relieving pain and preventing further injury. Decreasing activity with partial weight bearing or non-weight bearing on the affected leg should be used.[4] Oral analgesics or nonsteroidal anti-inflammatory drugs (NSAIDs) may be prescribed and the patient referred to an orthopedic surgeon.

Posterior Hip Dislocation

Posterior hip dislocations account for the majority of hip dislocations. The classic example of this injury is when a force is applied to the knee with the hip flexed and adducted, such as when the knee strikes the dashboard during a motor vehicle collision. The femoral head is driven posteriorly out of the acetabular socket (Figure 6-15). Sciatic nerve injury is often associated with posterior hip dislocation, as is the disruption of the blood supply to the femoral head. Osteonecrosis is a fairly common complication, occurring in up to 40% of posterior hip dislocations[8]; femoral neck fractures occur in approximately 7% to 10% of dislocations.[8,32] With significant dislocation, the hip is flexed, adducted, and internally rotated.

Abduction, extension, and external rotation of the leg are difficult or impossible for the patient to manage. The patient may note "fullness" in the buttock, and a mass (the femoral head) may be palpable on the ilium.

The patient should be immobilized and transported to an emergency department as soon as possible. Prompt reduction of the dislocation decreases the incidence of complications such as osteonecrosis and damage to the sciatic nerve or its peroneal branch.

Anterior Hip Dislocation

Any injury to the hip that causes forced abduction, external rotation, and flexion of the joint can result in anterior dislocation of the hip. For example, this type of injury can occur when a person's leg strikes a fence post while horseback riding. The fence post acts as a fulcrum that forces the femoral head anteriorly out of the acetabulum into the obturator foramen of the pelvis. It is unusual to see this injury in a primary care setting, since most patients are evaluated and treated in an emergency department.

Injury to the hip's obturator nerve can occur, resulting in weakness of the hip adductors. Associated damage to the femoral artery or vein can also occur. The possibility of vascular injury must be carefully assessed with an anterior dislocation of the hip. Reduction is performed under intravenous sedation or general anesthesia. Neurovascular status should be reevaluated after reduction, after which posttraumatic arthritis of the hip is not uncommon.

SOFT-TISSUE INJURIES

Quadriceps Muscles

Thigh injuries, especially in athletes, are common. The anterior thigh muscles, specifically the quadriceps, are frequently involved in injury. Fortunately most injuries to the quadriceps are relatively minor—primarily strains or contusions. Complete rupture of the quadriceps muscles, a more serious injury, is less common but fairly dramatic in its clinical presentation. Risk factors for muscle strains are believed to include muscle fatigue, inadequate warm-up and stretching exercises, and muscle imbalance between the quadriceps and hamstring muscles.[25]

Strains are classified into three categories, based on the severity of injury. Grade I involves stretching or tearing of muscle fibers, but the fascia and muscle function remain intact. Tearing the muscle fibers, resulting in significant hemorrhage, is a grade II injury. Grade III strains involve damage to the fascia and significant injury to the muscle fibers, resulting in obvious deformity and loss of muscle function. The rectus femoris is most susceptible to a strain, because it crosses both the hip and knee joints.

Contusions are usually the result of a direct blow to the anterior thigh. Although common in sports, contusions are also the result of falls and occupational injuries. These injuries may or may not result in obvious deformity over the muscle. Deeper muscular structures are affected by contusions rather than by strains.

Rupture of the quadriceps occurs when the contracted muscle is forced into flexion (i.e., the hip and knee are extended, and then the knee is forced into flexion). The most common scenario is a fall onto an extended leg, resulting in forced flexion of the knee. Rupture of the muscle most often occurs at its distal portion, immediately superior to the patella.

History

Patients with a quadriceps strain typically describe a "pulled" muscle. Often onset of symptoms is associated with a specific activity but not necessarily with a single incident. Contact sports such as martial arts and running sports (e.g., soccer, lacrosse, football, field hockey) predispose the muscles to forced stretching of a contracting muscle when a kick or cut is missed or when an on-field collision occurs. Pain is exacerbated by any activity that causes increased tension on the muscle.

Contusion of the quadriceps causes an immediate onset of pain. Intensity of pain usually correlates with the severity of the contusion. Decreasing ROM, especially at the knee, occurs as bleeding and inflammation inhibit muscle contraction.

Rupture of the quadriceps is almost invariably the result of a single, specific incident. Pain is intense, swelling is rapid, and the patient is unable to extend the ipsilateral knee. Pain is usually localized to the knee and structures immediately superior to it.

Physical Examination

Obvious deformity over the anterior thigh, combined with discoloration and tenderness to palpation, is the initial presentation of significant strain or contusion of the quadriceps muscles. Within the first 24 hours after the injury, a palpable defect may be present in the muscle. Once hematoma formation and swelling progress, this finding may be obscured.

A complete tear of the quadriceps usually has a palpable, painful defect, in spite of a hematoma formation. When palpating the quadriceps, a defect in the suprapatellar area is commonly felt. The defect is often described as "mush" at the distal quadriceps muscles.

In a rectus femoris strain, flexing the hip and knee causes greater pain than flexing the hip and extending the knee. This is because the rectus femoris crosses both the hip and knee joints, and pain is increased when both joints are stressed.

Quadriceps contusions are suggested on the basis of history and confirmed on examination by the presence of localized swelling, tenderness, and ecchymosis. Edema and ecchymosis tend to migrate in a dependent direction. Pain is usually localized to the area of ecchymosis. Knee examination is rarely abnormal.

Diagnosis

Diagnostic plain films are rarely useful for soft-tissue injuries unless a fracture is also suggested. Palpable tendon defect or tenderness over bony prominences may be an indication for radiologic evaluation. MRI provides the greatest detail for evaluating tendon rupture, but the diagnosis remains primarily clinical.

Treatment

Differentiation of strains, including rupture, and contusions is important because the treatment for each is different. Complete rupture of the quadriceps muscles requires surgical repair and immediate referral to an orthopedic surgeon.

Treatment of strains and contusions initially involves efforts to limit swelling and hemorrhage, as well as to decrease pain. The method of rest (ambulation with crutches), ice, compression, and elevation (RICE) is used for the acute phase, usually the first 24 to 48 hours after injury. NSAIDs are also useful for decreasing inflammation. Once the acute phase is over, treatment of strains involves gradually increasing ROM and strength. A formal physical therapy program is appropriate to meet the goals of a return of motion, strength, and endurance. Straight leg raising exercises should be initially avoided, because of the strain they place on the rectus femoris muscle. Return to normal activity may take several weeks.

Treatment of contusions also consists of therapy after the acute phase. However, flexion exercises seem to result in a quicker recovery than extension exercises. Full extension of the knee is usually the last movement to be regained. Delaying the patient's return to sporting activities may be difficult, but overusing the affected muscle will prolong rehabilitation beyond the usual 2 to 3 weeks.

Hamstring Muscles

Posterior hip pain, especially among physically active patients, is often the result of a hamstring injury. Three muscles, the semimembranosus, semitendinosus, and biceps femoris, make up the hamstrings (Figure 6-16). Of these, the semimembranosus forms most of the muscle mass, extending from the ischial tuberosity to the posteromedial tibia. The semitendinosus and biceps femoris muscles also originate at the ischial tuberosity, but the former inserts medial to the semimembranosus. The biceps femoris, which has two heads, has an additional origin on the posterolateral femur; the muscle obliquely crosses the posterior femur and inserts on the proximal fibula.

Activities that require bursts of speed or sudden acceleration, such as tennis, track and field, lacrosse, soccer, football, and rugby, are often associated with hamstring injuries; even cheerleading activities can result in an injury of the hamstring. The most common injury is a strain, commonly called a "pulled" muscle. Avulsion fractures can also occur with hamstring injury. Risk factors are thought to be fatigue, muscle strength imbalance, improper stretching, and poor flexibility.[24] The exact pathophysiology that causes hamstring injuries is not clearly understood, but increasing age and past thigh or knee injury may predispose one to this problem.[42] The injuries usually involve a tear in the muscle near the musculotendinous junction and are often recurrent. Stretching the hamstrings seems to improve their extensibility by increasing their stretch tolerance. Stretching may decrease the risk of injury.

History

Patients frequently report suddenly feeling or hearing a painful pop or tearing in the posterior thigh during an activity. Pain does not necessarily preclude further activity, but left untreated the pain tends to worsen and stiffness of the thigh may develop. Initially pain is present primarily with activity but may progress to being present even at rest.

Avulsion of the hamstring muscles from the ischial tuberosity is more common in adolescents than adults. In adolescents the ischial apophysis can be avulsed when there is significant pulling stress. In adults the apophysis has fused; but, when injured, it requires more aggressive treatment. The patient may have buttock pain and difficulty walking, standing, squatting, or flexing the ipsilateral knee.

Physical Examination

No gross anatomic abnormality is usually noted, but ecchymosis distal to the posterior ischial tuberosity is common. Having the patient stretch the hamstrings by attempting to touch the floor with the fingertips while standing with knees straight frequently elicits complaints of tenderness. It may be difficult to palpate any defect in the hamstring muscles unless there is an avulsion from the ischium.[5]

When the ischial apophysis in an adolescent is avulsed, there is usually point tenderness over the ischial

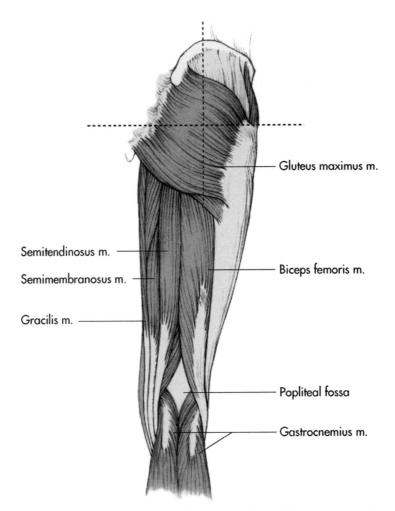

Gluteus maximus m.

Semitendinosus m.

Semimembranosus m.

Biceps femoris m.

Gracilis m.

Popliteal fossa

Gastrocnemius m.

Figure 6-16   Three Hamstring Muscles. The distal portions of the muscles form the medial and lateral borders of popliteal fossa. (From C.L.A.S.S.: *Clinical anatomy principles*, St Louis, 1996, Mosby.)

tuberosity and sitting may be uncomfortable. There may be some palpable asymmetry of the hamstrings.

Diagnosis

History and physical examination are the primary diagnostic tools for hamstring injuries. In the adolescent with a suggested avulsion of the ischial apophysis, a simple anteroposterior (AP) x-ray film of the hemipelvis will reveal the avulsed fragment (Figure 6-17). If the presentation of hamstring injuries in an adult indicates

significant trauma, sonography is a low-cost alternative to MRI for diagnosing complete muscle-tendon avulsion ruptures.

Treatment

Although no consensus exists on optimal treatment, simple hamstring strains are usually treated with RICE and NSAIDs. Rest includes restricting any activities that stretch the hamstrings. Compression with an elastic bandage may decrease the amount of swelling. Once

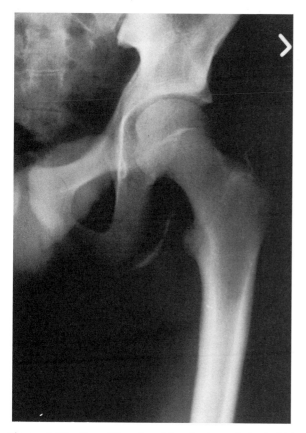

Figure 6-17 X-ray film of avulsion fracture of the ischial apophysis in an adolescent male patient.

acute symptoms subside, usually within 7 to 10 days, the patient can begin physical therapy (PT) exercises designed to stretch and strengthen the muscles.

Avulsion injuries in adolescents can also be treated conservatively. The patient should not return to sports until the fracture has healed—a process that normally takes 6 weeks. Healing progress can be monitored with plain x-ray films. An ischial avulsion in an adult requires immediate referral to an orthopedic surgeon for surgical repair, if the best chance for full recovery is to be provided.

Bursitis

As previously noted, the hip area contains multiple bursae; four of primary clinical interest are the iliopsoas, ischiogluteal, and the trochanteric bursae—subgluteus medius, subgluteus minimus, and subgluteus maximus (Figure 6-18). These bursae are classified as "constant" bursae (i.e., they are formed during normal embryonic development). Bursae, as mentioned, are saclike structures that function as gliding mechanisms to decrease friction between structures. They contain synovial cells that secrete synovial fluid. Any mechanism that causes inflammation or irritation of these sacs can result in bursitis.

Trauma to a bursa is a well-known cause of bursitis, but other conditions are also associated with bursal inflammation. These include degenerative arthritis, lumbar spondylosis, obesity, fibromyalgia, and neurologic problems. Hip replacement surgery can also bring about bursal inflammation. An underlying condition such as arthritis is often associated with development of iliopsoas bursitis. Pressure or compression on adjacent anterior hip structures may cause symptoms of arthritis, venous obstruction, ureteral displacement, or other vague symptoms that may delay diagnosis of bursitis.[18] Examination may reveal tenderness and/or a palpable mass at the femoral triangle, just lateral to the femoral artery.[3]

The incidence of trochanteric bursitis peaks between the fourth and sixth decades of life and is more common in women than men. Onset may be acute or insidious, and the condition may be chronic. Bursitis may be inflammatory, hemorrhagic, infectious, or calcific. Inflammatory bursitis is more common in the hip than the other forms.

Pain is usually a chronic, localized aching over the lateral portion of the hip. Pain may occasionally extend into the low back or knee and is exacerbated by certain movements.

History

Most patients relate a history of progressive, localized, deep aching over the lateral hip. Pain may be intermittent or constant. A history of trauma may or may not be present. Inability to lie on the affected side is one of the most common complaints. External rotation and abduction of the hip (e.g., getting in or out of a vehicle) frequently exacerbates pain, as does climbing stairs or prolonged standing. In the younger patient, running or jogging causes pain.

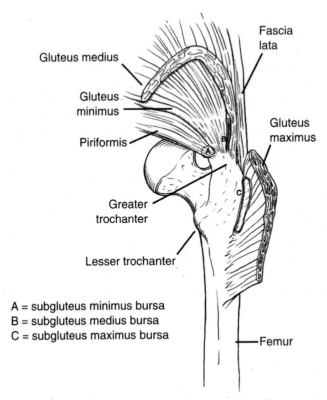

Gluteus medius

Gluteus minimus

Piriformis

Fascia lata

Gluteus maximus

Greater trochanter

Lesser trochanter

A = subgluteus minimus bursa
B = subgluteus medius bursa
C = subgluteus maximus bursa

Femur

Figure 6-18 **A-C**, The three major bursae around the greater trochanter. The subgluteus maximus (**C**) is most often affected by bursitis.

Often patients ingest acetaminophen or over-the-counter NSAIDs to relieve pain. Some improvement in symptoms is common, but the pain does not completely abate with such therapy.

Pain does not involve numbness, tingling, or weakness. The presence of neurologic complaints or muscular weakness should alert the practitioner to possible lumbar neuropathy, vertebral disk disease, or femoral head or neck pathologic abnormalities.

Physical Examination

Localized tenderness or pain over the greater trochanter is the cardinal symptom of trochanteric bursitis. Erythema is usually absent, and swelling is difficult to palpate in this area. Painless flexion and extension of the hip helps differentiate bursitis from diseases of the hip joint. Iliopsoas bursitis may manifest as weakness with

active external rotation and hip flexion. Passive rotation of the hip is painless.[34]

Diagnosis

Clinical examination is the basis for diagnosing trochanteric bursitis. X-ray films have little or no value unless there is suggested associated arthritis. Diagnosis of iliopsoas bursitis may require further imaging studies such as ultrasound or MRI to differentiate it from other conditions.

Treatment

NSAID therapy alone is inadequate treatment. Injection of a local anesthetic combined with a corticosteroid is often an effective treatment. After one or more corticosteroid injections, most patients will have relief of symptoms, although recurrence is common. Adjuvant

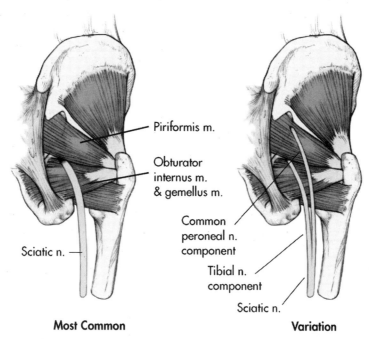

Piriformis m.

Obturator
internus m.
& gemellus m.

Common
peroneal n.
component

Tibial n.
component

Sciatic n.

Sciatic n.

Most Common   **Variation**

Figure 6-19   Two Variations in Anatomy of the Sciatic Nerve. When the tibial branch exits through the piriformis muscle, contraction of the muscle exerts pressure on the nerve, causing pain. (From C.L.A.S.S.: *Clinical anatomy principles,* St Louis, 1996, Mosby.)

treatment with NSAIDs and a program of PT (including ultrasound) may increase the efficacy of local injection.

Piriformis Syndrome

An increasingly recognized cause of buttock and sciatic nerve pain is the pressure that can be placed, when the piriformis muscle contracts, on the nerves that pass though the piriformis or through the sciatic notch (Figure 6-19). When this occurs, it is known as piriformis syndrome.

The most common path of the sciatic nerve exits the gluteal area below or anterior to the piriformis muscle. Anatomic variations of the sciatic nerve also allow the peroneal and tibial portions to pass over and through the piriformis or entirely through the muscle. As a result, the clinical manifestations of piriformis syndrome are very similar to those of sciatica. The last two arrangements may make an individual susceptible to developing piriformis syndrome.

History

Buttock pain, with or without radiation into the leg, is the cardinal symptom of piriformis syndrome. The pain itself is not diagnostic, but pain that worsens with prolonged sitting or after activities that require hip abduction and internal rotation suggests the likelihood of the syndrome.

Physical Examination

Unless there is recent trauma, bruising or soft-tissue swelling is not usually present. Tenderness to palpation is common from the sciatic notch to the greater trochanter. Sometimes there is palpable muscle spasm, which is described as a "spindle-shaped mass." Lower-extremity neurologic testing is generally normal, but straight leg raising may be positive. Pain tends to increase with resisted hip flexion, adduction, and internal rotation (FAIR test).

Abnormal biomechanics of the foot, such as excessive pronation or subtalar instability, may cause internal rotation of the knee and hip during the push-off phase of walking. A reactive correction of the hip's external rotators, including the piriformis, may result in the development of piriformis syndrome.

Diagnosis

History and physical examination are the primary factors leading to a diagnosis of piriformis syndrome, which is one of exclusion.[35] If there is any question of active lumbar disk disease, the patient should be referred to an orthopedic surgeon or neurologist. A positive FAIR test seems to correlate with the presence of piriformis syndrome and may be useful in predicting response to treatment.[10] Nerve conduction studies may help pinpoint the cause of pain.

Treatment

Once the diagnosis of piriformis syndrome has been established, conservative treatment is initiated. Ultrasound, coupled with PT to stretch the muscle and correction of poor posture or associated foot and ankle problems, helps in most cases. Once the patient is discharged from a formal PT program, stretching exercises and local application of ice can continue to relieve symptoms. NSAIDs will help relieve inflammation of the muscle and nerves. Nonnarcotic or oral narcotic analgesics may be necessary to control pain during an acute episode.

If the patient's symptoms do not improve, he or she should be referred to an orthopedic surgeon for possible corticosteroid injection. Intramuscular injection of botulinum toxin type A, performed under fluoroscopic and electromyographic guidance, also appears to reduce pain.[6,11] A patient who fails to respond to up to three injections may be a candidate for surgical release of the muscle.

Avascular Necrosis (Osteonecrosis)

Osteonecrosis of the femoral head is a serious complication of hip trauma, but it can also occur without trauma. When blood flow through the artery of the ligamentum teres (a branch of the obturator artery) is interrupted, the bone of the femoral head dies. Previously called avascular necrosis (AVN), osteonecrosis is the preferred term since it encompasses conditions other than vascular problems. Generally, there are two etiologies of osteonecrosis: traumatic and nontraumatic.[22,41] In adults, trauma, especially femoral neck fracture, is the most common cause of this condition.

In children, osteonecrosis of the femoral head is called Legg-Calvé-Perthes disease. The exact cause of Legg-Calvé-Perthes is not fully known. A slipped capital femoral epiphysis, a condition usually requiring surgical intervention, can also cause osteonecrosis in children and adolescents. As noted earlier, both femoral head fractures and posterior hip dislocations are associated with the development of osteonecrosis and injury to an artery of the ligamentum teres with osteonecrosis of ischemic origin. Individuals with sickle-cell disease, coagulopathy, gout, Gaucher's disease, lupus, and high radiation exposure may be at increased risk for nontraumatic osteonecrosis. Patients ingesting high-dose corticosteroids and those with a history of excessive alcohol intake have an increased frequency of osteonecrosis because alcohol may have a direct effect on bone. The net effect of osteonecrosis is progressive destruction of the femoral head, resulting in pain, limp, femoral head collapse, and severe arthritis (Figure 6-20).

The basic pathology of osteonecrosis is interruption of circulation to and increased hydrostatic pressure in the bone. Inflammatory exudates, vascular insufficiency, and microvascular thrombotic and fat emboli have been implicated.[19,22,41] When vascular insufficiency becomes vascular occlusion, both osteocyte and marrow-cell necrosis ensues within hours to days.[22]

History

Most patients with osteonecrosis are between 30 and 50 years old and complain of hip pain and limp. If there is no remote or recent trauma, there is often a history of chemotherapy, high-dose radiation, steroid treatment or excessive alcohol intake. Pain is often described as a deep ache, but it may also occur as groin pain with walking. Pain may have persisted for months or years before the patient seeks help. As the disease progresses, coughing may exacerbate hip pain.

Physical Examination

The patient complains of pain (often in the groin), has difficulty walking, and usually limps. Weight bearing

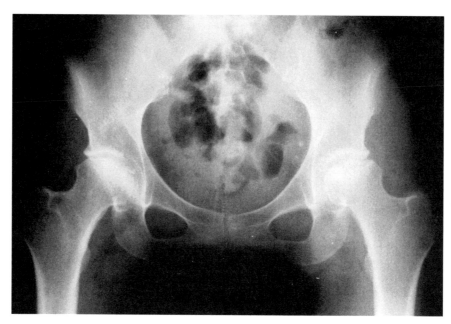

Figure 6-20   Bilateral Osteonecrosis of the Femoral Heads. Note the flattened appearance of the superior portion of the femoral heads. (From Loth TS: *Orthopaedic boards review II: a case study approach,* St Louis, 1996, Mosby.)

worsens complaints. ROM at the hip may be limited and painful at the extremes of movement, especially internal rotation and flexion. Sometimes a fairly forceful blow directed upward on the bottom of the heel will cause hip pain. There are no specific laboratory tests for osteonecrosis.

Diagnosis

Diagnosis is made by imaging studies. Late in the disease process, plain x-ray films (AP and frog-leg views) will show a grossly deformed, flattened femoral head with joint space narrowing. MRI is better at visualizing earlier changes of osteonecrosis that occur in the marrow. The marrow becomes necrotic before the trabecular architecture of the bone changes. Bone scanning is also used to visualize osteonecrosis, but the intensity of uptake does not correlate with severity or progression of the disease.

Treatment

Orthopedic referral is indicated for suggested or confirmed osteonecrosis. Although early osteonecrosis may

improve with the use of crutches and a decrease in weight-bearing activities, most cases require surgical intervention. During the early stages of osteonecrosis, core decompression of the femoral head may revascularize the area. More advanced stages require bone grafting or even joint replacement.

DEGENERATIVE AND DEVELOPMENTAL CONDITIONS

Osteoarthritis

One of the most frequently encountered causes of hip pain in adults is osteoarthritis (OA). The morbidity associated with OA is significant, considering the degree to which it limits normal activity. OA typically affects weight-bearing joints—the hip, the knee, and the spine are common sites.

The exact pathophysiology of the cause of OA is not known, but alterations in biomechanical and biochemical factors affecting the articular cartilage are involved.[1]

Trauma, infection, and obesity may predispose an individual to the development of OA.[24,29] The course of the disease is highly variable, and radiographic appearance of the joint does not necessarily correlate with clinical symptoms.

There is no known cure for OA, but appropriate primary care management can often decrease pain and disability while maintaining and even improving joint function. When conservative measures are no longer effective, total joint arthroplasty may be indicated.

History

OA tends to be associated with the older population, but it is not uncommon in middle-aged adults, particularly those with a history of remote trauma or aggressive physical activity such as football. Onset is usually insidious. One of the most common presenting complaints is limited motion, often accompanied by pain. Pain is usually in the groin area, although it is sometimes present in the anterior or lateral thigh. Some patients complain of hip stiffness in the morning, usually less than 1 hour in duration. Stiffness, sometimes called "gelling," usually decreases with activity. Any recent trauma should be noted since trauma, even relatively minor, tends to exacerbate symptoms. A thorough history will help focus the diagnosis. It is important to differentiate OA from periarticular disorders, such as muscle strains, bursitis, or back problems.

Patient-instituted therapies and their success are important components of the history. Pain associated with OA is not always caused by inflammation, and temporary relief of symptoms with over-the-counter analgesics such as acetaminophen may preclude the necessity of NSAID therapy.

The extent to which pain and stiffness limit the patient can provide clues on how aggressively to treat the symptoms. Difficulties walking, standing after sitting, and climbing stairs are common. A patient with a positive family history of degenerative joint disease is more likely to develop a similar problem.

Physical Examination

Typically, OA does not cause erythema, warmth, soft-tissue swelling, tenderness to palpation, or significant effusion. The presence of these findings is more indicative of an acute inflammatory process, such as septic arthritis or an acute rheumatoid flare.

The hallmark of OA is decreased ROM, especially internal rotation. Not uncommonly, either active or passive movement of the hip may cause palpable crepitus. Passive movement of the hip is usually painful at the extremes of motion. Joint loading, or compression, also usually causes pain. Joint compression is performed by having the patient lie in a supine position with the affected hip and knee flexed to 90 degrees. The practitioner then applies downward pressure on the knee; pain in the hip or groin area suggests degenerative changes within the joint.

Diagnosis

Diagnosis of hip OA is fairly straightforward when based on the criteria of the American College of Rheumatology. In a patient older than age 50, hip pain and the presence of at least two of the following symptoms lead to a diagnosis of OA: a radiographic joint space narrowing, the radiographic presence of femoral or acetabular osteophytes, or an erythrocyte sedimentation rate less than 20 mm per hour.[2]

Because OA is more of a degenerative than an inflammatory process, there are no specific laboratory tests for OA. Diagnosis of rheumatoid disease, on the other hand, can be augmented by several serologic laboratory tests.[24] If there is doubt regarding the diagnosis, these tests can assist in differentiating the two types of disease; however, as a rule, laboratory studies are of little help in positively diagnosing OA.

Plain x-ray films of the hip remain the standard for diagnosing OA. Typical findings include asymmetric joint space narrowing, subchondral cystic changes and sclerosis, and the presence of osteophytes. Although radiologic findings do not necessarily correlate with the severity of a patient's symptoms, there is some evidence that plain films can be used to monitor progression of the disease.[7]

Treatment

Nonsurgical management of OA is designed to optimize function and prevent or decrease pain. A number of nonpharmacologic therapies can alleviate or reduce symptoms. Often local branches of the Arthritis Foundation offer exercise programs. Water aquatics programs, PT and occupational therapy, local application of moist heat, and regular telephone contact to monitor patient status have all been shown to improve function.[2] Patient education is important in allowing the patient to maintain a sense of control, as well as improving compliance and function.

Assistive devices such as a cane held in the opposite hand of the affected side and padded insoles or shoe orthotics may reduce the amount of stress placed on the affected joint. Home devices such as grab bars in the tub enclosure or raised toilet seats can also help maintain a patient's independence. Weight loss is recommended for obese patients; many patients with end-stage OA of the hip have a high body mass index.[29] Nutraceuticals, nutritional supplements such as glucosamine and chondroitin, may provide some symptomatic relief of OA.[30]

Pain in OA is associated with aging, increased morbidity and mortality, depression, and greater dependence on others.[2] When nonpharmacologic therapies fail to reduce pain or when pain becomes problematic to the patient, analgesics should be used. Although NSAIDs are a mainstay of therapy, acetaminophen in divided dosages of up to 4000 mg per day is used as first-line treatment. Generally a trial of 2 weeks provides adequate information about whether analgesia alone is sufficient. Other nonopioid analgesics, such as tramadol, alone or in combination with acetaminophen, can be used before prescribing NSAIDs.

Instituting NSAID therapy must be considered in association with the patient's other medications and his or her physical condition. Although NSAIDs are generally safe, the gastrointestinal and renal side effects of these drugs increase with the age of the patient. Newer agents such as celecoxib, rofecoxib, and valdecoxib specifically inhibit the cyclooxygenase-2 enzyme, do not significantly affect platelet function or bleeding time, and appear to have fewer gastrointestinal side effects than traditional NSAIDs.[15,38] Therapy with nonprescription NSAIDs for a 4-week trial can be tried before prescription NSAIDs. Intermittent use of NSAIDs, alternating with acetaminophen or with entirely medication-free periods, may provide adequate pain relief with fewer side effects.

Narcotic analgesics can be used when NSAIDs are no longer effective. Unfortunately there are a number of side effects, such as drowsiness, respiratory depression, and constipation, which may limit their usefulness, particularly for the older patient.

Patients with significant radiographic changes, decreased function, or severe pain should be considered for joint replacement and referred to an orthopedic surgeon. Over 90% of older patients with severe rheumatoid or osteoarthritic hip or knee disease may expect significant improvement in pain and movement after total joint replacement.[24]

Osteoporosis

In its simplest terms, osteoporosis is a bone disease caused by an imbalance in bone formation and resorption. It is characterized by decreased bone mass and increased susceptibility to fracture. Hip fractures caused by osteoporosis are the most severe; vertebral fractures are the most common. The disease affects women twice as frequently as men.

There are three primary types of osteoporosis: postmenopausal (type I), senile (type II), and secondary (type III). Type I osteoporosis is related to osteoclast activity and is related to gonadal function. Fractures primarily involve trabecular bone. Type II is associated with advancing age and reduced osteoblast function. Both trabecular and cortical bone are affected. Type II affects women more often than men. Secondary osteoporosis affects either sex and is associated with a number of medical conditions, including rheumatoid disease, renal failure, stroke, liver disease, endocrine disease (e.g., hyperthyroidism, hyperparathyroidism, hyperadrenocorticism, diabetes), malabsorption syndromes, and malignancies. Long-term use of corticosteroids, phenytoin, ethanol, barbiturates, heparin, and high-dose thyroxine are also associated with secondary osteoporosis.[12]

Risk factors for osteoporosis are well documented. Small body frames in Caucasian or Asian women, a positive family history of the disease, cigarette use, early menopause, inadequate weight-bearing exercise, fracture as an adult, lack of estrogen replacement in postmenopausal women, and insufficient calcium and vitamin D intake are all associated with the development of osteoporosis.

Normal bone remodeling is the result of complex interplay among hormones (estrogens, androgens, parathyroid hormone), osteoblasts and osteoclasts, cytokines, genetics, and other factors.[5,13,26] Concomitant diseases also play a role in the development of osteoporosis. In addition to hormonal regulation, dietary calcium intake is crucial to maintain adequate serum and bone levels. Absorption of dietary calcium can be adversely affected by low serum vitamin D, high intake of phosphates (found in soft drinks), high fat intake, malabsorptive diseases, and certain medications (tetracycline, phenytoin, corticosteroids, and heparin).

To recognize the differences in the types of osteoporosis, an understanding of some basic bone biology is necessary. Osteoblasts are the cells responsible for bone formation; they eventually end up in the bone matrix as osteocytes. The osteocytes, in turn, communicate with the outer bone surface through a network of microcanaliculi that are crucial to maintaining the balance between serum and bone calcium levels. Osteoclasts resorb bone at sites along the bone surface called Howship's lacunae, through a process of bone acidification.

Bone resorption tends to occur before formation, a process called remodeling. After bone is resorbed, osteoblasts move into the areas of resorption and fill the cavities with new osteoid, which later becomes mineralized. Normally, bone remodeling in healthy adults occurs at an annual rate of 2% to 3% for cortical bone and 25% for trabecular bone. Trabecular bone, which has the appearance of a dry cellulose sponge, is found in the spine, the distal radius, and the calcaneus (Figure 6-21). It has a greater surface area-to-volume ratio than does cortical bone. Cortical bone has a more compacted, orderly appearance than does trabecular bone. The shafts (metaphyses) of long bones are made up of cortical bone. Bone remodeling occurs on the surface of the bone; as a result, trabecular bone with its greater surface area is affected by remodeling to a greater extent than cortical bone. Bone strength depends on an appropriate ratio of trabecular to cortical bone.

Although osteoporosis affects both types of bone, there seems to be an affinity tendency in the horizontal trabeculae for lysing. Radiographically this results in the appearance of preserved vertical trabeculae. Approximately 30% of bone mass must be destroyed before changes become apparent on plain x-ray films.

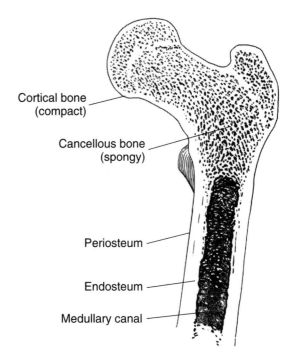

Cortical bone (compact)

Cancellous bone (spongy)

Periosteum

Endosteum

Medullary canal

Figure 6-21   Longitudinal cross section of the femur showing normal appearance of trabecular (cancellous) and cortical bone.

Type I, or postmenopausal, osteoporosis is sometimes termed high-turnover osteoporosis because osteoclastic activity rapidly resorbs bone. Shortly after menopause, the overall rate of bone turnover greatly increases, but the rate of resorption outpaces that of formation. This appears to be caused by an increased number of osteoclasts and the loss of a protective mechanism as estrogen levels decrease. It has been suggested that changes in pineal function may also play a role.

Osteoblast-mediated osteoporosis, also known as type II or senile osteoporosis, affects both cortical and trabecular bone and is characterized by an inadequate supply of osteoblasts relative to the demand for them. It is related to aging, decreased bone mass, and chronic calcium deficiency. Prevention, detection, and treatment of this type of osteoporosis is important in the primary care setting

Decreased femoral bone strength and increased risk of hip fracture are part of the net result of either type of osteoporosis. Other factors associated with hip fracture include poor nutritional status (especially low serum albumin), low body weight, and falls. Estrogen replacement, calcium and vitamin D supplementation, fall prevention, and exercise programs are often employed as preventive measures to decrease the incidence of hip fracture caused by osteoporosis.

Physical activity during growth periods has been shown to increase bone mass, but the effect of exercise on the mature skeleton is not yet fully documented. It has been shown that women who exercise moderately (not to the point of amenorrhea) tend to have greater bone mass than either those who are amenorrheic because of exercise or those who do not exercise but have menstrual cycles. Although prevention remains the best choice for a cost-effective approach to the disease, it remains clinically imperative to recognize and treat the estimated 28 million people in the United States affected by osteoporosis or low bone density.

Although predominantly a woman's disease, men are also affected by osteoporosis. Secondary osteoporosis is more common in men. Risk factors for men are not as well known, but low physical activity, hypogonadism, alcoholism, previous radiation or chemotherapy, current smoking, and inadequate calcium intake are associated with lower bone mass.[14,37] Diseases such as hyperthyroidism and hyperparathyroidism can lead to osteoporosis in men.

History

The presence of any risk factors for osteoporosis in a woman aged 50 or older should raise the suggestion of osteoporosis. Risk factors include nontraumatic fracture, early menopause (natural or surgical), prolonged amenorrhea, height loss of at least 2 inches, scoliosis, estrogen deficiency, or family history of osteoporosis. Other considerations associated with osteoporosis include sedentary lifestyle, thin body build, cigarette smoking, and excessive alcohol intake.

Physical Examination

A fracture may be the presenting sign of osteoporosis. Pain, bruising, and limited movement of the affected area are typical of a fracture. In the case of osteoporosis, the wrist, spine, and hip are most often affected.

Repeated compression fractures of the vertebrae may result in kyphosis. In nontraumatic fractures it is critical to rule out malignancy or other bone tumor before deciding the fracture is attributable to osteoporosis. Once tumor or malignancy have been ruled out, further evaluation can proceed.

Imaging studies are crucial to making the diagnosis of osteoporosis. Although plain x-ray films can visualize an osteoporotic fracture, bone density is necessary to evaluate bone mass accurately. The most commonly used method of measuring bone density is dual-energy x-ray absorptiometry (DXA). This scanning modality is a rapid, noninvasive, low-radiation exposure test. Since DXA provides a calculated value of bone mass (g/cm^2), it tends to overestimate true volumetric (g/cm^3) bone density.[17]

Diagnosis

Diagnosis of osteoporosis (and osteopenia) is based on the patient's bone density as measured against standards set by the World Health Organization (WHO).[21] Osteoporosis is defined as bone mineral density (BMD) levels ≥2.5 standard deviations (SD) below the mean bone density of young-normal controls. Osteopenia is defined as a BMD >1 SD but <2.5 SD below the young-normal mean.

Laboratory

Biochemical "markers" that measure bone resorption and bone formation are also being used to evaluate for osteoporosis. Urinary pyridinoline cross-links and plasma tartrate-resistant acid phosphatase correlate well with bone resorption rates, a marker for osteoclastic activity. Urinary pyridinoline cross-links and N-telopeptides are simple first- or second-morning void specimens that are sent to a laboratory for direct measurement of the markers by enzyme-linked immunosorbent assay. Laboratory testing time is 2 to 3 hours, and the cost is significantly less than serial DXA scans. Bone formation markers include serum bone-specific alkaline phosphatase, osteocalcin, and procollagen I extension peptides. Although these tests are an accurate reflection of bone metabolism, they provide little information about bone quality. Biochemical assays may have their greatest utility in rural or remote areas where access to DXA scanning is limited or difficult.

Treatment

Calcium and vitamin D supplements are useful for premenopausal women. For adult women, the U.S. National Institute of Health recommends a daily calcium intake of 1000 to 1500 mg in combination with 400 to 800 international units of vitamin D. Postmenopausal women should have their daily calcium increased to 1500 mg per day. Regular weight-bearing exercise for 30 minutes, three to five times a week, helps maintain bone density. Removal of loose throw rugs, use of grab bars in the bathroom, and adequate nighttime lighting around the house can help prevent falls. The use of hip protectors has been shown to decrease the incidence of hip fracture.[21] In selected patients, hormone replacement therapy is still recommended for prevention of postmenopausal bone loss.

Once BMD is more than 2.5 SD below WHO standards or a fracture is present, therapy with a bisphosphonate (e.g., alendronate or risedronate) should begin. Both alendronate and risedronate may be given as daily or once-weekly doses. Bisphosphonates are administered on an empty stomach, with a full 8 ounces of water in the morning, 30 minutes before taking any food, drink, or other medication. The patient must also remain upright for 30 minutes after taking the medication. Parathyroid hormone, injected subcutaneously on an intermittent basis, has been shown to increase bone formation.[27,36]

DIFFERENTIAL DIAGNOSIS OF HIP PAIN

Evaluation of hip pain should first focus on serious abnormalities such as malignancy, fracture, dislocation, or nerve injury. Most acute, serious hip injuries are the result of high-energy trauma and therefore are not routinely encountered in a primary care setting.

Malignancy and nerve (especially lumbar) injury, however, can begin insidiously and progress steadily. Neoplasms of the pelvis, acetabulum, or femur can all cause hip pain, and a careful history and physical examination are necessary to identify these problems.

Assessment of physical activity and sports training may alert the practitioner to muscle strain that may or may not have become a tear. Post-activity pain and swelling near the site of muscle attachments suggest a tear or even an avulsion fracture at the site of a ligamentous attachment.

Once the history is obtained, observing the patient's stance, walk, and limb position can provide clues to the areas of malrotation, shortening, or guarding. Palpation of the groin while the patient coughs can help differentiate an inguinal hernia from lumbar disk disease. Nontraumatic trochanteric pain and tenderness with palpation is suggestive of bursitis. Movement of the joint with attention to ROM, crepitus, and pain can provide clues about arthritic disease and hip stability. Pain with active but not passive movement suggests a muscle or other soft-tissue injury rather than a joint abnormality.

Diagnosis of a discrete problem in the patient who complains of only hip pain can be challenging. Posterior hip pain may be caused by sciatica, gluteal or other muscle strain, or ischial bursitis. Sciatic nerve pain typically extends from the buttock and goes down the posterior thigh to the posterolateral aspect of the leg, around the lateral malleolus, and into the lateral dorsum and the sole of the foot. Pain is exacerbated by coughing or with Valsalva's maneuver, and there is tenderness to palpation at the sciatic notch.

Gluteal muscle or hamstring strain pain is usually associated with activity. Movements that increase stress on the muscle will intensify pain. Moist heat tends to decrease symptoms. Pain is fairly well localized to the specific muscle or muscle-tendon site.

Ischial bursitis, also known as weaver's bottom, tends to be an unrelenting pain that, with coughing, may extend down the posterior thigh to the knee. Sitting aggravates pain, but a hard seat is more comfortable than a soft one. Often affected are operators of farming or other heavy equipment with seats that vibrate significantly. The ischial tuberosity is exquisitely tender to palpation.

Posterior hip pain should be further differentiated from buttock pain. The latter is associated with herniated intervertebral disks, spinal cord tumor, lumbosacral disease, spondylolisthesis, and thrombophlebitis. Increased pain with percussion over the spine is suggestive of spinal cord tumor. Lumbosacral disease or a herniated disk will have a negative Flexion, Abduction, External Rotation (FABER) test. Spondylolisthesis can be diagnosed with plain x-ray films.

Muscle strains, inguinal or femoral hernias, prostatitis, testicular problems, urinary tract infection, or kidney stones can cause anterior hip pain. Most of these can be discerned by means of a careful history and physical examination. Once a clinical diagnosis has been made, confirmatory evaluation can be ordered. Imaging studies play a major role in evaluating pathologic hip abnormalities.

EVALUATION MODALITIES

X-Ray Films

Plain radiographic films remain one of the simplest, most cost-effective tools for evaluating hip joint abnormalities. Dislocations and significant fractures of the femoral head, acetabulum, femoral neck, femoral trochanters, and femoral shaft are readily seen on plain films. Hip x-ray studies are usually ordered in two views: internal and external rotation. Internal rotation of the hip allows better visualization of the lesser trochanter, whereas external rotation highlights the greater trochanter. Lateral hip x-ray films are also useful in providing additional information regarding the acetabulum. If there is concern about one hip joint, an AP view of the pelvis allows comparison of acetabulae and proximal femurs.

Scintigraphy

Stress fractures or acute septic joints are poorly visualized on plain films. Bone scintigraphy provides better information regarding subtle changes caused by cumulative bone trauma. One drawback of bone scanning is its lack of specificity, which can make differentiation of bone infection, neoplasm, and stress fracture difficult to interpret. Accurate results of bone scans are also dependent on the radiologist's expertise.

Computed Tomography

Computed tomography (CT) is the best imaging tool for evaluating bony abnormalities of the hip, particularly in the case of trauma. Helical CT has the advantage of creating overlapping images without overlapping radiation exposure; it is therefore faster than conventional CT. Examination of the acetabulum and femoral head using helical CT lasts only 30 to 40 seconds. CT is also useful in rendering three-dimensional reconstructions that can help with fracture identification.

Magnetic Resonance Imaging

MRI is the standard diagnostic tool for evaluating osteonecrosis of the femoral head, musculoskeletal tumors, and osteomyelitis. It is also an excellent modality for assessing trauma and bone marrow processes.[9] Compared with other studies, the improved sensitivity and specificity of MRI is valuable in improving the accuracy of diagnosis, including those of femoral neck stress fractures.[9] Although more expensive than either bone scanning or CT, MRI is advantageous in sorting out processes at or near the osseous–soft tissue border, determining the extent of osteonecrosis, evaluating bone tumors and cysts, and localizing tendon abnormalities.

INDICATIONS FOR REFERRAL

See the Red Flags box for referral information.

Red Flags *for Hip and Thigh Disorders*

Patients with these findings may need to be referred for more extensive work-up.

Signs and Symptoms	Response
Inability to bear weight; affected leg appears shortened and is externally rotated from the contraction of the iliopsoas and gluteus maximus muscles	Possible femoral neck fracture; urgently refer to orthopedic surgeon for reduction and surgical fixation
Radiographic image shows fracture involving shaft (metaphysis) of femur (or suggestion of such fracture)	Intertrochanteric femur fracture; urgently refer to orthopedic surgeon for surgical fixation, typically with sliding hip screw or intramedullary nail
Hip abducted, femur externally rotated; weight bearing difficult or impossible	Possible subtrochanteric femur fracture; immediately refer to emergency department or orthopedic surgeon; surgical fixation may be necessary
Hip is flexed, adducted, and internally rotated; "fullness" in buttock may be noted; mass (femoral head) may be palpable on ileum	Possible posterior hip dislocation; immediately immobilize patient and transport to emergency department
Presenting symptom of significant trauma to hamstring in adult patient	Possible avulsion fracture of the ischial apophysis; refer to orthopedic surgeon for surgical repair to provide best chance for full recovery.
Buttock pain, with or without radiation into the leg; pain worsens with prolonged sitting or after activities requiring hip abduction and internal rotation; may be tenderness to palpation from sciatic notch to greater trochanter; sometimes palpable muscle spasm described as "spindle-shaped mass"; straight leg raising may be positive; pain tends to increase with resisted hip flexion, adduction, and internal rotation	Possible piriformis syndrome; refer to orthopedic surgeon or neurologist if any question of lumbar disk disease; if patient's symptoms do not improve with conservative treatment, refer to orthopedic surgeon for possible corticosteroid injection; failure to respond after three injections may require surgical release of muscle

Signs and Symptoms	Response
Patient is between 30 and 50 years old and has pain and limp; deep ache or groin pain when walking may have persisted for months or years; coughing may exacerbate hip pain; ROM of hip may be limited and painful at extremes, especially external rotation and flexion; plain x-ray films may show grossly deformed, flattened femoral head with joint space narrowing; MRI may show marrow that has become necrotic before the trabecular architecture of the bone changes	Possible osteonecrosis; refer to orthopedic surgeon for possible surgical intervention; check for history of remote or recent trauma; if negative, there may be history of steroid treatment or excessive alcohol intake
Patients with OA of hip with significant radiographic changes, decreased function, or severe pain	Possible need for joint replacement; refer to orthopedic surgeon

ROM, Range-of-motion; *MRI,* magnetic resonance image; *OA,* osteoarthritis.

REFERENCES

1. Aigner T, McKenna L: Molecular pathology and pathobiology of osteoarthritic cartilage, *Cell Mol Life Sci* 59:5, 2002.
2. American College of Rheumatology Subcommittee on Osteoarthritis Guidelines: Recommendation for the medical management of osteoarthritis of the hip and knee, *Arthritis Rheum* 43:1905, 2000.
3. Arromdee M, Matteson EL: Bursitis: common condition, uncommon challenge, *J Musculoskel Med* 17:213, 2001.
4. Browning KH: Hip and pelvis injuries in runners, *Physician and Sportsmed* 29(1):23, 2001.
5. Chan GK, Duque G: Age-related bone loss: old bone, new facts, *Gerontology* 48:62, 2002.
6. Childers MK et al: Botulinum toxin type A use in piriformis muscle syndrome: a pilot study, *Am J Phys Med Rehabil* 81:751, 2002.
7. Dougados M et al: Radiological progression of hip osteoarthritis: definition, risk factors and correlations with clinical status, *Ann Rheum Dis* 55:356, 1996.
8. Egol KA, Koval KJ: Hip: trauma. In Koval KJ, editor: *Orthopaedic Knowledge Update 7: Home Study Syllabus,* Rosemont, Ill, 2002, American Academy of Orthopaedic Surgeons.
9. Erb RE: Current concepts in imaging the adult hip, *Clin Sports Med* 20:661, 2001.
10. Fishman LM et al: Piriformis syndrome: diagnosis, treatment, and outcome—a 10-year study, *Arch Phys Med Rehabil* 83:295, 2002.
11. Fishman LM et al: BOTOX and physical therapy in the treatment of piriformis syndrome, *Am J Phys Med Rehabil* 81:936, 2002.
12. Fitzpatrick LA: Secondary causes of osteoporosis, *Mayo Clin Proc* 77:453, 2002.
13. Francis RM: Androgen replacement in aging men, *Calcif Tissue Int* 69:235, 2001.
14. Geier KA: Osteoporosis in men, *Orthop Nurs* 20:49, 2001.
15. Hawkey C et al: Comparison of the effects of rofecoxib (a cyclooxygenase-2 inhibitor), ibuprofen, and placebo on the gastrointestinal mucosa of patients with osteoarthritis: a randomized, double-blind, placebo-controlled trial, *Arthritis Rheum* 43:370, 2000.
16. Hewitt JD et al: The mechanical properties of the human hip capsule ligaments, *J Arthroplasty* 17:82, 2002.
17. Hunter DJ, Sambrook PN: Epidemiology of bone loss, *Arthritis Res* 2:441, 2000.
18. Johnson CA et al: Iliopsoas bursitis and tendinitis: a review, *Sports Med* 25:271, 1998.

19. Jones JP Jr: Risk factors potentially activating intravascular coagulation and causing nontraumatic osteonecrosis. In Urbaniak JR et al, editors: *Osteonecrosis: etiology, diagnosis, and treatment,* Rosemont, Ill, 1997, American Academy of Orthopaedic Surgeons.

20. Reference deleted in proofs.

21. Kannus P et al: Prevention of hip fracture in elderly people with use of a hip protector, *N Engl J Med* 343:1506, 2000.

22. Lieberman JR et al: Osteonecrosis of the hip: management in the twenty-first century, *J Bone Joint Surg (Am)* 84(A):834, 2002.

23. Linville DA II: Osteoporotic fractures, *South Med J* 95:588, 2002.

24. Lozada CJ, Altman RD: Osteoarthritis. In Robbins L et al, editors: *Clinical care in the rheumatic diseases,* ed 2, Atlanta, Ga, 2001, American College of Rheumatology.

25. Mair SD et al: The role of fatigue in susceptibility to acute muscle strain injury, *Am J Sports Med* 24:157, 1996.

26. Manolagas SC et al: Sex steroids and bone, *Recent Prog Horm Res* 57:385, 2002.

27. Maricic MJ, Gluck OS: Osteoporosis: therapeutic options of prevention and management, *J Musculoskel Med* 18:415, 2001.

28. Reference deleted in proofs.

29. Marks R, Allegrante JP: Body mass indices in patients with disabling hip osteoarthritis, *Arthritis Res* 4:112, 2002.

30. McAlindon TE et al: Glucosamine and chondroitin for treatment of osteoarthritis: a systematic quality assessment and meta-analysis, *J Amer Med Assoc* 283:1469, 2000.

31. No author: Prevention of pulmonary embolism and deep vein thrombosis with low dose aspirin: Pulmonary Embolism Prevention (PEP) trial, *Lancet* 355:1295, 2000.

32. Pape HC et al: Hip dislocation in patients with multiple injuries: a follow-up investigation, *Clin Orthop* 377:99, 2000.

33. Ray N et al: Medical expenditures for the treatment of osteoporotic fractures in the United States in 1995, *J Bone Miner Res* 12:24, 1997.

34. Reginato AM, Reginato AJ: Periarticular rheumatic diseases. In Robbins L et al, editors: *Clinical care in the rheumatic diseases,* ed 2, Atlanta, Ga, 2001, American College of Rheumatology.

35. Rodrigue T, Hardy RW: Diagnosis and treatment of piriformis syndrome, *Neurosurg Clin North Am* 12:311, 2001.

36. Roe EB et al: PTH-induced increases in bone density are preserved with estrogen: results from a follow-up year in postmenopausal osteoporosis, *J Bone Miner Res* 15(suppl 1):S193, 2000 (abstract 1221).

37. Seeman E: Pathogenesis of bone fragility in women and men, *Lancet* 359:1841, 2002.

38. Simon LS et al: Anti-inflammatory and upper gastrointestinal effects of celecoxib in rheumatoid arthritis: a randomized controlled trial, *JAMA* 282:1921, 1999.

39. Stevens JA, Olsen S: Reducing falls and resulting hip fractures among older women, *MMWR Recommendations and reports* 49 (RR02):1, 2000.

40. Tan V et al: Contribution of acetabular labrum to articulating surface area and femoral head coverage in adult hip joints: an anatomic study in cadavera, *Am J Orthop* 30:809, 2001.

41. Urbaniak JR, Barnes CJ: Meeting the challenge of hip osteonecrosis in adults, *J Musculoskel Med* 18:395, 2001.

42. Verrall GM et al: Clinical risk factors for hamstring muscle strain injury: a prospective study with correlation of injury by magnetic resonance imaging, *Br J Sports Med* 35:435, 2001.

Chapter 7

Knee and Leg

Among the most common orthopedic complaints seen in primary care are problems of the knee and its supporting structures. Although both stable and flexible, the knee joint is not exceptionally strong. Knee strength depends on the support of intraarticular and extraarticular ligaments, tendons, and muscles. Dependence on supporting structures makes the knee susceptible to injury.

Although not usually subject to chronic degenerative processes, the diaphyses (i.e., shafts of the long bones) of the leg are still sites of wear and tear. Trauma, overuse injuries, residual effects of surgery, neurologic processes, and vascular disease all affect the leg. Patients with complaints related to any of the previously mentioned abnormalities are treated in primary care settings.

Extending from the knee to the ankle, the leg contains two bones, thirteen muscles, multiple nerves, and several important blood vessels. Some leg muscles cross both the knee and ankle joints and are therefore involved in movement of either or both joints. Walking (e.g., up and down inclines), dorsiflexing the foot, standing on the tips of the toes, and running from a standstill or starter's block are all possible because of the structures of the leg. Stability of the ankle joint is also largely attributable to normal integrity of leg structures.

ANATOMY

BONY STRUCTURES

The knee is a complex, modified hinge joint whose three articulations include each femoral condyle with the tibial plateau and patellofemoral joint. The tibiofemoral joint is the largest in the body. The arrangement of three articulations allows a combination of rolling, gliding, translation, and rotation in addition to flexion and extension. Although attached to the lateral tibia, the fibula does not articulate with the knee joint.

The distal femur widens into two condyles that are separated by an intercondylar notch or fossa. Anteriorly, the condyles are joined by a fairly shallow groove that extends downward and backward into the intercondylar notch (Figure 7-1). The condyles are more prominent posteriorly. The medial surface of the lateral condyle is the attachment point for the anterior cruciate ligament (ACL); the posterior cruciate ligament (PCL) attaches to the anterior portion of the medial condyle (Figure 7-2).

Second in length only to the femur and articulating with it, the tibia (specifically the tibial plateau) forms the primary articulation of the knee. The tibial plateau is formed by two smooth, slightly concave surfaces that are separated by the tibial spine, which in turn is situated

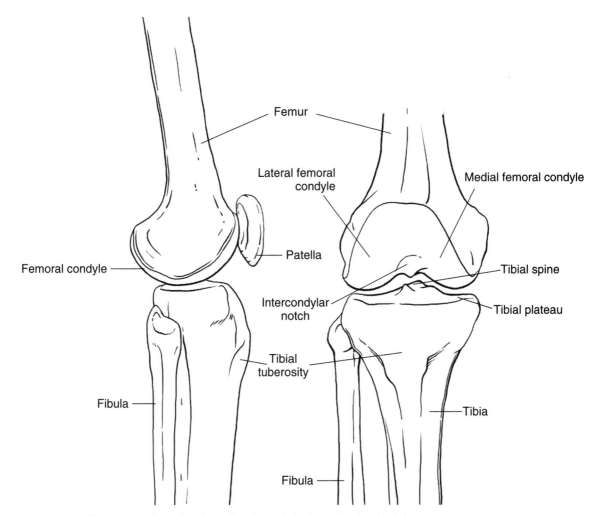

Figure 7-1   Lateral and anterior views of the knee showing basic bony anatomy.

slightly posteriorly. In front of and behind the spine is a rough depression, the point at which the ACL and PCL attach. The superior anterior portion of the tibial plateau is flattened to form a single surface. Posteriorly, a shallow popliteal notch separates the tuberosities of the tibial plateau. Each femoral condyle articulates with the corresponding surface of the tibial plateau.

The patella is the largest sesamoid bone in the body and completes the three principle osseous structures of the knee. Two primary functions of the patella are: (1) protecting the anterior joint, and (2) increasing the

leverage of the quadriceps muscle. Anteriorly the surface of the bone is fairly rough because of the presence of numerous nutrient vessels. The quadriceps tendon anchors the patella superiorly; inferiorly the patellar tendon stabilizes the bone. The posterior surface of the patella forms a ridge that allows it to articulate with the femur in its medial groove. The patella becomes "locked" into the medial groove of the femur at approximately 30 degrees of flexion. Occasionally, bony development occurs from two centers and the patella may ossify as two pieces, a condition known as a bipartite patella.

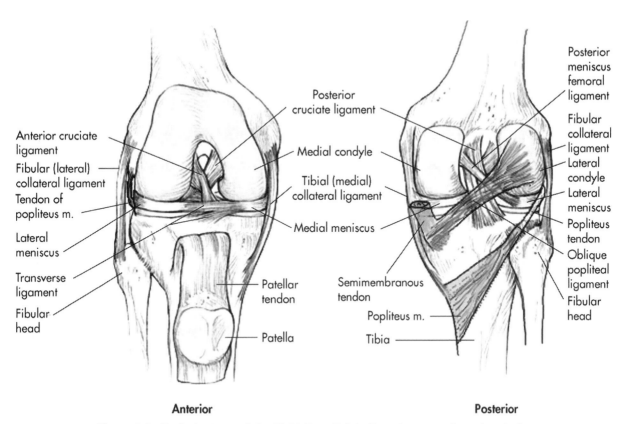

Anterior cruciate ligament

Fibular (lateral) collateral ligament

Tendon of popliteus m.

Lateral meniscus

Transverse ligament

Fibular head

Posterior cruciate ligament

Medial condyle

Tibial (medial) collateral ligament

Medial meniscus

Patellar tendon

Patella

Posterior meniscus femoral ligament

Fibular collateral ligament

Lateral condyle

Lateral meniscus

Popliteus tendon

Oblique popliteal ligament

Fibular head

Semimembranous tendon

Popliteus m.

Tibia

Anterior

Posterior

Figure 7-2   Basic Anatomy of the Right Knee Joint. The primary anterior and posterior soft-tissue structures are shown. (From C.L.A.S.S.: *Clinical anatomy principles*, St Louis, 1996, Mosby.)

There are two bones in the leg, the tibia and fibula (Figure 7-3). After the femur, the tibia is the second largest and longest bone in the body. During walking, running, jumping, and standing, the tibia bears the brunt of forces on the leg. Serving primarily as a muscle attachment, the fibula plays a role in locomotion, balance, and ankle stability but has no part in movement of the knee.

As the tibial shaft (or diaphysis) progresses distally, it becomes almost triangular on cross section. The sharp anterior ridge of bone is the shin, occasionally called the tibial crest. The shin begins just above the lateral border of the tibial tubercle and extends to the anterior margin of the medial malleolus.

At its distal end, the tibia terminates in a widened, flattened horizontal surface with an inferiorly directed process on the medial portion. This process is called the medial malleolus, which, in turn, forms the medial aspect of the ankle joint.

The fibula is the smaller of the two lower leg bones and attaches to the lateral edge of the tibia both proximally and distally. Proximally the fibular head attaches below the level of the knee joint and therefore has no involvement in the movement of the knee. Extending inferiorly from the fibular head, the bone tapers somewhat, forming the fibular neck. The shaft has a rough surface, providing attachment for nine muscles. Distally the fibula terminates in the lateral malleolus, a pyramid-shaped, somewhat flattened bone. The lateral malleolus, which forms the lateral part of the ankle joint, extends distally farther than the medial malleolus. The two primary functions of the fibula are: (1) forming the lateral malleolus, and (2) serving as a muscle attachment.

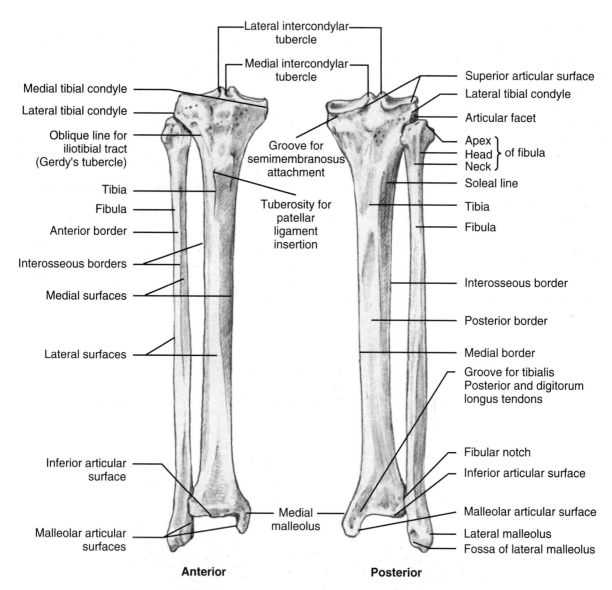

Lateral intercondylar tubercle

Medial intercondylar tubercle

Medial tibial condyle

Lateral tibial condyle

Oblique line for iliotibial tract (Gerdy's tubercle)

Tibia

Fibula

Anterior border

Interosseous borders

Medial surfaces

Lateral surfaces

Inferior articular surface

Malleolar articular surfaces

Groove for semimembranosus attachment

Tuberosity for patellar ligament insertion

Medial malleolus

Superior articular surface

Lateral tibial condyle

Articular facet

Apex ⎫
Head ⎬ of fibula
Neck ⎭

Soleal line

Tibia

Fibula

Interosseous border

Posterior border

Medial border

Groove for tibialis Posterior and digitorum longus tendons

Fibular notch

Inferior articular surface

Malleolar articular surface

Lateral malleolus

Fossa of lateral malleolus

Anterior   **Posterior**

Figure 7-3   The Right Tibia and Fibula. The tibia is the main weight-bearing bone of the leg. Although primarily a muscle attachment, the fibula is responsible for carrying approximately 30% of the weight placed on the leg. (From C.L.A.S.S.: *Clinical anatomy principles*, St Louis, 1996, Mosby.)

SOFT-TISSUE STRUCTURES

Synovium

The synovium is a saclike structure that lines the knee joint. Its main functions are to form part of the joint capsule and secrete the viscid fluid that contains albumin, fat, mucin, and mineral salts, which lubricate and provide nutrition to the joint. The synovium of the knee is large, extending to and communicating with several of the bursae and pouches around the joint. Within the knee, however, the synovium does not encompass the cruciate ligaments. In turn, the joint capsule surrounds the synovium. Because of this arrangement, differentiating intraarticular from extraarticular swelling can be difficult. A weakness in the posterior capsule will allow herniation of the synovium into the popliteal fossa, forming a Baker's (or popliteal) cyst.

Muscles

Most of the muscles involved in the movement of the knee originate in the thigh and cross the knee joint before attaching on the tibia. The muscles are grouped according to their location: anterior, posterior, and medial (Table 7-1). The lateral thigh area has no real muscle group; it mostly contains a long tendinous structure known as the iliotibial band (ITB).

Anteriorly the quadriceps muscles (i.e., vastus medialis, vastus intermedius, vastus lateralis, and rectus femoris) cross the knee and extend it. Unlike the vastus muscles, the rectus femoris crosses both the hip and knee joints. The sartorius muscle, which flexes both the knee and the hip, also crosses both joints.

Posteriorly the hamstring muscles act to flex the knee. The semimembranosus, the semitendinosus, and the biceps femoris with both its short and long heads cross both the hip and knee joints. These muscles and their tendons form the superior margins of the popliteal fossa. The semitendinosus and semimembranosus muscles become the medial border, and the biceps femoris (i.e., both heads) attaches to the fibular side, forming the lateral edge (Figure 7-4).

Medially the sartorius, gracilis, and semitendinosus muscles cross the knee joint and attach on the anteromedial surface of the proximal tibia. Although knee flexion is one primary movement, the gracilis muscle also medially rotates the knee.

Laterally the ITB, described as a thickened band of fascia, extends from an area near the greater trochanter to the lateral tibial condyle. It extends from the iliac crest across the knee joint anteriorly to the lateral femoral condyle and inserts in the lateral tibial tubercle. The ITB is an additional extraarticular knee stabilizer that also reinforces the joint capsule.[71] It serves as an attachment for the gluteus maximus posteriorly and for the tensor fascia lata muscle anteriorly (Figure 7-5). Each muscle exerts roughly equal pull on the ITB, keeping it in its lateral position and effectively allowing it to become the lateral muscle of the thigh. Its primary function is to help stabilize the patella against valgus forces. The ITB assists in both flexion and extension of the knee. As a result, it can be injured by overuse or trauma in either movement.

Twelve muscles attach to the tibial plateau and metaphysis. Most of these muscles serve to move the knee and ankle. The muscles of the leg play an important role in walking and maintaining an erect posture. The muscles lie in four compartments: the superficial posterior, the deep posterior, the anterior, and the lateral. Each muscle in each compartment is encased in a tough fibrous covering called the fascia (Figure 7-6). Figure 7-7 shows detail of the relationship of various leg structures as visualized with magnetic resonance imaging (MRI).

The superficial posterior compartment contains the gastrocnemius, soleus, and plantaris muscles. The gastrocnemius is the most superficial of these three muscles, forming what is commonly called the calf. The primary functions of these three muscles are extending the foot at the ankle and raising the heel (and entire body) off the ground during walking. In addition, they stabilize the leg on the foot during standing. The plantaris can extend the knee if the foot is free or help flex the knee if the foot is planted on the ground.

Four muscles, the popliteus, the flexor hallucis longus, the flexor longus digitorum, and the tibialis posterior, lie in the deep posterior compartment (Figure 7-8).

TABLE 7-1	Primary Muscles Involved in Knee Movement	
Movement	**Muscles**	**Location**
Flexion	Hamstrings (semimembranosus, semitendinosus, biceps femoris)	Posterior thigh
Extension	Quadriceps (vastus medialis, vastus intermedius, vastus lateralis, rectus femoris)	Anterior thigh
Medial rotation	Gracilis; sartorius	Anteromedial thigh

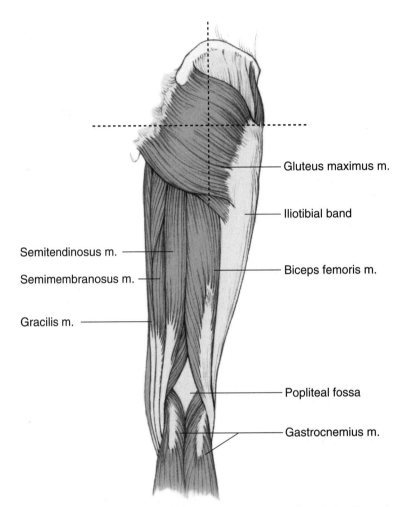

Semitendinosus m.

Semimembranosus m.

Gracilis m.

Gluteus maximus m.

Iliotibial band

Biceps femoris m.

Popliteal fossa

Gastrocnemius m.

Figure 7-4 The Hamstrings and Their Relationship to Other Major Posterior Leg Muscles. The hamstrings form the medial and lateral borders of the popliteal fossa. (From C.L.A.S.S.: *Clinical anatomy principles*, St Louis, 1996, Mosby.)

They serve to inwardly rotate the tibia (popliteus), extend the foot at the ankle joint and assist with ankle inversion (tibialis posterior), and flex the toes and assist in extending the foot on the leg and standing on the tips of the toes (flexor longus digitorum and flexor longus hallucis). These actions are important in bending the knee and walking.

Dorsiflexion of the ankle and toes is primarily attributable to the action of the four muscles in the anterior compartment (Figure 7-9). The tibialis anterior and per-oneus tertius dorsiflex the foot; inversion of the foot is partly attributable to the action of the tibialis anterior. The extensor hallucis longus dorsiflexes the great toe, whereas the extensor digitorum longus dorsiflexes the second through fifth toes. The anterior compartment is most often affected by trauma-induced compartment syndrome.

The lateral compartment contains the peroneus longus and peroneus brevis muscles (Figure 7-10). These muscles assist in plantar flexion of the foot. The per-

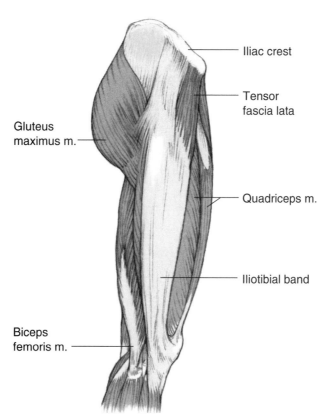

Figure 7-5 The Iliotibial Band. This tendinous band extends the length of the lateral thigh, attaching to the lateral tibia. It assists with both flexion and extension of the knee. (From C.L.A.S.S.: *Clinical anatomy principles*, St Louis, 1996, Mosby.)

oneus longus also everts the foot and helps maintain the position of the leg when standing on one leg. (The normal tendency is to turn the leg inward when supporting the body's weight, but the peroneus longus contracts on the lateral leg, thus maintaining proper alignment.) Table 7-2 summarizes the myofascial compartments of the leg.

Knowledge of the muscles in each compartment and their actions can assist the practitioner in evaluating injury or disease processes of the leg. Each compartment also contains tendons, nerves, and blood vessels that are affected by injury or disease.

Tendons and Ligaments

The knee is the most stressed joint in the body and depends on supporting tendons and ligaments for stabil-

ity and strength. The patellar tendon attaches to the inferior portion of the patella and inserts on the anterior tibial tuberosity. The quadriceps tendon runs along the longitudinal axis of the patella and attaches to it superiorly. Clinically, the term patellar tendon frequently but incorrectly refers to both the quadriceps and patellar tendons as a single unit (Figure 7-11). One of the primary functions of the patellar and quadriceps tendons is ensuring that the patella tracks normally in the patellar groove of the femur. As the knee is flexed, the patella slides downward into the patellar groove of the femur, normally locking into the groove at about 30 degrees of flexion. When the knee is fully extended, the quadriceps muscle contracts, moving the patella upward to a position just superior to the top of the femoral condyles.

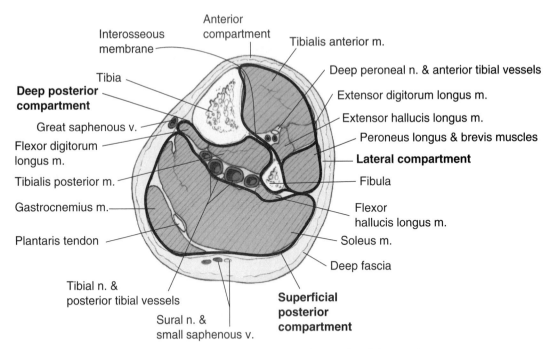

Anterior
compartment

Interosseous
membrane

Tibialis anterior m.

Deep peroneal n. & anterior tibial vessels

Tibia

**Deep posterior
compartment**

Extensor digitorum longus m.

Extensor hallucis longus m.

Great saphenous v.

Peroneus longus & brevis muscles

Flexor digitorum
longus m.

Lateral compartment

Tibialis posterior m.

Fibula

Gastrocnemius m.

Flexor
hallucis longus m.

Plantaris tendon

Soleus m.

Deep fascia

Tibial n. &
posterior tibial vessels

Sural n. &
small saphenous v.

**Superficial
posterior
compartment**

Figure 7-6   The Four Compartments of the Leg. The muscles of the anterior compartment dorsiflex the foot. Foot eversion is due to the muscles in the lateral compartment. The muscles of the superficial posterior compartment plantor flex the foot while flexion of the toes is provided by the muscles within the deep posterior compartment. (From C.L.A.S.S.: *Clinical anatomy principles*, St Louis, 1996, Mosby.)

Stability of the knee is attributable in large part to its numerous intraarticular and extraarticular ligaments (Figure 7-12, *A-C*). The primary functions of ligaments are to stabilize and guide the bones of a joint during range of motion (ROM).[81] The two major ligaments of the knee are the ACL and the PCL. Their main function is to prevent excessive anterior and posterior movement, or translation, of the tibia on the femur. These ligaments also help stabilize the knee during internal rotation. Although the cruciate ligaments lie in the center of the knee joint space, they are not technically within the joint because the synovial membrane does not encompass them.

The ACL extends from the medial surface of the lateral femoral condyle to the anterior intercondylar area on the tibial plateau. When the knee is extended the ACL

prevents excessive anterior translation of the tibia on the femur. When the knee is flexed, the ligament is lax.

The PCL crosses behind the ACL. As it extends from the lateral surface of the medial femoral condyle to the posterior intercondylar ridge of the tibia, the PCL prevents excessive posterior movement of the tibia on the femur. The PCL is lax when the knee is extended.

Extraarticular knee ligaments include the medial collateral ligament (MCL), the lateral collateral ligament (LCL), and the transverse ligament. Collectively, they function to reinforce the joint during range of motion (ROM) and stabilize it against outside forces. The MCL and LCL constitute the knee's primary extraarticular ligaments.

The MCL is also known as the tibial collateral ligament. It attaches to the medial femoral condyle and inserts about 4 cm below the medial tibial joint line. At

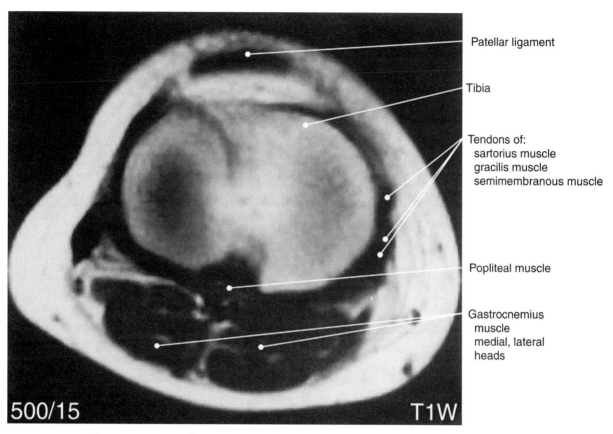

Patellar ligament

Tibia

Tendons of:
  sartorius muscle
  gracilis muscle
  semimembranous muscle

Popliteal muscle

Gastrocnemius
  muscle
  medial, lateral
  heads

500/15   T1W

Figure 7-7   Magnetic Resonance Image of the Left Leg. (From C.L.A.S.S.: *Clinical anatomy principles*, St Louis, 1996, Mosby.)

its midsection the MCL attaches to and stabilizes the medial meniscus. Stabilization of the knee joint against medially directed lateral forces (valgus stress) is one of the predominant functions of the MCL. Sports that require quick turns and cuts, such as football, soccer, and lacrosse, can place a great amount of stress on the MCL. The MCL is also a secondary restraint to anterior translation of the tibia, an important function if the ACL is torn. The MCL exerts most of its stabilizing effect at 25 to 30 degrees of knee flexion.[36] Structurally the MCL is a broad but relatively thin ligament; it is injured more often than the LCL.

The LCL is a tough, cordlike structure that extends from the lateral femoral condyle to the anterior fibular head. Also known as the fibular collateral ligament, it is

relatively stronger than the MCL and is therefore less frequently injured. The LCL also has further protection, because the biceps femoris muscle covers the ligament.

Two other structures, the lateral and medial retinacula, are also worth noting (Figure 7-13). The patellar retinacula are bands of tissue that help hold the patella in place, reducing medial and lateral malalignment. The retinacula arise from the vastus medialis and lateralis muscles, forming part of the knee joint capsule. The lateral retinaculum attaches obliquely at the anterior lateral tibial condyle. It helps stabilize the patella during movements of the knee. Occasionally the lateral retinaculum may be unusually tight, pulling on the patella and contributing to lateral patellar subluxation. The medial retinaculum also stabilizes the

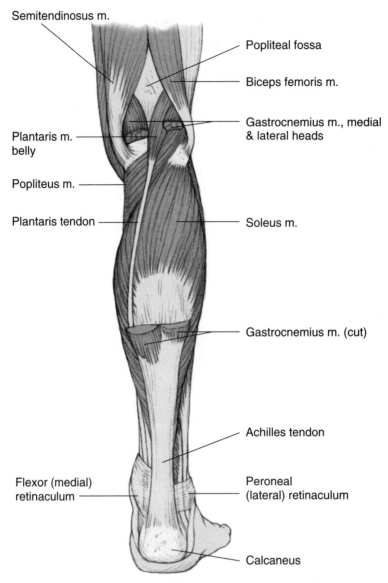

Semitendinosus m.

Popliteal fossa

Biceps femoris m.

Gastrocnemius m., medial
& lateral heads

Plantaris m.
belly

Popliteus m.

Plantaris tendon

Soleus m.

Gastrocnemius m. (cut)

Achilles tendon

Flexor (medial)
retinaculum

Peroneal
(lateral) retinaculum

Calcaneus

Figure 7-8   Muscles in the Deep Posterior Compartment. The muscles of the superficial compartment, the gastrocnemius and soleus, have been cut. (From C.L.A.S.S.: *Clinical anatomy principles*, St Louis, 1996, Mosby.)

patella before inserting into the medial condyle of the tibia.

All of the ligaments supporting the knee are susceptible to stretching, tearing, or complete rupture. If a ligament is not totally ruptured, it has the ability to repair and heal itself. When injured, ligaments heal by laying down scar tissue. Although normal strength can return after a ligament strain, the strength is attributable to a large quantity of poor-quality scar tissue. As a result, the normal resilience of the ligament may be decreased.

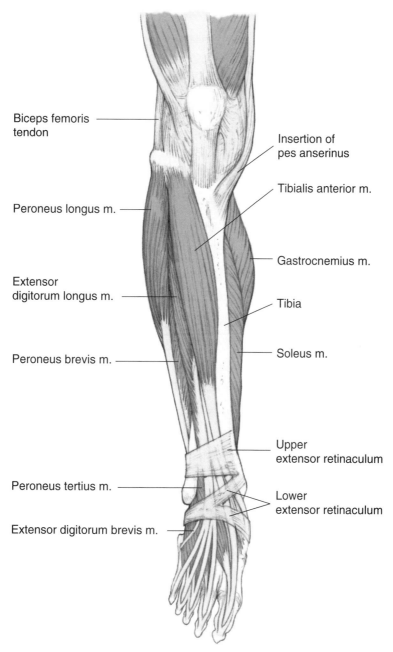

Figure 7-9   Muscles in the Anterior Compartment. Note that the tendons cross the ankle joint and extend along the dorsum of the foot, allowing movement of the ankle and toes. (From C.L.A.S.S.: *Clinical anatomy principles*, St Louis, 1996, Mosby.)

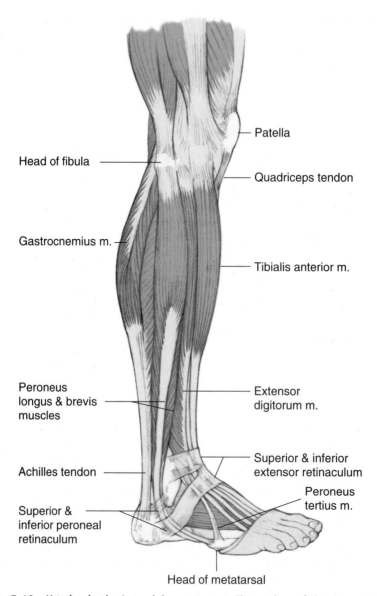

Head of fibula

Patella

Quadriceps tendon

Gastrocnemius m.

Tibialis anterior m.

Peroneus longus & brevis muscles

Extensor digitorum m.

Achilles tendon

Superior & inferior extensor retinaculum

Peroneus tertius m.

Superior & inferior peroneal retinaculum

Head of metatarsal

Figure 7-10   Muscles in the Lateral Compartment. The tendons of the peroneus longus and brevis can become inflamed as a result of overuse or overstretching, causing lateral ankle and leg pain. (From C.L.A.S.S.: *Clinical anatomy principles*, St Louis, 1996, Mosby.)

Simultaneous injury to more than one ligament can lead to a poor clinical outcome.

Each muscle of the leg has a tendinous attachment; generally, the tendons bear the same name as their associated muscles. The gastrocnemius and soleus muscles share a common tendon, the Achilles' tendon (Figure 7-14). Beginning about the middle of the leg and extending approximately 6 inches in length, the Achilles' tendon is the thickest and strongest in the body, inserting into the lower part of the posterior calcaneus. This tendon allows

TABLE 7-2	Leg Muscle Compartments and Primary Muscle Action(s)	
Compartment	**Muscles**	**Muscle Action(s)**
Superficial posterior	Gastrocnemius	Plantar flexes foot; raises heel from ground during walking; helps flex knee
	Soleus	Steadies leg on foot when standing to prevent falling forward
	Plantaris	Plantar flexes ankle if foot is free; flexes knee if foot is fixed
Deep posterior	Popliteus	Assists in flexing leg on thigh; posterior internally rotates tibia
	Tibialis posterior	Plantar flexes foot at ankle; inverts foot; helps maintain arch of the foot
	Flexor digitorum longus	Flexes toes two through five; assists in plantar flexion of foot
	Flexor hallucis	Flexes great toe; assists in plantar flexion of foot; helps maintain perpendicular alignment of leg on ankle joint
Anterior	Tibialis anterior	Dorsiflexes foot; assists with inversion of foot
	Peroneus tertius	Dorsiflexes foot; assists with eversion of foot
	Extensor hallucis longus	Dorsiflexes great toe; strengthens ankle joint
	Extensor digitorum longus	Dorsiflexes toes two through five; strengthens ankle joint
Lateral	Peroneus longus	Plantar flexes foot; everts foot
	Peroneus brevis	Plantar flexes foot; everts foot

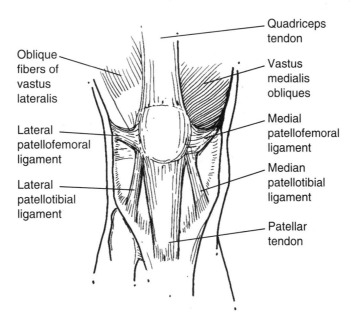

Figure 7-11   The Quadriceps and Patellar Tendons. These tendons stabilize the patella during flexion and extension of the knee. Patellofemoral and patellotibial ligaments provide additional stability. (From walsh WM: patellofemoral joint. In DeLee JC, Drez D Jr, editors: *Orthopaedic sports medicine: principles and practice*, ed 2, vol 2, Philadelphia, 2003, WB Saunders.)

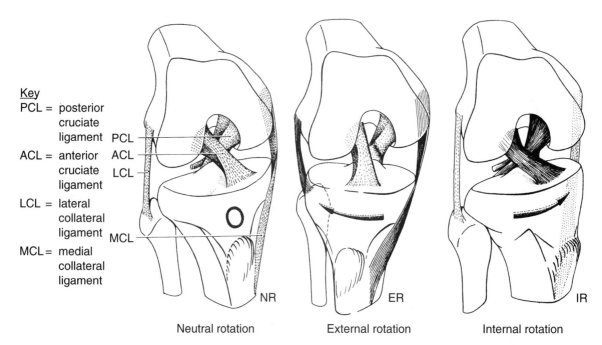

Key
PCL = posterior
      cruciate
      ligament   PCL
ACL = anterior   ACL
      cruciate   LCL
      ligament
LCL = lateral
      collateral
      ligament   MCL
MCL = medial
      collateral
      ligament

NR   ER   IR

Neutral rotation   External rotation   Internal rotation

Figure 7-12   Four Primary Stabilizing Ligaments of the Knee and Their Function During Rotation of the Knee. A, In neutral rotation, all the ligaments are under normal tension. **B,** The medial and lateral collateral ligaments tense during external rotation to prevent excessive rotation. **C,** During internal rotation, the cruciate ligaments wind around each other and become tense to prevent unusual rotatory stress on the knee joint. (From Canale ST, editor: *Campbell's operative orthopaedics*, ed 10, vol 3, St Louis, 2003, Mosby.)

plantar flexion of the foot. Just medial to the Achilles' tendon is the much thinner plantaris tendon. Although the plantaris tendon is not nearly as strong as the Achilles' it also assists in plantar flexion of the foot.

In addition to assisting inversion and plantar flexion of the foot, the tibialis posterior tendon is important in maintaining the bony arch of the foot. Injury to the muscle or tendon may manifest as a unilateral flatfoot. The flexor hallucis longus muscle and its tendon begin on the lateral portion of the leg, but the muscle passes obliquely across the back of the leg. The tendon lies in a groove posterior to the medial malleolus and talus, finally inserting into the base of the distal phalanx of the great toe. The flexor digitorum longus tendon remains on the medial side of the leg until after it passes the medial malleolus. It extends distally and laterally to the four lesser toes of the foot.

Menisci

The menisci are two of the most important structures in the knee. The knee contains both a medial and a lateral meniscus. They act as shock absorbers when walking, running, or jumping. They also provide joint congruity and increase contact area between the femur and tibia, help protect the articular cartilage and evenly distribute load-bearing forces, assist in proprioception, and help distribute synovial nutrients to the articular cartilage.[85]

The menisci are two crescent-shaped pieces of fibrocartilage that are attached to the outer rim of the tibial plateau (Figure 7-15). Compared with the hyaline cartilage covering the articular surfaces of the femur and tibia, the menisci are more similar to the composition of the cartilage of the nose or external ear. Wedge-shaped on cross section, the outer edge is thicker and has a vascular supply that allows the periphery to be called the

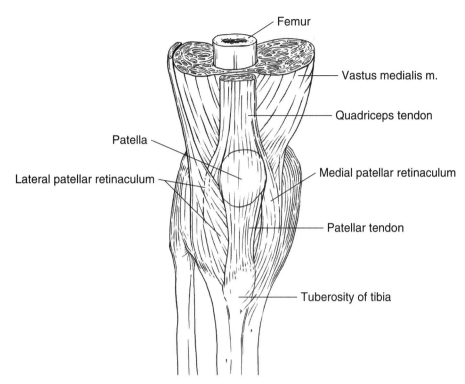

Figure 7-13 Retinacular System of the Knee. An imbalance in retinacular function, especially tightness of the lateral retinaculum, can result in patellar subluxation.

"red zone." This vascularized area is 10% to 30% of the peripheral medial meniscus and 10% to 25% of the lateral meniscus periphery.[89] Toward the inner edge the menisci taper and are not attached to the tibial plateau. The inner portions (70% to 90%) of the menisci are essentially avascular and rely on synovial fluid for their nutrients. As vascular supply declines, the meniscus grows pale toward the center, becoming a "red-white zone" and then a "white zone." Injuries in the red-white or white zone have poor healing potential.

The medial meniscus is larger and more firmly attached to the tibial plateau and joint capsule than the lateral meniscus.[51] When the knee joint extends from a flexed position, both menisci move posteriorly—the lateral meniscus more than the medial. Because the medial meniscus is in a more fixed position, it is more susceptible to injury than the lateral meniscus.

Bursae

Bursae, which are padlike sacs containing both a synovial lining and synovial fluid, function to reduce friction between tendon and bone, between tendon and ligament, or even between two ligaments (Figure 7-16). As many as eleven bursae have been identified around the knee,[16] but those most commonly inflamed are the pes anserine, prepatellar, and infrapatellar bursae.

Neurovascular Structures

Branches of the femoral, popliteal, and lateral circumflex arteries supply the knee joint. Five branches of the

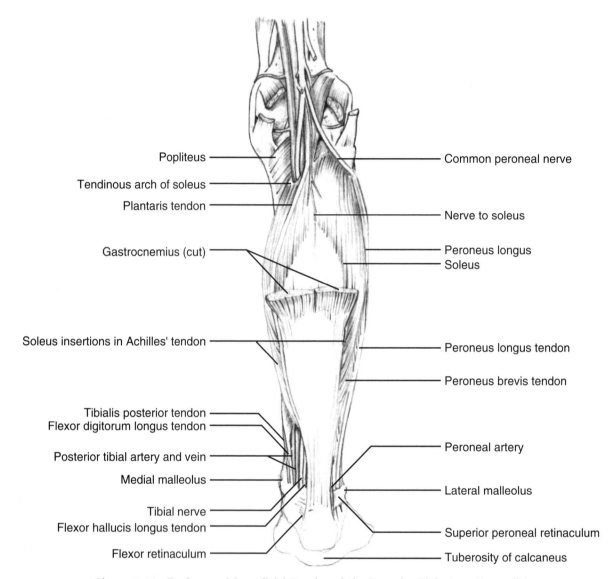

Figure 7-14 Tendons and Superficial Muscles of the Posterior Right Leg. The medial and lateral heads of the gastrocnemius muscle have been cut to show the soleus muscle and plantaris tendon. (From C.L.A.S.S.: *Clinical anatomy principles*, St Louis, 1996, Mosby.)

popliteal artery and two major branches of the femoral artery supply the knee.

Innervation of the knee is from branches of the femoral and saphenous nerves. The tibial and common peroneal nerves are also located posteriorly around the knee joint.

Innervation of the leg muscles begins in the lower lumbar and first sacral nerve roots (i.e., the upper portion of the sacral plexus). By the time the branches of the sciatic nerve divide to supply the leg, there are two main nerves—the tibial and peroneal nerves; they sup-

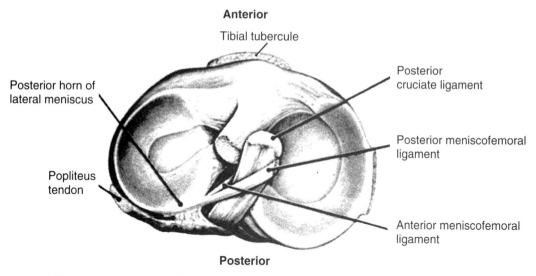

Anterior

Tibial tubercule

Posterior horn of
lateral meniscus

Posterior
cruciate ligament

Posterior meniscofemoral
ligament

Popliteus
tendon

Anterior meniscofemoral
ligament

Posterior

Figure 7-15   Superior View of the Left Tibial Plateau. The cruciate ligaments and menisci
are shown. The fibrocartilagenous menisci serve several functions in protecting the knee joint.
(From Canale ST, editor: *Campbell's operative orthopaedics*, ed 10, vol 3, St Louis, 2003, Mosby.)

ply most of the leg. Generally, these divisions occur proximal to the leg. The tibial division is the larger of the two.

Coursing down the posterior aspect of the tibia, the tibial nerve progressively becomes more superficial as it descends. The nerve supplies the muscles of the superficial and deep posterior compartments. At its more distal portions, smaller branches of the tibial nerve divide and supply part of the ankle, heel, and medial aspect of the sole of the foot.

The peroneal nerve begins in the distal posterior thigh, but then it courses anterolaterally at the fibular head. In fact, the nerve has been described as "wrapping itself around the fibular neck."[66] From the fibular head it travels inferiorly, further dividing into the superficial and deep branches of the peroneal nerve. The superficial branch is the more lateral of the two, providing cutaneous innervation to the lateral leg, as well as to the dorsum of the foot and lateral toes. Three small branches supply portions of the knee. The deep branch supplies the muscles of the anterior compartment, part of the anterior and lateral ankle joint, and the medial side of

the dorsum of the foot. Injury to the peroneal nerve, described as "foot drop," is not uncommon with trauma to the proximal fibula.

The leg has a rich blood supply to its muscles. The popliteal artery is essentially an extension of the femoral artery. Most of the major arterial supply to the leg comes from branches of the popliteal artery (Figure 7-17). Its location is almost in the center of the popliteal fossa and its lack of muscular support makes the popliteal artery susceptible to shear forces and direct trauma. Hyperextension or even extreme forced flexion of the knee may damage the vessel.

In the deep posterior compartment lie the posterior tibial artery and veins. A branch of the posterior tibial artery, the peroneal artery, also lies in the deep posterior compartment. The peroneal artery closely follows the fibula and can be injured with trauma to the proximal fibula. The anterior compartment contains the anterior tibial artery and vein. The sural arteries are in the superficial posterior compartment. Laterally the anterior tibial artery (i.e., a branch of the popliteal artery) lies against the medial aspect of the fibular head.

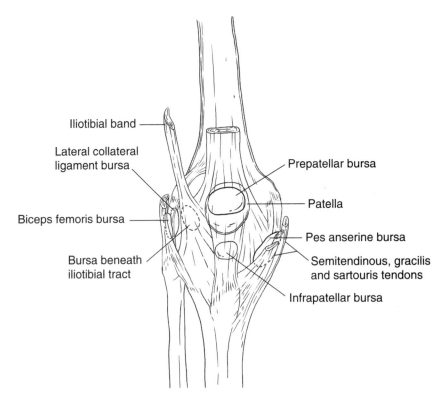

Iliotibial band

Lateral collateral ligament bursa

Biceps femoris bursa

Bursa beneath iliotibial tract

Prepatellar bursa

Patella

Pes anserine bursa

Semitendinous, gracilis and sartouris tendons

Infrapatellar bursa

Figure 7-16 **Bursae around the Knee Joint.** Those most frequently affected by bursitis are the prepatellar, infrapatellar, and pes anserine bursae.

This artery, too, can be affected when there is trauma to the proximal fibula.

EXAMINATION

KNEE

The complexity of the knee joint can make examination of it a daunting task. Together, a careful history and examination can lead the practitioner to a more accurate diagnosis.

Initially, any obvious swelling, discoloration, or malalignment should be noted. Anterior knee swelling is more easily detected if compared with the contralateral joint. Flexion of the knee can be limited by either intra-

capsular or extracapsular swelling. Intraarticular swelling tends to limit full extension, as often seen in meniscal tears. Extracapsular swelling, as seen in bursitis, does not usually limit extension. Clinically, limited extension of the knee is usually more significant than limited flexion. Swelling in the joint does not usually cause visible discoloration. Ecchymosis is usually the result of direct trauma to the knee. Obvious erythema can be attributable to infection or inflammation. Observing the patient's stance and gait serves to initially assess alignment.

With the patient standing with the patellae facing forward and the knees and ankles as close together as possible (preferably touching), genu valgum (i.e., "knock knees") and genu varum (i.e., "bow legs") can be evaluated (Figure 7-18). Genu valgum is present if the knees

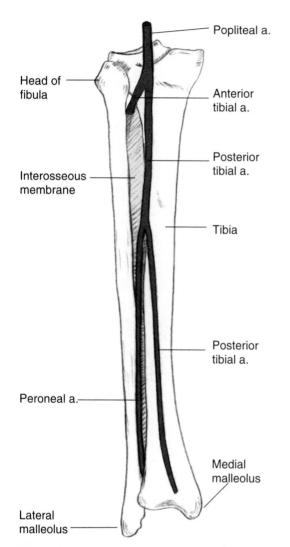

Popliteal a.

Head of
fibula

Anterior
tibial a.

Posterior
tibial a.

Interosseous
membrane

Tibia

Posterior
tibial a.

Peroneal a.

Medial
malleolus

Lateral
malleolus

Figure 7-17   Major Branches of the Popliteal Artery.
These vessels supply most of the blood to the leg. (From
C.L.A.S.S.: *Clinical anatomy principles,* St Louis, 1996, Mosby.)

pensation for excessive lumbar lordosis. Genu recurvatum is not uncommon in women and may measure as much as −15 degrees.

With the patient still standing, the popliteal fossae can also be compared for abnormal color or swelling, such as a Baker's cyst. Most Baker's cysts are not obvious to visual examination and are only rarely palpable.[39]

Once the patient is on the examining table, the knees can be viewed from the lateral position. Anterior knee swelling is sometimes more apparent when viewed laterally. Occasionally an unusually high-riding patella (i.e., patella alta) can be seen when viewed laterally. One deformity is called a "camel sign" because the infrapatellar fat pad appears more prominent when the patella sits above the femoral condyles.

Once an initial visual inspection is made, active ROM can be measured. Beginning with the fully extended knee at 0 degrees, normal flexion is approximately 135 degrees. Flexion is stopped by the contact of the calf and posterior thigh muscles. Knee extension may extend beyond 0 degrees in individuals with ligamentous laxity (genu recurvatum). Because it is confusing to describe limited extension in terms of "having only 10 degrees of extension," it is often more clinically useful to indicate "the patient lacks 10 degrees of full extension." Muscular inability to extend the knee against resistance is a classic sign of a quadriceps muscle tear. If there is any abnormality of active ROM, the practitioner should then assess passive ROM.

The tibiofemoral joint allows approximately 20 degrees to 30 degrees of both internal and external rotation, but external rotation of up to 40 degrees is still considered normal. Tibial rotation is best evaluated when the patient is sitting on the edge of the examining table. Neutral rotation is present when the anterior tibial spine faces forward as the patient sits with his or her legs over the edge of the table. Tibial rotation can also be assessed when observed during passive ROM. The practitioner stabilizes the distal femur with one hand and grasps the posterior calcaneus and ankle with the other and rotates the tibia.

Once the patient is supine on the table, the quadriceps angle, or Q angle, can be measured. The Q angle refers to the angle of the patella's position relative to both the femur and tibia. Measured with a goniometer,

touch but the ankles do not. Genu varum is present when the ankles touch but the knees do not. Varus deformity of the knee is often seen in degenerative osteoarthritis (OA). Another abnormality of knee alignment is hyperextension of the knee joint, or genu recurvatum. This deformity is frequently associated with generalized ligamentous laxity or may be a sign of com-

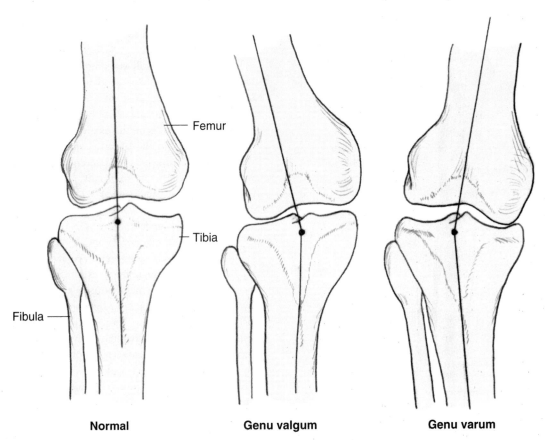

Normal Genu valgum Genu varum

Figure 7-18 Varus and Valgus Deformities of the Knee. Compared with normal alignment of the knee (*left*), both varus and valgus deformities cause uneven wearing of the articular cartilage and predispose the joint to early degenerative changes. Note the asymmetry
of the joint space. (From C.L.A.S.S.: *Clinical anatomy principles*, St Louis, 1996, Mosby.)

normal Q angle in men is approximately 10 degrees; up
to 15 degrees in women is acceptable because of the
wider pelvis. An increased Q angle can be associated
with patellar subluxation, femoral anteversion, external
tibial torsion, and pes planus.

To measure the Q angle, a point in the center of the
patella is located, then an imaginary line is drawn up to
the anterior superior iliac spine. Another imaginary line
extends from the center of the patella down to the anterior tibial tubercle. The angle is then measured at the
intersection of these two lines (Figure 7-19).

Palpation of the knee is performed to assess the joint,
its ligaments and tendons, the muscles, and the menisci.

If there is swelling, the presence of patellar ballottement
can help differentiate intracapsular from extracapsular
fluid. With the patient supine on the examining table,
the practitioner gently "milks" the knee toward the
femur and then briskly taps the patella down against the
femoral condyles. A palpable "clunk" as the patella
strikes the condyles is a positive ballottement test and is
indicative of excessive fluid within the joint.

Next, the bony landmarks of the knee—the femoral
condyles, patella, and femoral and lateral joint lines—
are palpated for any pain or tenderness. These areas are
more easily palpated if the knee is flexed to 90 degrees.
The femoral condyles are located adjacent to the patella;

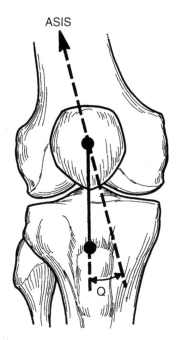

ASIS

Q

Figure 7-19 Measurement of the Q Angle. The angle is formed by the intersection of imaginary lines from (1) the center of the patella to the tibial tuberosity and (2) the center of the patella to the anterosuperior iliac spine. The angle is measured from the center of the patella. Normal Q angle in men is 10 degrees or less. In women an angle up to 15 degrees is considered normal, since the female pelvis is wider than the man's. (From Canale ST, editor: *Campbell's operative orthopaedics*, ed 10, vol 3, St Louis, 2003, Mosby.)

the medial condyle is more easily felt because the patella covers a greater portion of the lateral joint. Localized tenderness over these osseous structures can be caused by a fracture, bone contusion, or the presence of degenerative osteophytes.

The patella is fairly prominent and easily palpated. Tenderness along the superior or inferior border may indicate tendonitis. Point tenderness anywhere over the patella can be caused by fracture or contusion.

Palpating the inferior patellar border along the patellar tendon allows evaluation of its integrity and can localize pain associated with patellar tendonitis. The patellar tendon continues distally, attaching to the tibial tubercle (the bony anterior prominence on the proximal tibia). Localized pain and tenderness directly over the tibial tubercle are associated with Osgood-Schlatter (see Figure 7-38) disease or fracture. Diffuse anterior knee pain and swelling or anteromedial knee pain and swelling are often caused by bursitis.

The superior border of the patella is the attachment of the quadriceps tendon. Bogginess or a palpable defect in its normal cordlike quality may indicate rupture of the quadriceps. Inability to extend the knee against resistance is almost pathognomonic for a quadriceps rupture.

The patellar grind (or inhibition) test is useful in evaluating the quality of the articulating surface of the patella. With the patient supine, the practitioner manually moves the patient's patella distally and gently holds it in place. The patient is then instructed to tighten the quadriceps muscle. As the patella moves proximally, any pain, crepitus, or grinding is noted. If the patella does not move painlessly and smoothly, the patellar grind test is positive.

Stability of the MCL and LCL should be evaluated with the knee in both 0 degrees and 20 to 30 degrees of flexion.[89] Normally the knee can open medially or laterally up to 5 degrees. The MCL provides most of its stability against valgus stress when the knee is flexed from 20 to 30 degrees. If the MCL is stable at 0 degrees but unstable from 20 to 30 degrees of flexion, only the MCL is damaged. If the MCL is unstable at both 0 and 30 degrees of flexion, the MCL and possibly the posterior medial joint capsule have been damaged. Similarly, LCL instability at both 0 and 30 degrees indicates probable damage to the posterolateral knee capsule, as well as to the LCL.

To test collateral ligament stability, the patient should lie supine with the legs extended (Figure 7-20, *A, B*). The lower leg is secured by using one hand to grasp the patient's ankle. To test MCL stability, the practitioner's other hand is placed over the fibular head, and a medially directed (valgus) force is applied in an attempt to open the medial joint.

LCL stability is tested in a manner similar to the one testing MCL stability, but the hand near the knee applies a laterally directed (varus) force. If the practitioner is unable to apply adequate varus stress to the joint, an alternate method can be used. While one hand stabilizes

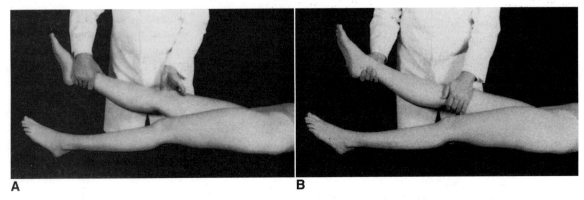

A   **B**

Figure 7-20   Testing Medial and Lateral Collateral Ligament Stability. A, The medial collateral ligament is tested by applying valgus stress to the knee while stabilizing the patient's ankle. **B,** Varus stress is applied to the knee joint to test the lateral collateral ligament. (From Evans RC: *Illustrated orthopedic physical assessment*, ed 2, St Louis, 2001, Mosby.)

the knee, the practitioner rests the elbow of his or her opposite arm on his or her own hip and grasps the patient's ankle. The knee joint acts as a fulcrum as the practitioner takes a step forward and turns toward the patient. With LCL instability, the lateral knee joint will open.

Joint opening can be classified as grades I to III, which correlate with the degree of ligament damage in MCL and LCL sprains. A grade I sprain correlates with microtears in the ligament and has 0 to 5 mm of laxity; the ligament has no increased joint opening when compared to the uninjured knee. Grade II sprains correspond with partial, larger tears of the ligament and have laxity ranging from 6 to 10 mm of joint opening with varus or valgus stress. Grade III injury has greater than 10 mm of laxity[89] and is associated with a complete tear in the ligament.

Stability of the cruciate ligaments should also be evaluated. There are three primary tests for assessing ACL integrity. They are the anterior drawer, Lachman's, and pivot shift tests. The latter is relatively difficult to perform correctly and is not discussed since anterior drawer and Lachman's tests, if positive, are sufficient to necessitate referral to an orthopedic surgeon.

The most commonly used test of ACL stability is the anterior drawer (Figure 7-21 *A-C*). The patient lies supine with the knees flexed to 90 degrees. The practitioner then sits on the patient's ipsilateral foot and places

his or her hands behind the patient's knee, over the medial and lateral hamstrings. The test is performed by pulling the tibia toward the practitioner. If the tibia moves forward, the test is positive and may indicate a torn ACL. It is important to check the unaffected knee for symmetrical movement because it is not uncommon to have some ACL laxity. Normal forward movement of the tibia (i.e., anterior translation) is 5 to 6 mm and should be equal bilaterally. If the test is positive, it should be repeated with the patient's leg internally and externally rotated to assess for additional damage to the posterolateral capsule (internal rotation) and posteromedial capsule (external rotation).

There are drawbacks to the anterior drawer test. First, it is not accurate if the patient has tight hamstrings since it is nearly impossible to overcome their resistance. In addition, it may be impossible to perform the anterior drawer test if there is significant fluid in the joint and the patient cannot flex her or his knees to 90 degrees.

Lachman's test is a more accurate assessment of ACL stability. This test is done by having the patient lie supine. The practitioner supports the patient's leg by grasping the proximal posterior calf and resting the patient's ankle on the examiner's hip. The patient's knee is flexed 20 to 30 degrees while the practitioner stabilizes the anterior thigh with the other hand. Using the hand that is supporting the calf, the lower leg is drawn anteriorly and the amount of forward sliding (i.e., anterior transla-

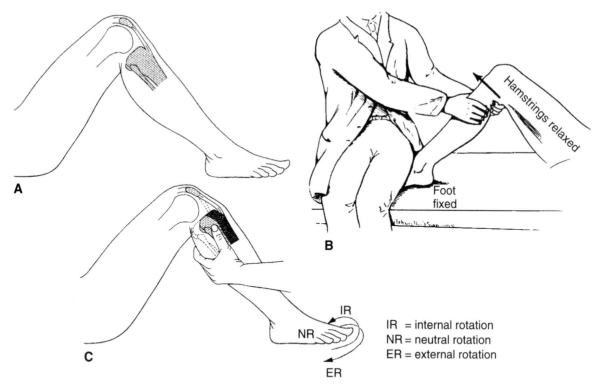

Figure 7-21   Anterior Drawer Test. A, The patient is supine with the hip and knee flexed. **B,** While the practitioner stabilizes the foot and distal tibia by sitting on the patient's foot, the practitioner firmly grasps the posterior proximal calf and pulls forward. **C,** While pulling forward on the tibia, the examiner notes any forward movement of the tibia. If movement is greater than 5 to 6 mm, an anterior cruciate ligament strain or tear is suggested. The anterior drawer test should be repeated with the foot in 30 degrees of internal rotation and then in 30 degrees of external rotation. (From Canale ST, editor: *Campbell's operative orthopaedics*, ed 10, vol 3, St Louis, 2003, Mosby.)

tion) of the tibia is noted (Figure 7-22, *A-C*). Again, a comparison with the other knee should be made. The advantages of the Lachman's test are that it can be performed in the presence of a large effusion, and there is no resistance from the hamstrings since they are not tensed at 30 degrees of flexion.

Posterior Cruciate Ligament

Injury to the PCL is less common than an ACL injury. The posterior drawer test is used to assess the integrity of the PCL. The test is performed with the patient supine, the knees flexed to 90 degrees, and the

sole of the foot flat on the examining table. While stabilizing the patient's foot by sitting on it, the practitioner firmly grasps the patient's proximal tibia and pushes it posteriorly. A positive test occurs when the tibia slides posteriorly against the femoral condyles. The examiner should compare the injured knee with the unaffected knee.

Another test, the tibial sag sign, is also suggestive of a PCL tear. When the supine patient's hip and knee are both flexed, a positive sign is present when there is a depression visible over the anterior proximal tibia when viewed laterally (Figure 7-23, *A-C*). Godfrey's test is also

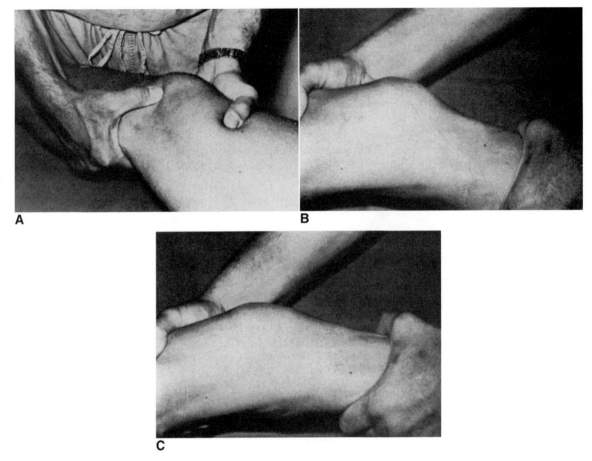

Figure 7-22 Lachman's Test. A, The correct hand position is shown for performing Lachman's test. **B,** Normal contour of the knee is 20 degrees of flexion. **C,** A positive Lachman's test shows loss of the normal patellar tendon silhouette as the tibia slides forward on the femur. This indicates a tear of the anterior cruciate ligament. (From Canale ST, editor: *Campbell's operative orthopaedics,* ed 10, vol 3, St Louis, 2003, Mosby.)

used for evaluating PCL injury. The patient is supine and both the hip and knee are flexed to 90 degrees. If necessary, gentle downward pressure can be applied to the tibia. In the presence of a PCL rupture, the normal patellar contour will not be visible when viewed laterally (Figure 7-24). If necessary, gentle downward pressure can be applied to the tibia. A positive Godfrey's test indicates a significant PCL injury and requires referral to an orthopedic surgeon.

Meniscus

Clinically, several examinations are used to evaluate damage to the meniscus. The simplest test is palpation of the tibial joint line; tenderness may indicate a tear of the meniscus, but it is not specific. McMurray's test is considered the standard for evaluating the meniscus. To perform this test, the patient is asked to lie supine with the knees extended but relaxed. The practitioner then cradles the patient's heel with one hand and rests the other

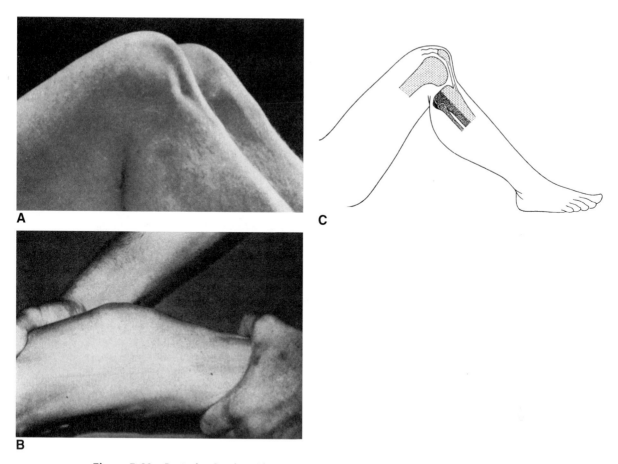

A

B

C

Figure 7-23   Posterior Cruciate Ligament Rupture. A, The right knee shows obvious laxity when flexed to 90 degrees. This is a positive tibial sag sign. **B,** Drawing shows posterior translation of the tibia on the femur. **C,** As the tibia is manually pulled forward, the normal contour returns. It is prevented from moving too far forward by an intact anterior cruciate ligament. (From Canale ST, editor: *Campbell's operative orthopaedics,* ed 10, vol 3, St Louis, 2003, Mosby.)

hand on the patient's knee with the fingers over the joint line. The practitioner then fully flexes the patient's knee. While passively extending the knee, the practitioner simultaneously rotates the leg, first internally and then externally (Figure 7-25, *A-C*). A palpable "clunk" or "click" over the joint line is the classic positive test. However, it is not unusual for pain to be the only symptom with McMurray's test.[50]

Apley's compression test is another maneuver used to assess the meniscus. To perform this test the patient is in a prone position with the affected knee flexed to 90 degrees. The practitioner then applies constant downward pressure on the patient's heel while rotating the tibia internally and externally (Figure 7-26, *A, B*). Pain with either medial or lateral rotation is suggestive of a corresponding meniscus injury.

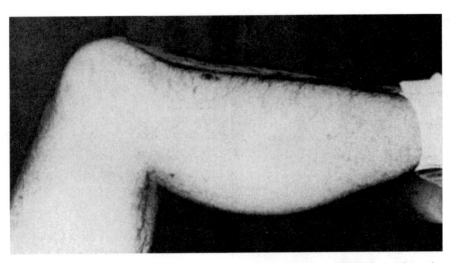

Figure 7-24 Godfrey's Test for Posterior Cruciate Ligament Disruption. When the patient's hips and knees are flexed to 90 degrees, there is noticeable sagging of the proximal right tibia, indicating a posterior cruciate ligament rupture. (From Canale ST, editor: *Campbell's operative orthopaedics*, ed 10, vol 3, St Louis, 2003, Mosby.)

LEG

Examination of the leg begins with visual inspection. The patient's gait and weight-bearing ability while standing should be noted. An antalgic gait or inability to bear weight on one leg may occur with fracture, tendonitis, muscle strain, or rupture. The location and size of bruising or discoloration should be noted. Apparent size of each leg, as well as any vascular problems such as varicosities or pitting edema, should be evaluated. Bilateral leg edema is common with circulatory or other chronic problems; unilateral swelling is suggestive of an acute process. Asymmetry of the leg muscles may indicate a congenital abnormality, disuse, or certain neurologic disease processes such as post-poliomyelitis syndrome. Tibial alignment should be evaluated by asking the patient to face the examiner directly. Malrotation of the legs can be attributable to valgus or varus deformities of the knee, fracture of the tibia, or developmental abnormalities such as tibial torsion or femoral anteversion.

Palpation of the leg can help diagnose fracture (point tenderness), vascular disease (temperature or color change), strain (diffuse muscle tenderness), sprain (tenderness over ligaments), and tendonitis (localized pain exacerbated by specific movements).

As with other areas of the body, examination should be guided by site-specific patient complaints and symptoms. Ankle and knee complaints should include adjacent areas of the leg to rule out associated pathologic conditions.

TRAUMA

FRACTURES

Fractures of the knee and leg include those of the tibial plateau, fibular head and shaft, and tibial pilon. Most, but not all, knee fractures are the result of fairly significant trauma and are often present in conjunction with injury to associated structures. Any suggested or documented fracture around the knee should be immediately referred to an emergency department or orthopedic surgeon.

Most fractures around the knee are associated with a large effusion. If the joint is tapped, the presence of

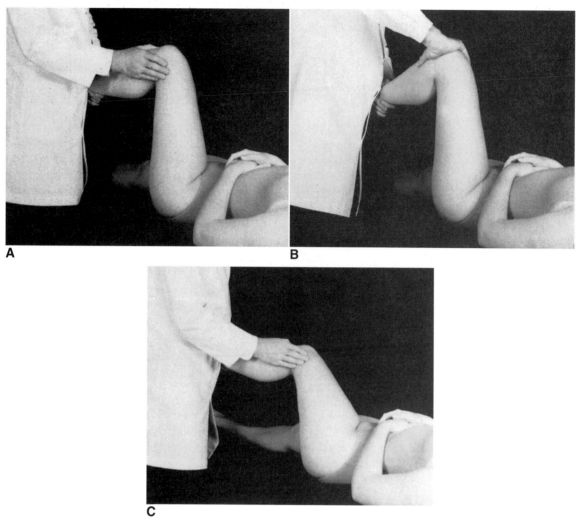

Figure 7-25   McMurray's Test. A, The patient's knee is flexed to varying degrees while the practitioner palpates the tibial joint line for tenderness. **B,** While placing his fingers over the area of joint line pain, the practitioner firmly grasps the patient's heel or ankle with the other hand. **C,** The patient's knee is extended, while the practitioner externally and internally rotates the leg. (From Evans RC: *Illustrated orthopedic physical assessment*, ed 2, St Louis, 2001, Mosby.)

hemarthrosis with fat globules is clinically indicative of a fracture. Initial treatment of a suggested or confirmed fracture begins with anteroposterior (AP) and lateral x-ray projections only if facilities are readily available; the primary care practitioner should not waste time sending the patient to a radiology facility. Initial treatment also includes immobilization, instituting nonweight-bearing status on the affected leg, and immediate orthopedic or emergency department referral. Application of ice may provide some pain relief, but analgesics are usually

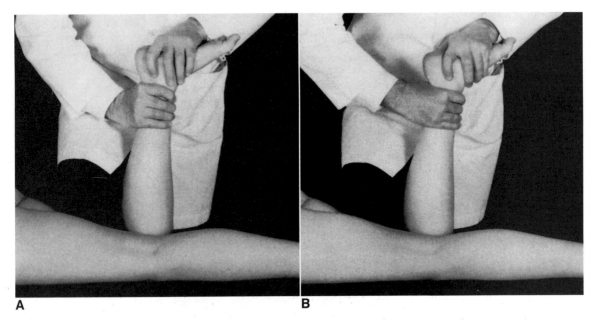

Figure 7-26   Apley's Compression Test. A, The practitioner firmly grasps the patient's ankle while applying downward pressure to the sole of the patient's foot. **B,** While maintaining downward pressure, the leg is firmly rotated both internally and externally. Pain with rotation in either direction is suggestive of a torn meniscus. (From Evans RC: *Illustrated orthopedic physical assessment*, ed 2, St Louis, 2001, Mosby.)

necessary. Nonsteroidal antiinflammatory drugs (NSAIDs) are not initially indicated, since their effect on platelet function may increase the hemarthrosis.

Patellar Fractures

Patellar fractures are usually the result of a direct blow from a blunt object or attributable to a fall or motor vehicle accident. Avulsion fractures from the superior or inferior pole can result from significant patellar or quadriceps tendon strain.[9] The patient with a patellar fracture is often unable to flex the knee or perform a straight leg raise. Marked joint effusion is generally present, and there is point tenderness over the affected portion of the patella. Transverse fractures can separate as the quadriceps and patellar tendons contract with flexion and extension. On plain x-ray films, a bipartite patella (most often present at the superolateral pole) may be difficult to distinguish from a fracture. Patients with a history of trauma, pain, and significant effusion

should have the knee immobilized in an extended position and be referred to an orthopedic surgeon for definitive treatment.

Distal femoral fractures include those attributable to osteochondritis dissecans, avulsion fractures of the lateral or medial femoral condyles, and epiphyseal plate fractures. In elderly patients, supracondylar femur fractures are not uncommon. For any of these fractures, weight bearing and knee flexion are usually painful and difficult. Joint deformity may be obvious. Any patient, especially young ones with still-open physes or elderly individuals, who has distal femoral tenderness or deformity after trauma should be referred to an orthopedic surgeon or an emergency department.

High-energy forces such as falls from heights and motor vehicle accidents are commonly associated with leg fractures. However, relatively minor trauma and repetitive stresses can also result in fractures.

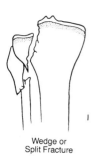
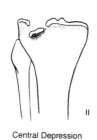
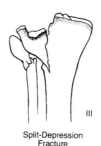
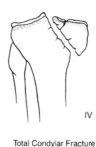
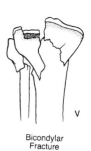

I	II	III	IV	V
Wedge or Split Fracture	Central Depression Fracture	Split-Depression Fracture	Total Condylar Fracture	Bicondylar Fracture

Figure 7-27   Types of Tibial Plateau Fractures. Mildly depressed fractures (grade II) can be easily missed on plain x-ray films. Computed tomography evaluation provides better detail for evaluating all types of tibial plateau fractures. (From Bucholz RW: *Orthopaedic decision making*, ed 2, St Louis, 1996, Mosby.)

Tibial Plateau Fractures

Tibial plateau fractures can be the result of either a fairly minor trauma or a significant impact. One of the most frequent cases of this type of fracture is that of a pedestrian struck by a car bumper. Other forces such as direct axial loading from landing on one's feet after a fall, or a shearing force from aggressive physical contact (e.g., football, soccer, lacrosse, rugby), can also fracture the proximal tibia. Injury caused by a high-energy force is usually seen and treated in an emergency department or orthopedic office. Less dramatic mechanisms of injury, such as landing on one's feet after a fall from a moderate height, may initially be overlooked. Patients who are osteopenic or osteoporotic are susceptible to low-energy tibial plateau fractures. In such instances the fractures tend to be depressed.

Knee pain and swelling after an injury should be considered signs of a potential tibial plateau fracture. Signs and symptoms may be subtle; when a fracture occurs near a ligamentous attachment, the injury may be mistaken for a sprain. Fractures of the anterior tibial plateau tend to occur when the knee is extended. Posterior tibial plateau fractures are more common when the knee is flexed. Figure 7-27 shows types of tibial plateau fractures.

One of the most important ramifications of failing to recognize or treat a tibial plateau fracture is the uneven joint surface that almost uniformly results. When this occurs, the relationship of the femoral condyles on the tibial plateau is affected, resulting in a "contact pressure overload" on one of the femoral condyles. In this situation, the articular cartilage wears unevenly and there is a high degree of associated posttraumatic OA. An uneven tibial plateau may also increase the likelihood of meniscal injury, since the meniscus becomes "caught" in the impacted or displaced tibial fragment(s). Ligamentous injuries are not uncommon in association with tibial plateau fractures.

Significant valgus stress to the knee can rupture the MCL. At the same time, enough force can also cause the lateral femoral condyle to impact the lateral tibial plateau, fracturing it. When this occurs, the LCL and MCL may be unstable on examination. LCL instability may actually be caused by displacement of the tibial plateau.

Injury to neurovascular structures occurs more often with high-energy injuries. Any evidence of neurovascular compromise necessitates immediate referral to an orthopedic surgeon or emergency department. If possible, the leg should be immobilized before transporting the patient.

History. Motor vehicle accidents, falls from either relatively low or great heights, pedestrian against car bumper collisions, and significant ligamentous injury to the knee have all been associated with tibial plateau fractures. After the initial insult the patient usually has knee pain or difficulty walking. Swelling occurs almost immediately, and bruising begins within hours of the injury. If he or she has been seen in an emergency department, x-ray films may have been reported as "negative," if a radiologist did not interpret them. Swelling and pain do not significantly diminish over the course of time. The patient may not seek additional treatment for a week or more after injury. The patient's age, general health, and mechanism of injury may raise or lower the practitioner's index of suspicion for fracture.

Physical Examination. A prominent knee effusion (usually a hemarthrosis) is common, and the knee area is tender or painful to palpation. Bony tenderness at the site of injury is typical, especially if the mechanism of injury was a valgus or varus force. Ligament pain may be present on the opposite side of the knee. Bruising around the proximal portion of the tibia is not unusual, especially if the joint capsule has also been disrupted.

Flexion and extension of the knee may be uncomfortable or painful. The presence of a hemarthrosis alone will make full flexion difficult. A positive McMurray's test is not unusual, since meniscal tears have been estimated to be present in one half of the cases of tibial plateau fractures.[53]

Diagnosis. History and physical examination are often nonspecific for tibial plateau fracture. The practitioner's suspicion of fracture may be increased if fat globules are visible in the presence of bloody aspirate drawn from the joint under aseptic conditions.

Plain x-ray films should be obtained to visualize the tibial plateau. Findings on AP and lateral views are frequently subtle and easily missed. An AP x-ray projection with a 15-degree caudal tilt better visualizes any tibial condyle depression. Unless familiar with this view, however, it may be difficult for the practitioner to detect abnormalities. Any suggestion of a tibial plateau fracture is adequate for referral to an orthopedic surgeon.

Computed tomography (CT) is the most accurate tool for determining the amount of tibial plateau fracture depression. Once the extent of depression or displacement is known, operative or nonoperative treatment can be planned.

Treatment. Surgical versus nonsurgical treatment of tibial plateau fractures remains controversial. Although the return to or maintenance of an intact weight-bearing surface is the goal of treatment, not every patient requires surgery. It should be noted that patients more than 50 years old tend to have poorer clinical recovery regardless of what treatment is chosen. Minimally depressed fractures (i.e., less than 1 cm) can

be treated without surgical elevation and fixation. Choice of treatment is the decision of the orthopedic surgeon.

In the primary care setting, appropriate initial treatment consists of stabilizing the knee with a splint or other immobilizer, keeping the patient from weight bearing, and referring him or her to an orthopedic surgeon. If x-ray facilities are available and films have not previously been made, radiographic films of the knee should be obtained. A CT scan of the knee can be obtained before referral to the orthopedic surgeon if immediate referral is not available. Referral, however, should not wait until a CT scan has been performed.

Proximal Fibula Fractures

Most proximal fibular fractures are the result of direct trauma to the lateral leg (Figure 7-28). Some fractures, however, can be the result of forces transferred from a lateral malleolar injury of the ankle, particularly if the deforming force is a combination of compressive and rotational trauma. In the presence of a lateral malleolar fracture, a proximal fibular fracture is clinically more important, because the distal fibula forms the lateral buttress of the ankle joint. In an isolated simple fracture of the distal fibula, the stability of the proximal fibula will usually maintain integrity of the ankle joint. If both the proximal and distal portions of the fibula are fractured, there will no longer be enough support to prevent lateral dislocation of the ankle joint. A similar problem can occur when concomitant severe ligamentous damage to the ankle accompanies a fracture of the proximal fibula.

Both the peroneal nerve and anterior tibial artery pass near the fibular head and neck. Injury to either of these structures is a serious complication of a proximal fibular fracture. Weakness in everting the foot, foot drop, or loss of the dorsalis pedis pulse may indicate neurovascular damage near the proximal fibula. If there is any suggestion of damage to a nerve or blood vessel, the patient must be quickly referred to an emergency department or orthopedic surgeon.

History. The mechanism of an isolated proximal fibular fracture is usually fairly easy for the patient to recall. Contact sports such as soccer, football, field hockey, rugby, and lacrosse are associated with blows to

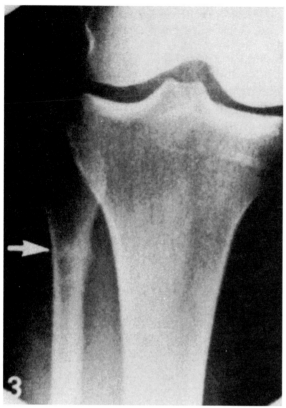

Figure 7-28 Typical appearance of a proximal fibular fracture.

only obvious finding on initial examination. Bruising may not occur for a few days and may be relatively faint. Palpable deformity at the site of tenderness is frequent. In the case of severe lateral ankle injury, it is prudent to quickly palpate the proximal fibula so as to not miss a fracture.

Diagnosis. Usually plain AP and lateral radiographic films will adequately show the fracture. Special tests are unnecessary unless there is associated neurovascular damage. In those instances, arteriography or nerve conduction studies may be indicated.

Treatment. An isolated nondisplaced fracture of the proximal fibula can often be treated with a compressive wrap such as an elastic bandage and the use of crutches. Casting is almost never indicated. Evaluation by an orthopedic surgeon is appropriate even with a simple fracture. More complicated injuries, especially when neurovascular compromise in known or suggested, must be referred to an orthopedic surgeon.

Midshaft Tibial and Fibular Fractures

Fractures to the midshaft of either leg bone are almost universally the result of significant, direct trauma. These fractures are frequently complex, inherently unstable, and often associated with an open wound. Initial treatment consists of maintaining nonweight-bearing status, splinting if possible, and immediate referral to an emergency department or orthopedic surgeon.

Stress Fractures

Stress fractures of the tibia most often occur at the junction of the middle and distal third of the bone along the posteromedial side. Stress fractures of the fibula are more common above the lateral malleolus. Pain in the distal portion of the posteromedial tibia is common in military recruits, joggers, and long-distance runners. In addition to running, other risk factors for stress fracture include poorly fitting footwear, excessive pronation of the feet, low fitness level, female sex, and Caucasian race.[12]

Stress fractures can be thought of as the end stage of a continuum that begins with shin splints. Initially, pain is intermittent and primarily occurs during the first portion of activity. As the condition progresses, pain occurs before, during, and after activity and becomes constant.

the lower extremities. Sometimes the patient will have heard or felt a pop or crack, followed by the onset of pain. Bruising may not become apparent for several days after the injury, but deformity is often soon apparent. Weight bearing is usually possible, but pain is worse especially when the affected leg is planted on the ground and the patient attempts to turn the body.

If there is a concomitant distal fibular fracture or significant ligamentous disruption of the ankle, pain with a proximal fibular fracture may be noticeable only with direct palpation or accidental bumping of the area. In these instances, the patient's primary complaint is usually ankle pain and an inability to bear weight on the affected leg.

Physical Examination. Although some swelling is usually present, tenderness to palpation may be the

If activity continues without allowing enough rest for bone repair, a break in the cortical bone will develop.

Even though there is an actual break in the bone, it is usually too small to be seen on plain x-ray films. A minimum of 2 weeks is necessary to allow sclerosis or enough callus formation to be visible over a fracture site. As a result, it can be difficult to differentiate a stress fracture from shin splints clinically.

History. Running and jumping activities are associated with both shin splints and tibial stress fractures. Cross-country athletes, cheerleaders, dance team members, and hurdlers are prone to stress fractures. Even recreational runners who may have recently increased their distance may be subject to stress fractures. There is rarely any specific incident associated with the onset of symptoms.

Dull, aching pain over the posteromedial tibia (i.e., usually the middle to distal third) tends to become more frequent and of longer duration with activity as the stress on the bone progresses. Pain is usually localized to one specific area. Intensity of pain is often variable but may increase in intensity and duration.

Physical Examination. Visual inspection of the affected leg usually reveals no abnormality. Palpation of the medial aspect of the tibia typically localizes the area of pain. Medial tibial pain may be either anteromedial or posteromedial.

Exacerbation of anteromedial pain can sometimes be accomplished by dorsiflexing the foot against resistance. Repeated toe raises can sometimes reproduce posteromedial tibial pain. Both tests involve using the muscles located near the site of pain and thus tend to exacerbate symptoms.

Percussing the tibia is one final test and is a key clinical tool in differentiating stress fractures from shin splints. Percussion is performed by tapping the tibia with the fingertips directly over or away from the area of tenderness. Pain with percussion away from the site of tenderness (remote percussion) is more indicative of a fracture than of shin splints.

Diagnosis. Once a history and examination are suggestive of a tibial stress fracture, imaging studies are used to confirm the diagnosis. Plain x-ray films are usually not helpful in making the initial diagnosis but are useful in ruling out larger fractures or other osseous processes. It may take weeks to months before callus formation is apparent on plain x-ray films.

In cases of persistent pain despite negative x-ray films, bone scanning and MRI are the diagnostic studies of choice. The high sensitivity of the bone scan and its relatively low cost make it the preferred test of many orthopedic surgeons. Bone scanning may become positive as early as 48 hours after the onset of symptoms. On a bone scan, a localized area of increased radionucleotide uptake is highly suggestive of a stress fracture. MRI is also extremely sensitive and can provide more detailed information about periosteal reaction and edema of the bone marrow. The primary limitation of MRI is its cost, two to three times higher than that of a bone scan.

Treatment. Rest, specifically cessation of those activities associated with pain, is the keystone of treatment. If there is no frank fracture line, partial weight bearing with the use of crutches for 3 to 4 weeks may be all that is necessary. If x-ray films or MRI confirms a cortical fracture, up to 12 weeks of rest may be necessary. Casting is rarely used unless a frank cortical fracture is present. NSAIDs are used for both their analgesic and antiinflammatory effects. Ice packs, whirlpool, and ultrasound treatments may also be beneficial in decreasing the amount of periosteal inflammation. A formal rehabilitation program is important to prevent recurrence of symptoms. Physical therapy (PT) with a cross-training program is useful in maintaining the patient's physical conditioning.[12] Orthotics may be indicated to correct overpronation of the foot and decrease stress on the posterior tibial and soleus muscle attachments.

Tibial Pilon Fractures

Significant injury to the distal end of the tibia (Figure 7-29) can occur with falls from great heights or from significant impact (i.e., motor vehicle crashes). Called tibial pilon or plafond fractures, these injuries are rarely seen in primary care. Extreme dorsiflexion of the ankle appears to be the common factor in these injuries. Because of the causes of these fractures, emergency departments and trauma centers tend to treat pilon fractures. Primary care providers need to be aware that recovery is prolonged, and residual pain and stiffness, as well as decreased function, are frequent sequelae.

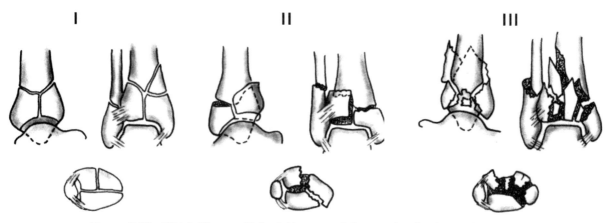

Figure 7-29 Tibial Pilon or Plafond Fractures. Injury to the distal end of the tibia caused by the direct axial loading of the leg requires immediate orthopedic surgical referral. Type I injuries are nondisplaced, type II fractures cause joint incongruity, and type III are crush-type injuries with displacement of the joint surface. (From Coughlin MJ, Mann RA: *Surgery of the foot and ankle,* ed 7, vol 2, St Louis, 1999, Mosby.)

SOFT-TISSUE INJURIES

Soft-tissue injuries are more frequently encountered in primary care than are fractures. Some soft-tissue injuries can be readily managed in a primary care setting; others require referral to an orthopedic surgeon.

Quadriceps Injuries

Quadriceps strains often occur in contact sports, and though pain is typically over the middle portion of the anterior thigh, partial or complete rupture of the muscle-tendon unit can also occur near the patella. Quadriceps tendon ruptures are more common in patients older than age 40. Patellar tendon ruptures occur more often in patients younger than age 40, and patients may have a history of patellar tendonitis or Osgood-Schlatter disease. In either case the history usually involves falling onto a partially flexed knee. The quadriceps tendon sustains the greatest stress at knee flexion angles less than 45 degrees; the patellar tendon is subject to the greatest force at 60 degrees of flexion.[59] As a result, ruptures of the quadriceps tendon tend to occur with the knee relatively straight, and ruptures of the patellar tendon are more likely to occur with the knee in flexion.

On examination, the patient will be unable to fully extend the knee against resistance (Figure 7-30). A palpable defect over either the quadriceps or patellar tendon is clinically diagnostic. When present, the defect is usually adjacent to the superior (quadriceps tendon) or inferior (patellar tendon) pole of the patella. On a lateral x-ray projection, an abnormally high-riding patella (patella alta) may indicate a rupture of the patellar tendon; an unusually low-riding patella (patella baja) may be present with a rupture of the quadriceps tendon. Treatment is immediate surgical correction. The patient should have the affected leg immobilized, and he or she should be referred to an emergency department or orthopedic surgeon. Earlier surgical correction is associated with better functional outcome.[26]

Patellar Malalignment

One of the most frequent causes of anterior knee pain is patellofemoral syndrome (PFS), also known as anterior knee pain syndrome. The term "chondromalacia patella" has been used in the past, but now refers to specific pathophysiologic changes of the cartilage.[26] Other common causes of anterior knee pain include a tilted patella and patellar subluxation.

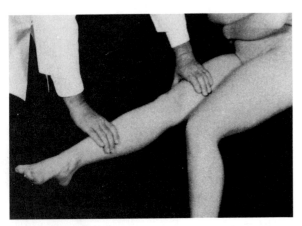

Figure 7-30 Testing Quadriceps Function. An inability to extend the knee against gravity is the predominant finding in a quadriceps rupture. Inability to extend the knee against resistance may indicate poor quadriceps tone or a partial rupture of the quadriceps tendon. (From Evans RC: *Illustrated orthopedic physical assessment*, ed 2, St Louis, 2001, Mosby.)

Several factors determine patellar alignment. Among them are overall muscle tone, femoral alignment, genu recurvatum, pelvic width, Q angle, and forefoot pronation. Anterior knee pain syndrome affects women more often than men, probably because of several factors. Women tend to have less developed vastus medialis muscles and a wider pelvis, which results in a greater incidence of genu valgus and an increased Q angle.[5] Women are also more prone to femoral anteversion. Adolescent girls are most commonly affected by patellar malalignment problems.

The medial patellofemoral ligament is the primary patellar stabilizer as the knee goes through its range of motion.[11] One of the primary functions of the quadriceps muscle and tendon is to ensure proper patellar tracking in the patellar groove, or trochlea, as the knee moves. When one of the quadriceps muscles is less developed than the others, it causes an imbalance in the group.

The medial and lateral retinacula also help stabilize the patella. The ITB is the primary origin of the lateral retinaculum, which is much stronger than the medial retinaculum. Portions of the vastus medialis muscle make up the medial retinaculum. The retinacula extend to the sides of the joint, forming part of the capsule and helping prevent the patella from displacing.

Normally the patella is fixed in the femoral trochlear groove when the knee is flexed from 20 to 30 degrees. During normal knee flexion and extension, the patella tilts slightly and rotates, in addition to moving superiorly and inferiorly.[5] With patellar subluxation the patella does not become centered in the groove until the knee is flexed to a greater angle. As a result, popping, snapping, or the sensation of the knee "popping out, then back in" occurs as the patella centers into the groove.

An increased Q-angle may exaggerate the normal tendency for the patella to laterally displace during walking and running. No definitive relationship between Q-angle and symptoms has yet been demonstrated.[5] Pronation of the forefoot intensifies any valgus deformity of the knee, again predisposing the patella to improper tracking. One result of patellar malalignment, regardless of cause, is an uneven wear on the retropatellar cartilage.

Repetitive mechanical stress on the patella's chondral surface can cause degenerative changes and anterior knee pain. The cartilage can become weakened, resulting in chondromalacia patella (which literally means softening of the patellar cartilage). PFS can also occur in patients with normal patellar tracking.

History. Onset of pain is usually gradual. Regardless of the specific cause, anterior knee pain that worsens when climbing stairs, kneeling, squatting, or sitting for prolonged periods is typical of patellar malalignment. Sometimes patients complain of aching with changes in the weather, feelings of instability, or a sensation of catching. Usually there is not one specific incident that has caused the onset of symptoms, though a recent increase in physical activity often precedes the patient's symptoms.

Physical Examination. Unless there is a history of recent trauma or significant patellar subluxation, there is rarely any discoloration of the knee. Swelling is not unusual. The patellar grind and patellar apprehension tests are usually positive in cases of patellar subluxation. The patellar apprehension test is easily performed by having the patient in a supine position with the legs relaxed and the knees in 20 to 30 degrees of flexion. The practitioner then gently pushes the patella laterally. If the patient feels as if the patella is going to pop out of position, she or he will contract the quadriceps to maintain the patella within the trochlear groove. This is a positive test.

Having the patient lie in a supine position and then raise the extended leg against the practitioner's hand evaluates quadriceps strength. Weakness can lead to patellofemoral pain. The patellar inhibition test is used to assess the retropatellar cartilage. After having the patient sit or lie with the legs extended and the quadriceps muscles relaxed, the practitioner uses one hand to inferiorly displace the patella (by pushing it toward the patient's foot, not into the patellar groove) and maintains this position. The patient then contracts ("tightens") the quadriceps muscle. Pain with quadriceps contraction is a positive test.

Although lateral patellar subluxation is more common, medial patellar subluxation can also occur. The patellar apprehension test for medial subluxation corresponds to the one for patellar subluxation: the practitioner pushes the patella medially.

Diagnosis. History, examination, and x-ray studies are used to diagnose patellar malalignment. AP, lateral, and sunrise (Merchant) views should be evaluated. The AP view allows visualization of patellar diameter but should not be used for assessing alignment, since any rotation of the leg during the x-ray procedure will distort apparent patellar position.

The lateral view allows measurement of the ratio between the patella and the patellar tendon (Figure 7-31). Normally the length of the patella from superior to inferior pole is at least 0.8 times that of the distance from the inferior pole to the patellar tendon insertion on the anterior tubercle. For example, a patellar length of 4.0 cm normally corresponds to a patellar tendon length of no more than 5.0 cm. If the patellar tendon length measures 6.8 cm, the patient has patella alta and is more likely to develop patellar subluxation.

The sunrise view allows visualization of the position of the patella within the trochlear groove. Normally the patella is centered in the groove (Figure 7-32). With patellar malalignment, there is a tendency for the patella to tilt laterally. On x-ray films, the lateral femoral condyle is more prominent than the medial condyle.

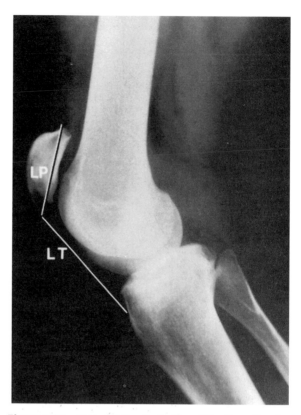

Figure 7-31   Lateral X-Ray Projection of the Knee Showing Patella Alta. This condition predisposes the patella to subluxation. *LP*, length of patella; *LT*, length of tendon.

Treatment. Exercise with emphasis on quadriceps strengthening is successful in treating most anterior knee pain problems. Some patients will progress better with a formal, supervised PT program. Both open- and closed-chain kinetic exercises can strengthen the quadriceps. Non-surgical treatment is effective in 80% to 85% of patients.[57] Exercises to stabilize the pelvis and correction of abnormal foot biomechanics, especially excessive pronation, are also useful.

Straight leg raising, consisting of raising the heel only 6 to 8 inches off the ground and holding for a count of five, is beneficial. The exercise should begin with ten repetitions twice a day and work up to three sets twice daily.

Riding a stationary or regular bicycle can be helpful if: (1) it is started after straight leg raising, since knee

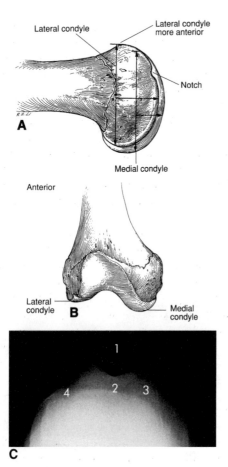

Figure 7-32 Sunrise View of the Patella Showing Normal Patellar Alignment. A, Lateral view of the femoral condyles, showing relative length and orientation. **B,** Anterior view of condyles. **C,** Sunrise view of patella, showing relationship to femoral condyles. (1) The patellofemoral joint space (2) is symmetrical, indicating the lack of any patellar tilt. The medial femoral condyle (3) is normally longer than the lateral femoral condyle (4). (**A, B** From Tria AJ, Klein AS: *An illustrated guide to the knee,* New York, 1992, Churchill Livingstone; **C** from C.L.A.S.S.: *Clinical anatomy principles,* St Louis, 1996, Mosby.)

flexion can aggravate symptoms; (2) the tension is adjusted to a very low resistance; and (3) the seat is high enough to allow nearly full extension of the knee on the down stroke.

Quadriceps setting exercises, consisting of isometric quadriceps contraction, have been shown to be particularly beneficial for strengthening the rectus femoris

muscle.[26] Again, the contracted muscle should be held for a count of 5 seconds, with ten repetitions twice daily, increasing to three sets of ten repetitions twice a day.

Patellar taping or a lateral patellar J-brace may also lessen symptoms.[64] This type of brace has a sewn-in buttress that prevents the patella from subluxating laterally. NSAIDs may provide some relief. If there is no improvement in symptoms with consistent exercise over a 4- to 6-week period, referral to an orthopedic surgeon is indicated. Surgical treatment may involve performing a lateral retinacular release or other realignment procedure.[76] Joint resurfacing has shown promise in treating PFS. Postoperatively, a course of PT is indicated to strengthen the quadriceps muscle and improve ROM.

Ligament Injuries

Medial Collateral Ligament

The MCL is the most frequently injured ligament in the knee; a sprained knee usually refers to an injury to the MCL. A common mechanism of injury is a direct blow to the lateral portion of the knee. MCL sprains are common injuries in contact sports such as football, rugby, and lacrosse. These injuries can also occur when there is sudden significant valgus stress to the knee, such as when cutting or turning to run when the knee is planted (as in basketball, soccer, or wrestling). In these instances there is usually associated meniscal damage. Cruciate ligament damage without meniscal injury can also occur with MCL rupture, particularly with extreme external rotation of the knee[75] (Figure 7-33 *A, B*).

The MCL extends from the medial femoral condyle to the medial proximal tibia, about 4 to 5 cm below the joint line. The ligament is situated slightly more posteriorly than anteriorly. The middle third of the knee joint capsule is formed by the MCL, which is also partially attached to the medial meniscus. The proximal and middle portions of the MCL are most frequently injured.

History. Typically a patient will describe a valgus force to the knee. It is not unusual to report hearing or feeling a pop or snap over the medial knee. Almost invariably there is medial knee pain. Occasionally the patient may describe the affected knee as having been bent inward or sideways. Often the patient will have fallen to the ground and will have had some difficulty

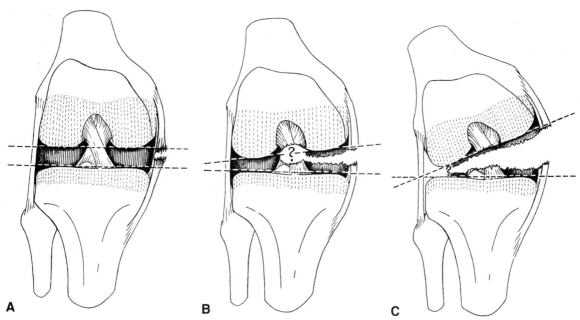

Figure 7-33   Examples of Ligament Damage. A, Isolated tear of the medial collateral ligament. **B,** Clinical examination of the medial collateral ligament with a possible injury of the anterior cruciate ligament showing medial laxity when the knee is tested in full extension. **C,** Severe injury with tearing of both anterior and posterior cruciate ligaments. (From Canale ST, editor: *Campbell's operative orthopaedics,* ed 10, vol 3, St Louis, 2003, Mosby.)

getting up or standing on the affected leg. Swelling is usually localized and may take an hour or more to be noticed by the patient. The knee may become stiff, if the patient has waited a few days to be examined.

Physical Examination. With an MCL injury the ligament is invariably tender to palpation. Localized spongy swelling over the ligament and even a mild joint effusion are not uncommon. In a thin patient the ligament may be visible when the knee is flexed 60 to 90 degrees. The presence of a large effusion suggests associated injury, such as a meniscus or cruciate ligament tear. Patients with a large effusion, gross knee instability, or a grade II or III injury should be referred to an orthopedic surgeon.

Degree of injury is assessed by applying valgus stress to the knee when fully extended and in 20 to 30 degrees of flexion. The grading of an injury is based on the degree of joint laxity or medial joint opening (see "Examination" earlier in this chapter). Grade I injuries

are tender to palpation, but the joint remains stable. Some palpable "give" with a definite end point (in addition to tenderness with palpation) indicates a grade II sprain. Grade III tears are associated with increased swelling and pain, and there is no definite end point with valgus stress. It is critical to compare the injured knee with the unaffected one because there is wide variation in normal ligamentous laxity.

Diagnosis. Diagnosis is based on history and physical examination. Plain x-ray films may show increased joint opening if taken while valgus stress is being applied. If the MCL has been injured at its proximal insertion, abnormal calcification may develop medial to the medial femoral condyle. This condition, known as Pelligrini-Stieda syndrome, may cause chronic medial knee pain. If an associated injury such as a torn cruciate ligament is suggested, MRI may be helpful. The cost of MRI, however, precludes its use for an isolated MCL injury.

Treatment. Most patients respond well to conservative therapy that includes rest, ice, compression, and NSAIDs for the first 1 to 3 days. Treatment of a grade I sprain includes ROM and quadriceps strengthening. PT combined with a program of "active rest" is beneficial for patients with a grade II or grade III sprain. Active rest involves weight bearing as tolerated, progressing over the first week from use of crutches to unassisted walking. Use of a hinged knee brace will improve medial stability of the knee while allowing full flexion and extension. In case of a grade III sprain, it is important to rule out an ACL tear. Surgical intervention is becoming less common for isolated MCL injuries.[74,82]

Grade I injuries generally heal sufficiently in 6 to 8 weeks, causing few, if any, residual problems. Return to sports should not be allowed until the patient has full ROM and muscle strength of the quadriceps and hamstrings is at least 90% that of the uninvolved side.[78] Recovery time until the patient can return to sporting activities can range between 6 weeks and 2 to 4 months.

Lateral Collateral Ligament

Normally the LCL prevents abnormal varus (bowlegged) deformity of the knee when medial force is applied to the joint. The LCL extends from the lateral femoral epicondyle and attaches on the fibular head. Unlike the MCL, the LCL is not attached to the meniscus. The LCL is a tough, cordlike structure that works in concert with several other structures to maintain lateral stability of the knee. As a result, it is injured less frequently than the MCL. When injured, the usual mechanism is a direct blow either to the medial knee or the anteromedial tibia with the knee flexed and the foot planted, causing hyperextension of the joint. Again, contact sports such as football, soccer, or rugby are often associated with LCL injury.

The LCL is one component of the area in the knee known as the posterolateral corner. Injury to this area often involves other structures, including the PCL. The LCL is also located fairly close to the peroneal nerve; associated injury to the nerve can cause motor and sensory problems of the lower lateral leg and foot.

History. The patient usually reports a history of direct trauma, but there may also be a history of the knee "bending out sideways" with a fall. Feelings of insta-

bility, especially when walking down an incline, are not uncommon, particularly if the PCL is involved.

Physical Examination. Pain, stiffness, and localized swelling are common with LCL injury. Varus stress testing of the knee in extension and 30 degrees of flexion will partially reveal the extent of LCL damage. LCL sprains are graded the same way as sprains of the MCL. In addition, with LCL injury the practitioner must carefully assess the peroneal nerve, since palsy can occur.

If present, peroneal damage is evident by weakness of foot dorsiflexion and eversion. There may be sensory deficit over the anterolateral portion of the lower leg or dorsum of the foot. Occasionally numbness in the web space between the great and second toes may be a sign of peroneal nerve involvement.

An additional test, the posterolateral drawer test, should be performed and interpreted by an orthopedic surgeon. Posterolateral rotatory instability (PLRI) may occur; if so, surgical repair may be indicated.[87] An orthopedic surgeon should perform evaluation of PLRI.

Diagnosis. A detailed history and careful physical examination are usually all that are required to diagnose injury to the LCL. Plain x-ray films may help rule out fractures of the fibular head or lateral femoral condyle, but they are not beneficial for assessing the LCL.

Treatment. Patients with a suggested diagnosis of LCL injury should be referred to an orthopedic surgeon. Surgical repair is more often appropriate in the case of LCL injury than in that of MCL sprains.

Anterior Cruciate Ligament Injuries

Lying in the center of the knee, the ACL extends from the posteromedial aspect of the lateral femoral condyle through the intercondylar femoral notch to the anterior border of the tibial plateau (see Figure 7-2). Its primary function is to prevent hyperextension and anterior movement (i.e., translation) of the tibia on the femur. It also assists in preventing varus and valgus angulation of the tibia, as well as reducing internal rotation of the tibia.[32,61]

The ACL can be injured by either a direct blow or indirect stress. Sports and activities that require a sudden change of direction in the weight-bearing knee are likely to cause ACL injury. Skiing, basketball, football, soccer, rugby, and volleyball are often associated with

ACL damage. Women who participate in basketball and soccer may be more likely to sustain ACL injury than men. Risk factors for ACL in women are not completely defined. However, the tendency of women to land from a jump with less knee and hip flexion and with a forward flexed lumbar spine seems to be a critical factor in causing ACL tears.[46] Women also tend to use their quadriceps rather than their hamstrings to counteract anterior translation, which provides less dynamic stabilization of the knee.[37] Sudden planting of the foot and stopping while running downhill can also adversely affect the ligament.

History. The most common complaints with acute ACL injury are immediate swelling and pain after sudden deceleration, cutting, or jumping. The patient may have felt something give or heard or felt a pop in the affected knee. The knee feels grossly unstable and weight bearing is exceptionally difficult. Swelling is rapid, often within an hour, and significant. Swelling with a cruciate ligament injury is usually more rapid than that associated with isolated collateral ligament or meniscal injuries. Recurrent instability of the knee when trying to change direction is also common. The patient may also feel that the joint slips out of place with walking.

Physical Examination. Knee swelling attributable to hemarthrosis is almost universally present. Pain may be felt to varying degrees. Pain and tenderness are commonly felt in the posterolateral area of the knee or near the tibial plateau, if there is associated LCL injury. Similarly, concomitant injury to the MCL results in medial tibial joint line pain. Meniscus tears are present in more than half of acute ACL tears.[31]

The most accurate clinical test for assessing ACL integrity is Lachman's test (see Figure 7-22). If there is a significant effusion, an anterior drawer test may be impossible to perform accurately because the knee may not be able to be flexed to 90 degrees.

Diagnosis. A positive anterior drawer (see Figure 7-21) or Lachman's test, combined with a history of trauma, is usually sufficient to diagnose an ACL injury.

Plain x-ray films may show an avulsion of the tibial insertion of the ACL. MRI, useful for a complete evaluation of the extent of ACL damage and the remainder of the joint, is often called for because of the high incidence of other knee injuries associated with ACL abnormality.

Treatment. Any patient with a suggested ACL injury, whether acute or chronic, should be referred to an orthopedic surgeon. Not all ACL injuries require surgical repair. Patients with a partial or isolated tear, or who have a fairly sedentary lifestyle and are both willing and able to participate in a PT rehabilitation program, may not require surgery. Prevention programs for ACL injuries have shown success in reducing the frequency of this problem.[40]

A complete tear of the ACL tends to result eventually in cartilage abnormalities and bony spurring. If there are associated meniscal or articular cartilage defects, degenerative changes of the joint are hastened.[31] Patients with a high level of activity tend to do better with surgical reconstruction.

Posterior Cruciate Ligament Injuries

The PCL is shorter and stronger than the ACL. It attaches to the back part of the depression behind the tibial spine and travels upward and anteriorly, crossing behind the ACL before inserting into the medial femoral condyle.

Functionally the PCL prevents posterior translation of the tibia on the femur. It also plays a role in stabilizing the knee against varus angulation and is a secondary restraint against external tibial rotation when the knee is flexed to 90 degrees.[74]

Injury to the PCL can occur when the knee is forcibly hyperextended (e.g., a fall or in gymnastics, football, and soccer) or when a direct blow is sustained to the anterior proximal tibia while the knee is flexed and the foot is planted (as in football, wrestling, or a dashboard injury in a vehicular accident).

Isolated PCL injuries are uncommon but not rare. Up to 70% of PCL injuries occur in combination with other knee injuries. This finding may be partially explained by the significant forces required to injure the PCL. When the PCL is injured, it is not uncommon to also have a knee dislocation that may have spontaneously reduced.

History. The patient with an isolated PCL injury may have vague symptoms of instability without significant pain or swelling. When present, pain may be described as a dull aching or stiffness. On careful questioning, a history of trauma to the anterior knee is usually noted.

Since a majority of PCL injuries occur in association with other knee injuries, especially an LCL sprain, it is important to obtain as much information as possible about the position of the knee and leg at the time of injury. Discovering the mechanism of injury is also important in determining the likelihood of an isolated PCL injury versus a combination injury. Treatment and prognosis of the two types of injury are different. As expected, combination injuries require more extensive treatment and have a more guarded prognosis.

Physical Examination. An examination begins with the patient lying supine with the legs semiflexed. The examiner inspects the knee for swelling, obvious injury, discoloration, or any abnormal alignment, comparing the injured knee with the uninjured one. A patient with a PCL injury may have only a mild effusion, but a moderate knee effusion is not unusual. Because of the force required to injure the PCL, anterior knee lacerations or contusions, indicating a significant force to the knee, are not uncommon. Lacerations around the knee, especially deep ones, should be suspected of communicating with the joint. An open joint is an orthopedic emergency, and these patients should be immediately referred. Bruising over the posterolateral knee may be present. Obvious unilateral malalignment of the knee indicates a serious pathologic condition, and the patient must be immobilized or limited to non–weight-bearing activities and immediately referred to an orthopedic surgeon.

Palpation of the knee is necessary to assess joint line, patellar, and ligamentous tenderness. If any of these structures are painful, additional injury may be present. Pain and swelling of the knee may make ROM difficult to evaluate.

Tests used to specifically evaluate the PCL include the posterior drawer, Godfrey's (see Figure 7-24), and quadriceps active tests. The posterior drawer test is the most accurate clinical test for identifying PCL injury.[25] This test is described earlier in this chapter in the Posterior Cruciate Ligament section.

The quadriceps active test is more difficult to interpret than the posterior drawer or Godfrey's test. Once again the patient is lying supine with the knee flexed to 90 degrees and the foot flat on the table. While the practitioner views from the side, the patient is asked to contract the quadriceps muscle. The quadriceps active test is

positive when there is visible anterior movement of the tibia on the femur. This movement occurs because the torn PCL cannot stabilize the knee against the force of the quadriceps contraction.

Diagnosis. A careful history regarding mechanism of injury, combined with physical findings, will provide most of the information necessary to diagnose a torn PCL. Plain x-ray films, including AP, lateral, and intercondylar notch views, will add information about bony avulsions or fractures near the knee.[25] A fibular head fracture may indicate injury to the joint capsule.

MRI is the best available test to evaluate the PCL itself. Other soft-tissue injuries, such as LCL or ACL tears and meniscal tears, are also visualized best on an MRI. The expense of MRI is its primary limitation.

Treatment. Treatment of an isolated PCL tear is controversial.[3,58,91] Many patients do well with conservative treatment and PT. However, the high incidence of associated injuries often makes surgical intervention the treatment of choice. Any significant bony avulsions should be surgically repaired. The choice of treatment options should be left to an orthopedic surgeon.

Rehabilitation after PCL repair should include quadriceps strengthening, power-enhancing exercises, and endurance training. Rehabilitation may take as long as six months. Residual PCL laxity may be present even after the person returns to activities and MRI appearance shows healing.[38] In a young, physically active patient, emphasis should be placed on any sport-specific skills the patient may request.

Meniscus Injuries

Tears to the meniscus frequently occur in activities that require twisting, jumping, cutting, and rapid deceleration. Football, soccer, basketball, lacrosse, skiing, and tennis are all commonly implicated as sports prone to causing meniscal damage. Most patients who sustain sport-related meniscus injuries are younger than age 40. Degenerative meniscus tears are more common in patients older than age 40.

Injury in either age group can occur with as simple an action as standing from a kneeling or squatting position. When the knee is rotated as it extends, the medial meniscus can become caught between the femoral condyles. Many different types of tears can occur (Figure 7-34, A-D).

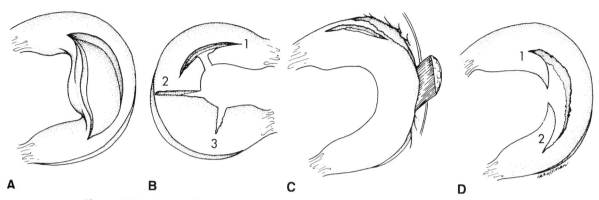

Figure 7-34   Types of Meniscus Tears. A, Bucket handle tear. **B,** Radial tears, including *(1)* "parrot beak" tear, *(2)* complete radial tear, and *(3)* incomplete tear. **C,** Peripheral tear. **D,** Oblique tears, including *(1)* posterior tear and *(2)* anterior tear. (From Canale ST, editor: *Campbell's operative orthopaedics,* ed 10, vol 4, St Louis, 2003, Mosby.)

Even though the lateral meniscus carries most of the knee load, the medial meniscus, which is responsible for distributing the load between the meniscus and articular cartilage, is more frequently injured. The posterior horn of the medial meniscus is the area most frequently damaged. Damage to the medial meniscus is often seen in conjunction with MCL injury, to which it attaches via the joint capsule. The lateral meniscus is not as firmly anchored and is thereby afforded some protection from the rotational forces that usually cause injury.

History.   Typically the predominant complaint after some type of twisting injury is knee pain. Pain is usually fairly well localized to the joint line. Swelling develops within the first 24 hours after injury, often within the first 4 to 6 hours.

OA of the knee is associated with degenerative changes of the menisci, and meniscal damage in the lateral compartment may be worse than damage to the corresponding articular cartilage.[6] Patients with degenerative tears may not have any particular incident that precedes the onset of symptoms. Pain and swelling tend to develop over several weeks to a few months.

Regardless of the cause of the injury, symptoms are usually of locking, catching, or a giving way of the knee.[85] Pain or a feeling of instability when descending stairs is not unusual. Climbing stairs is usually not as difficult as descending. Sometimes patients will feel a click in the knee, especially with certain movements. Activities associated with rotation or twisting of the knee, such as entering or exiting a vehicle or pivoting to turn with the foot of the affected leg planted on the ground, tend to exacerbate pain.

Locking of the knee occurs when a meniscal fragment or the flap of a tear becomes caught between the femur and tibia. When this occurs the knee cannot be flexed or extended.[75] Sometimes having the patient sit with the leg hanging over the edge of the table, then rotating the tibia back and forth, will release the fragment.[74] A "catching" of the knee also occurs when a fragment of meniscus is caught in the joint, but in this case it is not trapped. Giving way is not specific to meniscal injury but is commonly associated with it.

Symptoms of a torn meniscus may not improve; rather, they often increase over time. In individuals with OA of the knee, meniscal tears may be completely asymptomatic.[10] Many knee injuries, including collateral ligament sprains, tend to improve over a period of several weeks. Meniscus injuries, because of poor blood supply, may become more symptomatic and result in persistent, intermittent swelling in conjunction with pain.

Physical Examination.   The examination begins with the patient in a supine position. Both knees are examined, and any swelling or discoloration is noted.

The examiner will look for evidence of muscle asymmetry, because atrophy of the quadriceps, especially the vastus medialis, can quickly develop after knee injury. Measurement of quadriceps atrophy is performed by palpating the superior border of the patella, measuring upward 10 cm, and marking the distal thigh. At that mark the thigh circumference is measured. Any difference between the two thighs greater than 1.5 cm is significant. The practitioner also assesses collateral ligament stability, because the patient with an MCL sprain can have signs similar to those of the patient with a torn meniscus.

Palpation of the knee and its supporting structures will localize areas of tenderness and induration. Tibial joint line tenderness often indicates the location of a tear. With the patient supine and his or her knee flexed to 90 degrees with the foot flat on the table, the joint line is opened up, which makes pain in the tibial joint line easier to differentiate from pain in the femoral joint line. Caution must be exercised when interpreting the presence of joint line tenderness; pain with palpation over the medial tibial joint line also often occurs in the case of an MCL sprain.

Several more specific tests are commonly used to confirm a meniscal tear. McMurray's test (see Figure 7-25) is generally still considered the most important clinical test for meniscal injury.[75] Without some experience in performing these tests, the practitioner must review their interpretation cautiously. Even experienced surgeons can have difficulty clinically diagnosing meniscus tears.[50]

To test the lateral meniscus, the practitioner locates the most tender area of the lateral tibial joint line and rests his or her thumb there. McMurray's test is then performed, again repeating the test several times with varying degrees of flexion to allow evaluation of a greater area of the lateral meniscus.

Apley's (see Figure 7-26) compression test is also commonly used to test the meniscus. For this test the patient lies prone with the knee flexed to 90 degrees. The practitioner then applies downward pressure on the patient's heel while internally and externally rotating the tibia. The test is positive if knee pain occurs with tibial rotation.

Diagnosis. Patient history and a clinical examination are not always sufficient to accurately identify a meniscal tear. MRI is the diagnostic modality of choice for evaluating internal derangement of the knee. It is useful for evaluating cartilage, ligaments, and bone abnormalities. MRI is noninvasive and painless, but it is also expensive, and claustrophobic patients may have difficulty tolerating the closed area of conventional MRI. Other than the expense, perhaps the primary limitation of MRI is the radiologist's expertise in interpreting the images. MRI is not 100% accurate. Due to complex anatomy in the region, tears in the posterior horn of the medial and lateral menisci are often difficult to accurately visualize on MRI.[77]

Treatment. Referral to an orthopedic surgeon is necessary for treatment of a known or suggested meniscal tear. Surgical repair, usually performed arthroscopically, is the treatment of choice for most meniscal tears. There are a variety of repair techniques, including partial or total menisectomy, debridement, or suturing. Tissue engineering, using biological scaffolds, growth factor therapy, cell culture, and gene therapy present potentially revolutionary approaches to the treatment of meniscal tears.[52] If a tear is shown to be in the outer third, or the red zone, of the meniscus, the cartilage can be left to repair itself. However, most tears cross into the avascular portion of the meniscus and will not heal by themselves.

INFLAMMATORY CONDITIONS

TENDINOPATHY

Inflammation of the patellar or quadriceps tendons can be the result of either acute trauma or repeated overuse, but most overuse injuries result in degenerative changes to the tendon. Histopathologically there is an absence of inflammatory cells. The term *tendinopathy* encompasses both acute and chronic conditions.[71] The term *jumper's knee* is frequently used to describe an overuse tendinopathy. Tendinopathies affect the patellar more often than the quadriceps tendon. The patellar tendon near the inferior pole of the patella is the site most frequently affected, followed by the quadriceps tendon, and finally the patellar tendon at its attachment at the tibial tuberosity.[71]

Trauma in the form of a fall onto a hard surface with the knee flexed can result in local inflammation of the patellar tendon. Other causes of tendinopathy around the knee include malalignment syndromes, abnormal patellar location (i.e., patella alta or baja), and tightness of the quadriceps muscle. These conditions all increase stress forces on the patellar and quadriceps tendons.

History. Onset of pain is often insidious. Knee pain that is worse with climbing stairs, squatting, kneeling, and standing after sitting is the predominant complaint. Pain can range from occurring only after certain activities to being almost constant. A history of participating in sports that require sudden, forceful jumping such as ballet, soccer, or volleyball is not unusual. Jumping, kicking, and climbing activities also tend to affect the quadriceps tendon.[24] Little swelling is usually visible, but the patient may complain of a feeling of swelling or fullness.

Physical Examination. With the patient supine, the extended knees are evaluated for swelling, malalignment, or discoloration. Significant visible swelling is unusual in patellar and quadriceps tendinopathy; its presence may indicate a prepatellar bursitis or quadriceps tear. In quadriceps tendinopathy, resisted extension of the knee is painful and may be somewhat weak. The primary finding on examination is tenderness with palpation of the affected tendon; tenderness will increase when the affected tendon is stressed. A thickened patellar tendon may occasionally be palpable. Unless there is an associated injury, the remainder of the knee examination is usually normal.

Diagnosis. Physical examination and history are usually sufficient to make an accurate diagnosis. If symptoms are related to an acute injury, plain AP and lateral x-ray views can be used to rule out osteophytes or avulsion fractures of the patellar tendon insertion. Ultrasound can be useful in evaluating tendon pathology.[33,35] MRI can identify subclinical tears or degradation of the tendon.

Treatment. Treatment depends on the severity of symptoms. Mild cases of tendinopathy usually respond to rest, local application of ice after activities that exacerbate symptoms, NSAIDs, and stretching exercises. More severe forms of tendinopathy that interfere with normal daily activities require more involved treatment.

In these cases a formal PT program that stretches and strengthens the muscles should be employed, as well as isometric exercises and local measures to decrease pain. NSAIDs are also helpful in decreasing inflammation and pain. Recovery time is usually 3 to 4 weeks, but it may be longer depending on the patient's compliance and normal activities.

BURSITIS

Bursae are endothelial-lined, padlike sacs usually found near and sometimes communicating with nearby joints. Some bursae, called constant bursae, are formed during embryonic development and are lined with synovial cells. These bursae reduce friction by the secretion of a lubricating fluid called synovia. Bursae that form between areas of friction are called adventitious bursae. These types of bursae do not produce synovial fluid and are not lined with endothelial cells, but adventitious bursae also function to reduce friction.

Inflammation of the bursae can be the result of acute trauma (e.g., hemorrhagic bursitis), chronic irritation (e.g., as from kneeling or crawling), systemic illness (e.g., syphilis, scleroderma), infection, or crystal deposition (e.g., gout, rheumatoid arthritis, tuberculosis, thyroid disease). Numerous bursae are located around the knee (see Figure 7-16). The bursae most commonly affected by bursitis are the prepatellar and pes anserine bursae, and those of the MCL and the medial gastrocnemius and semimembranosus muscles. The latter two bursae are located in the popliteal space and are sometimes called popliteal cysts.

Prepatellar Bursitis

History. Prepatellar bursitis, often called housemaid's knee, is probably the most common bursitis of the knee. It is usually associated with repetitive kneeling and can be an acute or a chronic problem. The prepatellar bursa is often the site of a septic bursitis. Patients usually experience anterior knee swelling and pain with kneeling, squatting, or crawling. Unless there is a history of acute trauma, symptoms tend to begin insidiously. Some patients have minimal pain and instead may report a feeling of numbness. There may be warmth over the joint, and erythema is common. Increasingly noticeable swelling over the anterior knee and inability to kneel on the affected knee are the most common symptoms.

Prepatellar bursitis is more likely to become chronic than the other forms of bursitis of the knee. After one or more acute episodes, the bursa may become thickened and boggy to the touch. Continued pain with kneeling or crawling may become a major problem for tile and carpet layers, plumbers, electricians, and others whose jobs require squatting, kneeling, and crawling.

Hemorrhagic bursitis is most often associated with an acute trauma but can also be the result of chronic trauma. In the latter case, swelling and pain begin insidiously and progress over weeks to months. If the condition has persisted for some time, actual clots may form, producing the appearance of a soft-tissue mass.

Physical Examination. Anterior knee swelling is the cardinal sign of prepatellar bursitis. Swelling obliterates the normal anterior contour of the patella, but the superior patellar border is normal. Erythema and localized tenderness may be pronounced. The prepatellar bursa does not communicate with the knee joint, so movement of the knee does not increase pain, and ROM is minimally limited, if at all.

Diagnosis. In diagnosing prepatellar bursitis it is most critical not to miss a septic joint. For an experienced practitioner, history and physical examination are usually sufficient to make an accurate diagnosis. If there is any question regarding the diagnosis, the patient should be immediately referred to an orthopedic surgeon or emergency department.

Aspiration of the bursa will allow a preliminary differentiation between inflammatory, hemorrhagic, and septic bursitis. Inflammatory bursitis will produce a clear to slightly yellow or pink-tinged serous fluid. Hemorrhagic bursitis results in bloody (usually dark) fluid. Cloudy or purulent aspirate may indicate an infected bursa.

Treatment. If there is any suggestion of infection, the aspirate obtained is sent for Gram's stain and culture, and antibiotics that treat *Staphylococcus aureus* are prescribed; s*taphylococcus aureus* is the most common infecting organism in prepatellar bursitis.[21] The patient should be referred to an orthopedic surgeon or an emergency department for definitive treatment.

Sufficient treatment of a hemorrhagic bursa is usually provided by aspiration, followed by an application of a compression dressing, a short course of NSAIDs, and avoidance of kneeling, squatting, and crawling. Corticosteroid injection is generally not recommended for hemorrhagic bursitis.

Chronic bursitis may require surgical drainage if the blood cannot be aspirated. If pain and swelling have become chronic, surgical excision of the bursa can be performed to relieve symptoms.

Inflammatory bursitis can be treated with a corticosteroid injection after aspiration and a short course of NSAIDs. Extreme caution must be used in deciding whether to use a corticosteroid injection, because an infection will proliferate in the presence of a steroid. Patients requiring corticosteroid injection should be referred to an orthopedic surgeon.

Pes Anserine Bursitis

Pain and swelling over the medial knee below the tibial joint are typical of pes anserine bursitis. This type of bursitis is frequently associated with OA of the knee. Overweight, middle-aged women and athletes who run or jump are prone to pes anserine bursitis.

On examination there is swelling, pain, and tenderness over the anteromedial knee. Tenderness to palpation is present over the edematous area, usually 4 to 5 cm below the tibial joint line. Examination of the collateral ligaments helps differentiate between bursitis and an MCL injury.

Treatment begins with rest, application of ice, and NSAIDs. Stretching and strengthening exercises of the knee and hamstrings are helpful in avoiding future attacks. Corticosteroid injection usually alleviates most symptoms, but the proximity of the sartorius, gracilis, and semitendinosus tendons necessitates great caution[4] in administering an injection.

SEPTIC JOINT

Infection of any joint is an orthopedic emergency. If left untreated, some bacteria can destroy a joint within 24 hours. In the adult knee, two of the most common causes of infectious arthritis are an infected bursitis and a gonococcal infection. Acute open trauma can also cause joint infection. Persons with chronic joint inflammation (e.g., rheumatoid arthritis) or those who are immunocompromised are also at risk for joint infection. Mycobacteria, fungi, and bacteria may be responsible for a septic joint in the patient with human immunodeficiency virus. Symptoms may be minimal if the patient is already receiving NSAID therapy.

History. Acute onset of a red, painful, and swollen joint is the presenting symptom of nongonococcal infection of the knee. Systemic symptoms of fever, chills, nausea, and malaise are common. Recent infections, especially urethritis, cystitis, or a dental abscess, increase the likelihood of a septic joint. Gonorrheal infection should be suspected if there is a recent history of urethritis, salpingitis, or a vesicular skin rash.

Physical Examination. The patient usually has great difficulty bearing weight on the affected extremity. Inspection shows an inflamed, hot, erythematous, and acutely tender joint. ROM is frequently limited and pain is marked. Gonococcal infection often presents as a migratory arthritis, without overt findings of acute joint pathology.

Diagnosis. History and a physical examination form the basis of a presumptive diagnosis of a septic joint. Definitive diagnosis is made by joint aspiration. Fluid must be sent for immediate Gram's stain and culture. Synovial fluid should also be evaluated for cell count with differential, uric acid, glucose, and protein. A synovial white blood cell count of at least 50,000 mm^3 is highly suggestive of infection. Cultures of blood, sputum, urine, and any open wounds should also be obtained. If aspiration of the knee cannot be performed immediately, the patient should be referred to an emergency department or orthopedic surgeon.

Treatment. Once cultures of synovial fluid and other sites have been obtained, initial parenteral antibiotic therapy to treat staphylococcus and gonorrhea is prescribed. In-hospital treatment that includes intravenous antibiotics is often necessary. Daily joint aspirations for Gram's stain and culture should be performed.

POPLITEAL CYSTS

The bursa beneath the medial head of the gastrocnemius often develops a valve-type communication with the knee joint. This communication can result in popliteal swelling, a condition known as a Baker's cyst (Figure 7-35). A true Baker's cyst is located in the posteromedial area of the knee between the semimembranosus muscle and the medial head of the gastrocnemius muscle.[28] Commonly, however, the term "Baker's cyst" refers to any popliteal cyst.

Most popliteal cysts develop over time, but acute trauma has also been associated with their appearance. Cysts can vary from a single, fluid-filled cavity to a lobulated mass. Most Baker's cysts are associated with other knee abnormalities, especially medial meniscus tears; OA and, to a lesser extent, rheumatoid arthritis also frequently accompany them. Baker's cysts occur with higher frequency in the older adult, although they can also occur in children.[39]

Spontaneous rupture of a Baker's cyst is not uncommon. The result is intense pain, and it is often accompanied by swelling and bruising of the calf as fluid tracks along the myofascial planes. Although often frightening for the patient, spontaneous rupture of a Baker's cyst usually does not damage the structures of the knee. Treatment is symptomatic and focuses on relieving pain

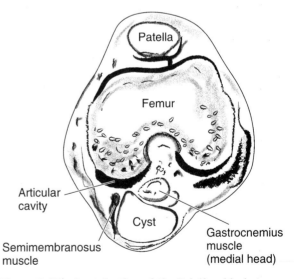

Figure 7-35 Cross Section of the Relationship between a Baker's Cyst and the Knee Joint. The cyst is more commonly found toward the medial side of the joint. (From Canale ST, editor: *Campbell's operative orthopaedics*, ed 10, vol 3, St Louis, 2003, Mosby.)

and decreasing activities until symptoms resolve. Pain gradually subsides over a few weeks.

The overall history and clinical appearance of a ruptured Baker's cyst is similar to a deep vein thrombosis (DVT). Differentiating these two entities is critical. Pain from a DVT is more likely to occur after immobilization or sitting for some hours. Pain from a ruptured Baker's cyst usually occurs with some activity, even walking. A positive Homans' sign, which consists of calf pain or tenderness when the foot is dorsiflexed while the knee is extended, is strongly suggestive of a DVT.

In the presence of a ruptured Baker's cyst, Homans' sign is usually negative. Unfortunately, Homans' sign is often subjective and therefore is not definitive for differentiating between a DVT and a ruptured popliteal cyst. Some patients with a ruptured cyst will report pain with Homans' sign. Objective differentiation, usually through ultrasonography, is necessary.

History. Most patients will report swelling, pressure or fullness behind the knee as their primary complaint. Pain may be present to varying degrees, and movement of the knee tends to increase symptoms. The size of the cyst may be more prominent after certain activities, such as prolonged walking, climbing, or descending stairs. Patients may express a concern about a tumor or a possible blood clot behind the knee.

Physical Examination. The appearance of popliteal cysts is highly variable, ranging from a normal-appearing area to a large, firm mass. Most popliteal cysts are not palpable. There is usually no significant discoloration, and tenderness may be more prominent over the proximal gastrocnemius muscles than over the popliteal fossa. Examination of the remainder of the knee may provide clues about additional pathologic conditions.

Diagnosis. Ultrasound is useful in differentiating a popliteal cyst from a DVT or thrombophlebitis. The test is relatively inexpensive, noninvasive, has a high degree of accuracy, and can distinguish complicated cysts from phlebitis.[39] If additional knee abnormality is suggested, MRI is useful. An arthrogram or a venogram can be performed, but they are invasive and can be painful for the patient. Another caution is that the dye itself may distend the normal bursa, causing a false-positive test. An MRI, though expensive, is noninvasive and better than arthrography for distinguishing cysts from tumors or effusion.

Treatment. Treatment of an isolated popliteal cyst is often benign neglect. The patient should be reassured that the cyst is not a tumor and that changes in size are normal. Aspiration or injection of corticosteroids into the cyst usually results in only temporary relief, and the cyst will often recur.

Treatment of a ruptured Baker's cyst is symptomatic: application of ice in the first 48 hours, use of mild analgesics such as acetaminophen or NSAIDs, and maintenance of mild physical activity. Pain and swelling generally resolve within 1 to 2 weeks. The patient should be cautioned that a Baker's cyst has a tendency to recur.

If additional knee abnormality is suggested or confirmed, the patient should be referred to an orthopedic surgeon. When repair of the underlying disorder is accomplished, the cyst usually resolves. Some surgeons may elect to repair the cyst at the time of arthroscopy for associated pathologic conditions.

ILIOTIBIAL BAND SYNDROME

Lateral knee pain, especially in athletes who participate in endurance sports such as running and cycling, may be attributable to ITB syndrome. The ITB is a tendinous band that extends from above the hip to below the knee (see Figure 7-5). Its function is to maintain lateral stability of the knee. When the knee is extended, the ITB is anterior to the lateral femoral condyle. As the knee is flexed beyond 30 degrees, the band moves from its anterior position to a position posterior to the lateral femoral condyle. Pain over the lateral femoral condyle with running, especially downhill, can be caused by irritation and inflammation from the band's friction over the lateral femoral condyle.[71] The ITB is also susceptible to sudden changes in tension as it is stressed by falls or twisting injuries; as a result, tendonitis can develop.

Patients with mild lower extremity malalignment or a tight ITB are more likely to develop ITB syndrome, since either condition increases the friction between the ITB and lateral femoral condyle. Malalignments may include genu varum, forefoot supination with compensatory pronation of the heel, or an unusually prominent lateral femoral condyle. Tightness of the ITB may arise from forces placed on it by its attached muscles. Weakness of the hip abductor muscles may cause ITB friction syndrome.[34] Proximally the gluteus maximus muscle, which attaches to the posterior side, and the tensor fascia lata muscle, which attaches anteriorly, keep the ITB in place by exerting opposite pulls on the band. The short head of the biceps femoris muscle has its origin at the distal aspect of the band. When one of these muscles exerts an abnormal pull or is strained, pain in the ITB can be the result.

History. Onset of pain is usually insidious but worsens progressively as endurance activities (especially running) continue. Running on banked surfaces or climbing stairs may aggravate symptoms. Pain is usually described as a burning or tightness localized to the lateral femoral condyle. There is no instability, locking, or catching of the knee. The patient rarely notices swelling, and there is usually no discoloration. Patients sometimes report grinding or snapping over the lateral knee.

Physical Examination. On examination, localized tenderness to palpation over the lateral femoral condyle is the predominant finding of ITB syndrome. The best place to palpate for pain is 2 to 3 cm proximal to the lateral joint line.

Ober's test is commonly used to test the tightness of the ITB (Figure 7-36, *A-C*). To perform the test, the patient should be lying on his or her side with the affected side up. The practitioner stands behind the patient and holds the hip in slight extension. With the knee flexed to approximately 90 degrees, the practitioner grasps the patient's ankle, places the upper leg into passive abduction and extension, and then slowly lowers the leg. If the ITB is tight, the hip will remain passively abducted; this is a positive Ober's test. Another test that may elicit pain symptoms is full weight bearing with the knee flexed to 30 degrees.

Another way to test the ITB is to have the patient supine while the practitioner places his or her thumb over the lateral epicondyle of the knee. The knee is actively flexed and extended by the patient while the practitioner palpates the lateral epicondyle. This test is known as Noble's compression test. Pain is usually greatest at 30 degrees of flexion.

Diagnosis. History and physical examination usually provide adequate information for diagnosis. Ultrasound or MRI can also be used to diagnose ITB syndrome, but these tests are generally not necessary.

Differential Diagnosis. Pain and tenderness extending more proximally over the lateral thigh may be caused by biceps femoris tendonitis. Care must be taken to rule out a nerve root irritation, especially at L5. Lateral subluxation of the patella, degenerative arthritis, iliotibial tract bursitis, and lateral meniscus injury can all cause lateral knee pain. With the exception of bursitis, the other abnormalities tend to cause pain at the knee joint rather than lateral to it. In the case of iliotibial tract bursitis, symptoms can be identical to ITB syndrome. Injection of a local anesthetic into the bursa, with or without a corticosteroid, can help differentiate the two.

Treatment. Rest, application of ice, NSAIDs, and PT to stretch the ITB usually have a favorable response. Ultrasound and electrical muscle stimulation can help improve blood flow to the area and promote healing. Once the acute phase has subsided, patient education is aimed at preventing recurrent episodes. Avoidance of downhill running, correction of excessive foot pronation, and proper footwear can reduce friction of the ITB over the lateral femoral condyle. If symptoms persist more than six months in spite of conservative therapy, surgery should be considered.[71]

OSTEOCHONDRITIS DISSECANS

The term *osteochondritis dissecans* literally means dry, inflamed bone. Although not an absolutely accurate term, osteochondritis dissecans generally refers to a lesion that involves separation of cartilage and subchondral bone on an articular surface.[83] The knee is the most frequent site of the disease. In addition to the knee, the condition can affect the elbow, the ankle, the femoral head, and the wrist. The exact cause is unknown but it may be related to cumulative microtrauma of the joint.[18]

There are two forms of osteochondritis dissecans (OCD)—adult and juvenile (JOCD). The distinguishing feature between the two is whether the epiphyseal plate is closed. The prognosis for JOCD is better than for the adult form.[18] The latter rarely heals without surgery.

The disease predominantly affects boys and men between the ages of 10 and 50. It seems to be more common among athletes.[17,18] It usually affects the lateral aspect of the medial femoral condyle; this area is in the intercondylar notch.

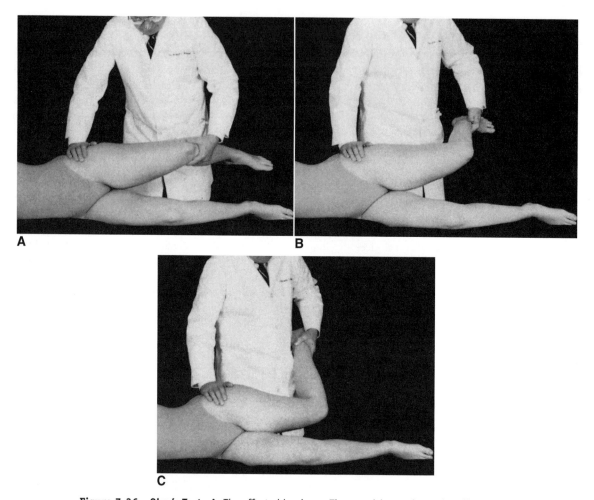

Figure 7-36   Ober's Test. A, The affected leg is up. The practitioner places the affected leg in abduction. **B,** With the knee flexed to 90 degrees, the practitioner extends the hip and asks the patient to adduct the leg. If the leg remains abducted, the test is positive for iliotibial band tightness. **C,** Normal (negative) Ober's test. The leg does not remain abducted. (From Evans RC: *Illustrated orthopedic physical assessment*, ed 2, St Louis, 2001, Mosby.)

History.   There is rarely any distinct event that precipitates the onset of knee pain, locking, and catching. Severity of symptoms is associated with how advanced the process is. For example, initial pain may be vague and intermittent. As the lesion progresses, a feeling of knee instability and swelling may occur. If a fragment has separated from the femur, the patient will usually have worsening symptoms and even complain of "something loose inside my knee." Sudden locking or catching of the knee in extension is a typical description of a loose body in the joint. Knee swelling with activity is not normal and may be an early sign of OCD. Symptoms are similar in both JOCD and adult OCD.

Physical Examination.   If the patient's medial femoral condyle is affected, the patient may walk with the corresponding leg externally rotated to decrease pain. Knee pain is usually diffuse. Unless there is a loose body within the joint, an effusion is rarely present. Loss of full extension can occur when there is a loose body within the joint. The knee may be somewhat warm to the touch, though discoloration is absent. Both the collateral and cruciate ligaments are usually stable to manual stress testing.

Diagnosis. Plain AP, lateral, and notch x-ray views of the knee will allow initial diagnosis of OCD. A small radiolucent area on the femoral condyle identifies the lesion. Usually there is a sclerotic rim around the lesion (Figure 7-37).

Further diagnosis and evaluation of the extent of the lesion is made by MRI. Some physicians will follow progression of the disease with serial bone scans.[17,18] Once an initial diagnosis of OCD has been made, the patient should be referred to an orthopedic surgeon for follow-up and definitive treatment.

Treatment. Adolescent patients are often treated conservatively with decreased activity (no running or jumping) and non–weight-bearing status (i.e., using crutches) for 6 to 8 weeks. During this time the lesion may heal spontaneously, but healing may take as long as 9 to 12 months.[18] The patient will require reevaluation in approximately 2 months to determine whether healing has occurred. Restriction of activity may be neces-

sary for up to a year. If the lesion does not improve, arthroscopic drilling of the lesion may be necessary.

The adult form of OCD is treated more aggressively; once the epiphyseal plates have closed, the odds of the lesion healing spontaneously are poor. Surgical therapy is indicated if there is a loose body in the knee joint.

Generally, arthroscopy is the preferred surgical approach. With arthroscopy, a free fragment can be removed, a partially separated fragment can be re-attached, and an intact area of OCD can be drilled to stimulate blood vessel growth. If the lesion is extensive, open repair may be necessary.

OSGOOD-SCHLATTER DISEASE

Nontraumatic anterior knee pain and swelling in adolescents, especially boys, is often the result of Osgood-Schlatter disease. The most common age for the disease to occur is between 10 and 15; in girls, it is most common between ages 11 and 13. Pain and tenderness over the tibial tubercle at the insertion of the patellar tendon is thought to be caused by excessive traction on an immature apophysis. Although usually unilateral, bilateral involvement can occur.

History. Symptoms tend to worsen with skating, gymnastics, running and jumping activities.[30] Growth

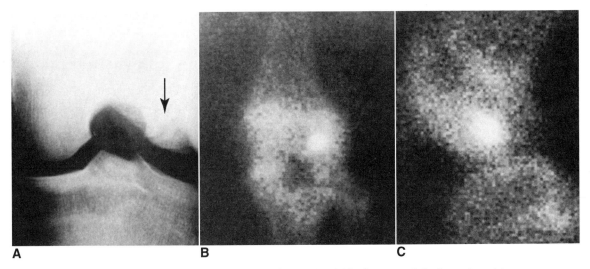

A   B   C

Figure 7-37 Plain x-ray and bone scan of osteochondritis dissecans of the femoral condyle.

spurts may also aggravate symptoms, because rapid bone growth places increased stretching force on the connective tissues around joints. Between episodes, the patient may have few, if any, symptoms. Aspirin or ibuprofen usually relieves pain.

Physical Examination. A prominent tibial tubercle is often present. Both the tibial tubercle and the patellar tendon are usually tender to palpation. Soft-tissue fullness or swelling may also be present. Discoloration, including erythema, is suggestive of a process other than Osgood-Schlatter disease.

Diagnosis. Clinical examination usually provides a presumptive diagnosis. A lateral x-ray film of the knee will confirm Osgood-Schlatter disease by the presence of a characteristic irregular ossification of the tibial tubercle. The tibial tubercle may appear to be separated from the tibial shaft, but it actually is not (Figure 7-38). If there are any angular or sharply defined areas over the tibial tubercle, the possibility of fracture cannot be ruled out. If there is any question about a possible fracture, the patient should be referred to an orthopedic surgeon.

Treatment. Symptomatic treatment during acute episodes consists of rest, application of ice, and sometimes over-the-counter NSAIDs. Physical therapy may be beneficial in maintaining flexibility of the quadriceps and hamstrings.[30] Reassurance of the patient and family is helpful in decreasing anxiety about growth abnormalities. The condition is self-limited, and symptoms will resolve when the tibial tubercle growth plate fuses, usually at about 15 years of age. Occasionally persistent symptoms necessitate surgical intervention.

OSTEOARTHRITIS

OA, the most common form of arthritis, affects more than 28 million people in the United States.[54] Once thought to be purely a degenerative process, the complex pathophysiology of OA involves disruption of colla-

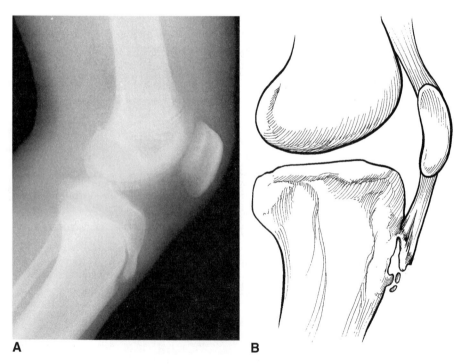

A   **B**

Figure 7-38 Lateral x-ray film and diagrammatic appearance of the knee showing prominent tibial tubercle in Osgood-Schlatter disease.

gen proteoglycans that comprise articular cartilage, followed by cartilage erosions, subchondral bone sclerosis and formation of osteophytes as the mechanical integrity of the joint breaks down.[14,80] Because of these pathophysiologic changes, OA is no longer considered a normal part of the aging process. The disease can affect any adult but is most common after age 50.

Degenerative changes of the knee joint visualized on x-ray films do not necessarily indicate the presence of OA. Most adults will eventually develop some degenerative change of the knees and other weight-bearing joints. Unless these changes are symptomatic, treatment is not specifically tailored for OA. The cause of OA is unknown, but a history of trauma, obesity or chronic valgus deformity of the joint tends to cause earlier onset of degenerative changes in the knee. Genetic factors also play a role.

Pain with weight bearing, which is relieved by rest, is a fairly succinct symptomatic description of OA. Morning stiffness, "gelling" of the knee, and cracking or grinding are also symptomatic of OA. Specific criteria for diagnosing OA of the knee have been established by the American College of Rheumatology.[41] The primary criteria necessary for a diagnosis of OA and subsequent treatment are knee pain and radiographic osteophytes and at least one of the following: an age over 50, morning stiffness lasting 30 minutes or less, or crepitus on motion. To make the diagnosis in patients younger than age 50, it is sufficient to establish the presence of knee pain, an age of at least 40, morning stiffness that lasts less than 30 minutes, and crepitus with movement.

OA of the knee may affect the medial or the lateral joint compartments, the patellofemoral joint, or any combination of these three areas. In the medial joint, degenerative changes cause a narrowing of the joint space, eventually resulting in a varus deformity. A valgus knee deformity occurs with lateral compartment involvement. The presence of more than 5 degrees of either knee deformity is associated with worsening disease and decreased physical function.[86]

History. The patient with OA usually has a long history of morning stiffness, crepitus with movement, and a gel-like feeling in the joints. Many patients do not seek treatment until pain becomes a problem. Unlike many knee complaints, the pain associated with OA is not always attributable to inflammation. Usually more than one joint is involved, since OA primarily affects weight-bearing joints. Before a diagnosis of OA is made, the patient's symptoms should correspond to the guidelines of the American College of Rheumatology.

Physical Examination. The knee joint appears large, but the increased size is usually caused by bony hypertrophy rather than by fluid or soft-tissue swelling. Bony hypertrophy is palpable at the knee joint. A painless effusion can occur. There is no discoloration or temperature difference unless the knee has also been subjected to some trauma, however minor. Limited ROM, most often flexion, is typical.

Crepitus with flexion and extension of the knee is one of the cardinal signs of OA. A positive patellar grind test, or shrug sign, occurs when there is knee pain when the patella is manually pushed against the femoral condyles as the patient contracts his or her quadriceps. A positive shrug sign is typical of patellofemoral arthritis.

Diagnosis. History, physical examination, and x-ray studies confirm the diagnosis of OA. Laboratory tests are usually normal. X-ray films that include an AP view and either a lateral or skyline view will show joint space narrowing and osteophytes (i.e., spurring) of the medial, femoral, or patellofemoral joints.[22] Persons over age 50 should have standing AP x-rays for more accurate visualization of the joint.[23] Several grading systems are used to stage progression of OA, but none is perfect. According to the most common system used today, which was proposed a half-century ago,[47] OA is categorized into four stages (Figure 7-39). Stage I is mild, with no osteophytes. The presence of bony sclerosis, osteophytes, and asymmetric joint space narrowing correlates with moderate (stage II) OA. Stage III shows moderately severe changes, including bone cysts and osteoporosis. In severe disease (stage IV), cartilage has eroded and there is bone-on-bone appearance on x-ray films. If unable to perform normal activities of daily living, patients with stage IV disease should be referred to an orthopedic surgeon for joint replacement.

Treatment. As yet, there is no cure for OA, so the goals of treatment are to reduce pain, maintain and/or improve joint mobility, and limit functional impairment.[4] Many patients with OA of the knee can be successfully managed with conservative treatment. Nonpharmacologic therapy and patient education are

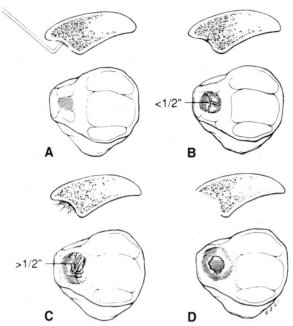

Figure 7-39   Staging of Osteoarthritis of the Knee. A, Stage I: mild OA with joint space narrowing noticeable. **B,** Stage II: moderate OA. Osteophytes are present and joint space narrowing is obvious. **C,** Stage III: moderately severe OA with bony sclerosis evident in addition to changes of stages I and II. **D,** Stage IV: severe OA with "bone-on-bone" appearance. (Modified from Tria AJ, Klein KS: *An illustrated guide to the knee,* New York, 1992, Churchill Livingstone.)

the keystones of therapy. In many communities the Arthritis Foundation sponsors self-help courses. Patients should understand the importance of remaining physically active and may benefit from a course of physical therapy to strengthen the leg muscles, especially the quadriceps. Aerobic activities such as bicycling, walking, or water aerobics programs have been shown to improve symptoms.[4] Weight loss (in overweight individuals), using assistive devices, bracing, occupational therapy, lateral-wedged insoles for correction of varus deformity, appropriate footwear, and patellar taping are all recommended interventions for OA of the knee. Application of cold or heat may reduce or relieve symptoms.

Intraarticular injection of corticosteroids can provide temporary relief of symptoms. Injections of hyaluronic acid into the joint to restore the viscosity of synovial fluid are useful in selected patients.[69] Care must be taken to ensure correct administration into the joint. Referral to a rheumatologist or orthopedic surgeon is appropriate for intraarticular injections.

According to the recommendations by the American College of Rheumatology, pharmacologic management of OA of the knee should be approached in a step-wise manner.[4] Initially, simple analgesics such as acetaminophen or tramadol should be used. Topical analgesics such as capsaicin cream can be added to acetaminophen or can be used as initial therapy in patients who do not respond to or cannot ingest oral therapy agents. Capsaicin cream causes joints to be insensitive to pain by depleting and preventing the accumulation of substance P in the peripheral sensory neurons. The cream should be applied to the symptomatic joint three to four times a day. Patients should be warned that a burning sensation after application is common. Avoiding application immediately after showering or shaving one's legs can reduce the burning sensation.

Nutraceuticals, such as glucosamine or chondroitin, have shown favorable outcomes in reducing pain, improving joint mobility, and slowing OA progression.[15,63,70,72] Other alternative therapies include S-adenosylmethionine (SAMe), ginger, dimethyl sulfoxide (DMSO), boron, and other dietary supplements. Most of these therapies have not been subjected to rigorous, scientifically controlled studies to evaluate their safety and effectiveness.[67]

NSAIDs, including cyclooxygenase-2 (COX-2)–specific inhibitors, are indicated if neither oral nor topical analgesics are successful in controlling symptoms. Opioid therapy may be necessary in some instances. Combination therapy with NSAIDs and analgesics is also appropriate.[4] Other interventions, such as tidal irrigations or other arthroscopic procedures are controversial.[13,29,43,68] Referral to an orthopedic surgeon is indicated if the patient is a candidate for joint replacement surgery.

ACUTE GOUT

Although the first metatarsophalangeal joint is the most common site of gout, the knee is another commonly affected site. With an acutely swollen, painful, erythematous joint, symptoms and signs of gout can easily be mistaken for those of a septic joint; this differential diagnosis is also the most critical one to make. Gout may also be associated with fever and malaise and can be difficult to distinguish clinically from a septic joint.[19,79] A septic joint is an orthopedic emergency. If there is any question whether a red, hot, painful joint is attributable to gout or to infection, the patient must immediately be referred to an emergency department or an orthopedic surgeon.

Hyperuricemia and gout are generally classified into three groups. Primary hyperuricemia is an inherited dis-order of uric acid metabolism. Secondary hyperuricemia occurs as the result of some other metabolic problem, such as glucose-6-phosphatase deficiency, reduced renal function from a number of causes, certain medications that block uric acid excretion, or neoplasms. The third category, idiopathic hyperuricemia, encompasses conditions that do not fit into either of the primary or secondary categories. The presence of hyperuricemia alone does not equal a diagnosis of gout, nor does a normal serum uric acid level exclude the diagnosis.

History. A history of alcohol consumption, lead exposure, obesity, hypertension, hyperuricemia, or use of thiazide diuretics, levodopa, nicotinic acid, low-dose salicylates, or diazoxide makes the diagnosis of gout more likely. Gout is more common among adults older than age 50. In fact, it is the most common inflammatory disease of men older than age 30. Postmenopausal women have a greater risk than younger women; the incidence of gout in postmenopausal women approaches that of men.

An initial gouty attack usually begins acutely, often at night, and awakens the patient with pain and swelling of the joint. The joint is exquisitely tender and even the weight of a sheet causes pain. The knee is red and hot. Weight bearing may also cause pain. The patient may describe a terrific pressure in the joint. Stresses such as recent trauma, significant emotional stress, medical illness, or surgery may be noted before the onset of symptoms. Chronic gout can lead to deposition of monosodium urate crystals in subcutaneous tissues, deposits known as *tophi.* Symptoms and clinical findings in chronic gouty arthritis can be similar to those in rheumatoid arthritis.

Physical Examination. An erythematous, swollen, hot, exquisitely tender knee is the presenting symptom of acute gout. Movement of the knee is often painful. Fever, headache, and tachycardia may be present. The clinical appearance of the joint with acute gout does not differentiate it from an acutely septic joint.

Diagnosis. The clinical suggestion of gout based on history is the first step in reaching a diagnosis. The presence of monosodium urate crystals in joint fluid remains the standard for diagnosing gout.[88] Unfortunately, aspiration of joint fluid is necessary to look for crystals, yet treatment may need to start before analysis. Colchicine or, preferably, an NSAID should be started as soon as possible, and, if warranted, the patient can be referred to a rheumatologist or orthopedic surgeon.

Typical radiographic changes occur with chronic gout, but they are generally absent with the first attack. When present, changes to the joint include an appearance of being "punched out," or of "Mickey Mouse ears," because urate crystals replace bone. There is a narrowing of the joint space, and calcific deposits may form in the meniscus cartilage.

Treatment. Local application of ice can reduce pain and inflammation.[84] High-dose NSAIDs are the treatment of choice for acute gout. An acute gouty attack usually responds to NSAID treatment within 48 to 72 hours. Indomethacin is commonly used, ingested on a schedule of 50 mg three to four times a day until acute symptoms subside. Other NSAIDs, including sulindac, ibuprofen, naproxen, and ketoprofen, have successfully been used. The gastrointestinal and renal side effects of NSAIDs must be considered, especially in the older patient.

Colchicine is prescribed less commonly because of its numerous side effects and narrow therapeutic range. Up to 80% of patients taking a full dose of colchicine will experience watery diarrhea, abdominal cramping, and nausea or vomiting.

Intraarticular corticosteroid injection is highly effective in treating acute gout. Unfortunately, the symptoms of acute gout and a septic joint can be similar enough to warrant extreme caution in considering joint injection. Corticosteroid injection into a septic joint is likely to have disastrous results.

Long-term dietary changes are often included in gout management. Patient consultation with a nutritionist is extremely helpful in planning weight loss and/or a low-purine diet that may decrease the incidence of attacks and should be considered as a first line of treatment.[73,93]

Pseudogout

The presence of calcium pyrophosphate dihydrate crystals in the knee's articular cartilage can cause symptoms almost identical to those of acute gout. The disease is also known as chondrocalcinosis because of its characteristic radiographic appearance. On x-ray films there are thin, linear calcifications visible in the cartilage.

Pseudogout is associated with a number of metabolic disorders, including hemochromatosis, hyperparathyroidism, and diabetes mellitus. There seems to be some familial tendency toward the disease. Treatment is a short course of high-dose NSAIDs or COX-2 inhibitors. Aspiration of the joint and injection of a corticosteroid is often useful in alleviating symptoms. Unlike true gout, the disease generally does not respond to colchicine.

SHIN SPLINTS

Periostitis of the tibia, commonly known as shin splints, is thought to be caused by inflammation at the site of muscle attachments on the tibia. A more specific term is *medial tibial stress syndrome* (MTSS), which is actually a stress reaction within the bone. Tibial stress injuries can be thought of as a continuum ranging from activity-associated pain ("shin splints") to an actual cortical fracture. In the anterior compartment the tibialis anterior, extensor hallucis longus, and extensor digitorum longus muscles eccentrically contract immediately after the heel strike in normal gait. The force of this type of contraction can cause microtears in the muscles and their attachments. The biomechanics of the feet in standing, walking, and running also influence the development and progression of shin splints, particularly in the posteromedial compartment. Training errors, improper footwear, and low bone mass are associated with development of MTSS.[7] Women tend to be more prone to stress fractures in general. The "female athlete triad" of disordered eating, amenorrhea, and osteoporosis may play a role in developing stress fractures.[20]

Individuals with either flat feet (pes planus) or unusually high arches (pes cavus) are more prone to developing shin splints. In the case of flat feet, the heel tends to be in a valgus position, causing an increased stretching of the posterior tibial muscle with walking or running. Excessive pronation of the feet and/or subtalar joint may predispose a person to MTSS.[6,27] Occasionally the foot has an exaggerated pronation with pes planus, and this, too, causes increased stretching of the posterior tibial muscle, resulting in posteromedial tibial pain. Pes cavus tends to be accompanied by a varus position of the heel, causing increased stretching of the peroneal and anterior tibial muscles resulting in anterolateral tibial pain.

Patients who participate in distance running, dancing, hiking, and track and field events such as hurdles or vaulting are prone to developing shin splints. Military recruits are also commonly affected because of the long distances and duration of marching and frequent running. Pain is usually more severe at the beginning of activity; then it tends to diminish as activity continues. Hours after cessation of activity, pain may return. Rest tends to relieve symptoms. Left untreated, stress on the bone can progress to a stress fracture or an actual cortical break.

History. Often patients will report a history of increased duration or intensity of activity before the onset of pain. Typically there is not one specific event that precedes the onset of symptoms. Pain is usually described as a dull, intermittent ache that becomes more constant over time. Obvious swelling, discoloration, numbness, and tingling of the leg are rare complaints. Pain is localized to the posteromedial or anterolateral border of the distal third of the tibia. Although pain is localized, point tenderness is uncommon unless there is a fracture.

Physical Examination. Inspection of the affected leg is usually normal. Soft-tissue swelling over the area of tenderness may at times be present. If swelling is present, comparison should be made with the contralateral leg and leg circumference should be measured. A circumferential difference of greater than 1 cm should be noted.

Exacerbation of symptoms can sometimes be demonstrated by stressing the muscles involved with the pain. In the case of posteromedial pain, the tibialis posterior muscle is involved. This muscle inverts and plantar flexes the foot. Having the patient perform these movements against resistance may reproduce the same pain the patient has with activity. Similarly, resisted dorsiflexion and inversion of the foot can reproduce symptoms over the anterolateral tibia attributable to the stretching of the tibialis anterior muscle.

Diagnosis. History and clinical evaluation are key to diagnosing MTSS. Symptoms are usually typical with regard to their onset and association with a specific activity. Clinical differentiation of MTSS and tibial stress fracture is difficult. A clinical test that may help is percussion of the tibia away from the site of pain. If pain occurs with this remote percussion, stress fracture is suggested. If pain does not occur, MTSS is more likely. Bone scan is extremely sensitive for detecting inflamma-

tion in both cases. A typical longitudinal uptake of tracer only on delayed images of a triple-phase bone scan is seen with MTSS.[27]

Treatment. Cessation of activities specifically associated with the onset of pain is often all that is necessary in cases of mild shin splints. Any abnormal biomechanics of the foot must be corrected to reduce symptoms.

Initially NSAIDs may be helpful in decreasing symptoms. Rest, ice, and elevation can also decrease pain. Application of ice to the affected area for 10 to 20 minutes after the activity often reduces pain. Stretching and strengthening the affected muscle groups while cross training is useful in maintaining conditioning. Swimming, bicycling, and stair stepping can be substituted for running while pain is acute. The patient can begin a gradual return to previous levels of activity 2 to 6 weeks after pain ceases.

Constant pain indicates progression to a stage that requires even greater restriction of weight-bearing activities. These patients can be treated with a combination of non–weight bearing (i.e., crutches), PT that includes ice massage and ultrasound, and NSAIDs. Persistent pain in spite of these measures is suggestive of a stress fracture, and a bone scan is indicated. Casting is sometimes used for MTSS.

Severe pain in the tibia is an appropriate reason for orthopedic referral. X-ray studies, though rarely helpful for identifying MTSS, are useful in ruling out bony abnormalities such as tumors. Surgical intervention may alleviate symptoms, but success is varied.[1,27]

Treatment of abnormal foot and ankle biomechanics is the critical issue in treating shin splints attributable to excessive foot pronation or supination or to pes planus or pes cavus. Referral for fabrication of custom orthotics to correct the underlying problem will usually correct shin splints. NSAIDs and PT with modalities such as ultrasound and phonophoresis, in addition to therapeutic exercise, are also helpful in reducing symptoms.

COMPARTMENT SYNDROME

One of the less common but more serious afflictions of the leg is compartment syndrome, a set of symptoms described as a condition in which increased interstitial pressure within a closed space compromises neurovascular and muscular structures within that space.[44,60] A tough, inelastic fascia covers the body's muscle compartments. When muscle swelling occurs in one of these compartments, the fascia restricts physical expansion and as a result, pressure within the compartment increases. Although compartment syndrome also occurs in the arm, hand, thigh, and foot, the leg is by far the most common site.

Increased pressure in a muscle compartment can be caused by decreased compartment size, brought about by overly tight dressings or casts or by prolonged limb compression; this can be the result, for example, of lying in an awkward position on a hard surface for an extended period of time. Increased compartmental pressure can also be attributable to fracture, hemorrhage, increased capillary permeability or increased capillary pressure, inflammation from venomous bites, crush injury, and even muscle hypertrophy.

Direct trauma to the leg is the most easily recognized cause of compartment syndrome. Even nontraumatic soft tissue swelling can result in compartment syndrome, although rarely.[92] Compartment syndrome can also occur after knee or leg surgery and can be either acute or chronic. In the primary care setting, chronic compartment syndrome is far more common than the acute form.

Exertional compartment syndrome (ECS) and march gangrene are common terms used to describe chronic compartment syndrome. Intensive exercise can cause muscle fiber swelling, increased intracompartmental blood volume, and capillary pressure in a muscle compartment, to the point that vascular and neurovascular function are compromised.

Vascular compromise is caused by increased pressure in the intracompartmental veins and the tissue around the veins. The net result is a decrease in the normal arteriovenous pressure gradient, thus reducing local blood flow. When local blood flow is reduced beyond the critical level, the tissue loses viability. Even under these circumstances, intracompartmental pressure usually remains less than arterial pressure. As a result, distal arterial blood flow and peripheral pulses are often intact.

Symptoms of compartment syndrome depend on which leg compartment is involved. Table 7-3 summarizes some of the key findings associated with various compartment involvement. The anterior compartment is most often involved in ECS.[45]

TABLE 7-3   Clinical Findings Associated with Compartment Syndrome

Compartment	Key Structures	Clinical Findings
Anterior	Deep peroneal nerve Tibialis anterior muscle Extensor hallucis longus muscle Extensor digitorum longus muscle Peroneus tertius muscle	Weak or no active dorsiflexion of foot Tender, tense anterolateral leg
Lateral	Superficial, deep peroneal nerves Peroneus longus, brevis muscles	Decreased plantar flexion of foot Decreased sensation over dorsum of foot and first toe web space
Superficial posterior	Tibial nerve Sural nerve Gastrocnemius and soleus muscles Plantaris muscle	Sensory deficit over lateral foot Pain with passive dorsiflexion and active plantar flexion of foot
Deep posterior	Tibial, saphenous nerves Tibialis posterior muscle Flexor digitorum longus muscle Flexor hallucis longus muscle	Pain with passive dorsiflexion of toes and ankle eversion Weak toe flexion Diminished sensation to plantar surface of foot Decreased flexion of the great toe

History. Traumatic injury resulting in significant soft-tissue damage or tibial fracture is often evaluated and treated in a facility other than a primary care setting. Chronic (exertional) compartment syndrome, frequently associated with exercise, is more often seen in primary care.

With ECS, a patient will typically relate a history of leg pain that is associated with running or prolonged, weight-bearing, physical activity. Often the pain is bilateral. Sometimes the patient will report a feeling of fullness along the middle to distal third of the leg or will have abnormal sensation over the dorsum or the plantar aspect of the foot. Pain is not usually debilitating, and activity may continue. After a period of inactivity, pain may subside only to recur several hours later. Pain is typically described as pressure or a deep throbbing or aching sensation.

Physical Examination. The cardinal finding on examination of acute compartment syndrome is a tense, tender, and swollen compartment. Passive movement of the muscles in the involved compartment increases pain.[66] In ECS, physical examination may be normal if the individual is not currently experiencing pain. The classic "six Ps" of compartment syndrome are:

1. Pain is out of proportion to the injury. This symptom is frequently overlooked, and the patient may be labeled as a symptom magnifier or be accused of drug-seeking behavior.
2. Paresis or paralysis of the muscles in the affected compartment may occur secondary to nerve damage or muscle necrosis.
3. Paresthesia of the area supplied by a specific nerve is a reliable finding if the patient is awake and can be examined.
4. Pulses are usually present unless major arterial damage has occurred.
5. Pallor of the digits is unusual unless arterial damage is also present.
6. Pressure in the compartment is the critical symptom. If compartment pressure cannot be measured in the primary care setting, the patient should immediately be referred to an emergency department.

Elevated compartment pressure is a surgical emergency. (The exact point at which intracompartmental pressure becomes dangerous is controversial.[42,65] Generally a compartmental pressure within 30 mm Hg of the patient's mean arterial pressure is significant enough to cause tissue damage.)

Diagnosis. Measurement of intracompartmental pressure is the standard for diagnosis and almost always requires referral to an emergency department or orthopedic surgeon. Diagnostic imaging and serologic testing are of little value in for diagnosing compartment pressure in the primary care setting.

Treatment. Acute compartment syndrome is treated by surgical decompression (i.e., fasciotomy) of the leg. Initially, chronic ECS can be conservatively treated if there is an obvious cause such as a tight cast, constrictive clothing, or brace. Any constrictive object is immediately removed, and the leg is placed at the level of the heart. Higher elevation of the leg will lower arterial pressure, further compromising circulation. Unless there is almost immediate resolution of symptoms after these steps, fasciotomy should be performed.

After a fasciotomy has been performed, the fascia itself is usually left open and only the subcutaneous and fatty tissues are closed. As a result, skin grafting is frequently required to cover the soft-tissue defect.

ACHILLES' TENDINOPATHY

A simple episode of overstretching or repeated, cumulative stress on the Achilles' tendon can result in inflammation that causes Achilles' tendonitis. Both tendonitis and tendinosis can result from overuse.

Measuring approximately 6 inches long, the Achilles' tendon is the longest in the body; it is also the strongest. Normal stress on the tendon can be up to ten times an individual's body weight. Although most common in runners, patients who walk for long distances wearing poorly fitting footwear or who wear footwear that has the heel lower than the toes are also subject to developing Achilles' tendonitis.

Typically Achilles' tendonitis is more of a chronic problem that progresses through several stages, although a single acute episode of overstretching can also inflame the tendon. The midportion of the tendon, which is 2 to 3 inches proximal to its insertion in the calcaneus, is most often affected. Less commonly, tendonitis occurs more distally. Inflammation of the tendon at its insertion site (i.e., insertional tendonitis) is associated with a prominent tuberosity on the superior border of the posterior calcaneus. This prominence is known as Haglund's deformity.

The first clinical stage of Achilles' tendonitis is pain and aching of the posterior heel when running or walking. Stage II is pain that is present at the beginning of activity but resolves during exercise, only to recur at rest. Continuous pain that worsens with running or walking is stage III. Pain that persists even during rest correlates with degenerative changes and, possibly, tears in the tendon; this is stage IV.

Tendinosis may be clinically asymptomatic or may result in decreased ankle motion. Tendinosis is a diffuse thickening of the tendon that may include nodules, but there is no histologic evidence of inflammation. Histologically the tendon shows collagen disorganization, increased ground substance, and calcification of focal necrosis without inflammatory cells.[49,62] The tendon becomes thickened due to fibrosis and calcification of the tendon in response to collagen degradation. Clinically, tendinosis is more common than tendonitis.

History. The predominant complaint is pain that occurs with running or walking and is felt over the posterior leg. Training errors, shoes with inadequate shock absorption, or abnormal foot biomechanics (particularly excessive pronation) can contribute to tendinopathy. Pain tends to correlate with the previously mentioned stages of tendonitis. Even with stage IV pain, night pain is unusual; resting decreases or resolves symptoms.

Occasionally the patient will note tightness, thickening, fullness, or stiffness over the Achilles' tendon. When any of these symptoms occurs, inflammation of the paratenon is the likely cause. The paratenon is the covering of the tendon; it is made up of several thin tissue layers containing mucopolysaccharides, which lubricate the tendon. Peritendonitis can be considered an early phase of tendonitis.

Physical Examination and Diagnosis. History and physical examination, combined with a reasonable degree of clinical confirmation, are essential to the diagnosis of Achilles' tendinopathy. Clinically, there is little difference in the presentation of tendinosis versus tendonitis. Ultrasound is a simple, noninvasive, and relatively inexpensive test that is accurate in diagnosing inflammation of the tendon. Plain x-ray films provide little assistance except for diagnosing calcific tendonitis, in which calcifications are visible on a lateral view. CT and MRI are expensive tests for a condition that usually responds to conservative therapy.

Treatment. Temporary cessation of the activities associated with pain is generally the first step in treating Achilles' tendonitis. If symptoms are not severe, decreasing activity may be the initial action. PT is useful in decreasing pain, improving mobility, and stretching the tendon. Eccentric exercises seem to provide greater improvement in symptoms than concentric exercises.[55] A PT program should consist of the application of ice, gentle stretching, massage, and electrostimulation. Use of a heel pad or lift can also be useful in reducing tension on the tendon. Return to normal activities ranges from 2 to 6 weeks for tendonitis and from 6 weeks to 6 months for tendinosis.[49] Since tendinosis is more common than tendonitis, and the former is not an inflammatory condition, NSAIDs are not indicated as initial therapy.[48]

Corticosteroid injections in and around the Achilles' tendon are not usually prescribed during the initial phase of treatment. Rupture of the tendon can occur after even a single injection. One problem associated with attempting injection is that the inflammation of the tendon is diffuse and a localized injection is unlikely to be sufficient to relieve symptoms. Another drawback to injections is the risk of the corticosteroid weakening the tendon if infiltration of the tendon occurs. Injection is not contraindicated in all cases, but an orthopedic surgeon may be more suited to make the decision.

Surgery to remove scar tissue from the tendon and paratenon is sometimes necessary if conservative therapy fails.[94] If symptoms are present for 6 months or more after initiation of therapy, surgery may be necessary to explore the tendon and repair any damaged tissue. After surgical intervention, a prolonged course of PT is usually necessary. Even after 6 months of postoperative therapy, strength may not yet be fully recovered.[2]

CALF PAIN

Trauma, overuse, and vascular and neurologic disorders can all cause calf pain. Strains of the gastrocnemius and soleus muscles occur in athletic and would-be athletic populations. Systemic or localized vascular disorders may be responsible for arterial occlusion, venous congestion, or DVT. Neurologic causes of calf pain can be referred from the spine, or they can be attributable to local injury.

The gastrocnemius and soleus muscles are subject to injury from indirect and direct forces; injuries range from contusions and hematoma formation to muscle strains and tears. Muscle contusions are generally straightforward in history, presentation, and treatment. Typically, a patient suffers a direct blow to the calf and develops stiffness or pain with bruising. Examination may or may not show swelling. There is usually tenderness with palpation of ecchymotic areas. Treatment is rest, application of ice, compression and NSAIDs. Cessation of aggravating activity and protected weight bearing (including use of crutches) for 1 to 3 weeks will reduce stress on the muscle. Early stretching and isometric exercises will aid recovery.

Hematoma formation is the result of a greater traumatic force, causing bleeding into the muscle tissue. Typically the patient will recall a forceful injury, sometimes involving associated joints. The joint complaint may be the primary presenting feature, with hematoma formation and pain noted hours later.

TENNIS LEG

Tennis leg is a term for a tear in the middle, or belly, of the gastrocnemius muscle. Most often the medial head is involved. Sudden onset of severe calf pain during strenuous activity, followed by an inability to actively dorsiflex the foot, is a typical history. Pushing a stalled vehicle, sprinting suddenly from a standing or crouched position, or a sudden directional change while running (as in tennis) are all common activities that precede the onset of symptoms.

An examination of the leg sometimes reveals calf swelling, but the key finding is pain without weakness during resisted plantar flexion of the foot on the affected side. As with other muscle tears, bruising may not become apparent for several days after injury. Weak dorsiflexion of the foot with the knee extended and normal dorsiflexion with the knee flexed differentiate a calf muscle tear from a high rupture of the Achilles' tendon or a ruptured plantaris tendon (Table 7-4).

A tear of the soleus muscle can also occur with strenuous running or pushing of a heavy object. Usually, soleus tears occur when there is also extreme dorsiflexion of the foot. Symptoms are similar to those of a gastrocnemius tear. In clinical practice the soleus and two heads of the gastrocnemius are grouped together as the triceps surae muscles.

TABLE 7-4   Clinical Findings Associated with Tears of the Gastrocnemius Muscle, Achilles' Tendon, and Plantaris Tendon

Location	Clinical Finding
Gastrocnemius muscle	Foot fixed in plantar flexion
	Pain, but no weakness with resisted plantar flexion of foot
	Spasm of gastrocnemius with passive dorsiflexion of foot
	Normal dorsiflexion of foot when knee is flexed; weak dorsiflexion when knee is extended
	Negative Thompson's test
Achilles' tendon	Foot in fixed plantar flexion
	Weakness with resisted plantar flexion of foot
	No muscle spasm with passive dorsiflexion of foot
	Positive Thompson's test
Plantaris tendon	Foot not fixed in plantar flexion; Achilles' tendon usually intact
	No pain or significant weakness with resisted plantar flexion of foot
	Possible swelling; tenderness to palpation just medial to Achilles' tendon

Diagnosis of a calf muscle tear is based primarily on history and physical findings. MRI is excellent for evaluating the extent of the tear and any associated soft-tissue abnormalities. In clinical practice, however, MRI is not always necessary to successfully treat the patient, since most calf muscle tears are relatively mild and respond to decreased activity, application of ice, NSAIDs, and a compressive dressing.

Treatment depends on the severity of injury, but usually it consists of resting the affected leg, often by using crutches for 1 to 2 weeks. Ice is applied several times daily for 15 to 20 minutes at a time. Antiinflammatory medications are also used in the acute phase. In mild-to-moderate injury, gentle ROM exercises may begin within 1 or 2 days of injury. It is important to keep the patient active while avoiding any activities that stress the calf. A suggested or obvious complete tear should be treated surgically. In those cases the patient should avoid weight bearing on the affected leg by using crutches and should be referred to an orthopedic surgeon.

NEUROVASCULAR PROBLEMS

DEEP VEIN THROMBOSIS

One of the more serious causes of calf pain is a DVT. Patients at risk for DVT include those with chronic venous insufficiency, women (especially cigarette smokers) on oral contraceptives, patients on prolonged bed rest, postsurgical patients, patients after stroke or myocardial infarction, or those with a history of trauma to the leg. Patients with concomitant chronic diseases such as blood dyscrasias, diabetes, and cancer are also at increased risk for DVT. Even healthy, active adults can be predisposed to a DVT if subjected to prolonged immobility of the legs, for instance when they are confined in a cast or kept in a dependent position on long automobile or airplane trips.

Symptoms may be subtle and include minimal warmth, swelling, and tenderness of the calf, or there may be an acute onset of calf pain, swelling, and a hot, erythematous calf. With a significant DVT, superficial veins may become dilated and appear quite prominent. Regardless of presentation, calf pain or discomfort tends to occur with walking or standing and is lessened by resting and elevating the leg.

On examination, the calf may appear minimally or significantly larger than the uninvolved, contralateral one. Swelling is usually at or below the site of the thrombus and may be pitting. Measuring calf circumference is helpful in objectively quantifying calf swelling, but it is rarely useful alone for diagnosing a DVT (Box 7-1). Peripheral pulses are usually present. A hard cord may be palpable in the presence of a significant DVT. Most DVTs, however, are not dramatic in presentation. Homans' sign (calf pain when the foot is dorsiflexed) is not a reliable indicator of the presence of a DVT. Some patients with DVT may not have pain or tenderness in the calf.

Diagnosis. A high index of suspicion for DVT is based on the patient's history, risk factors, and examination, but definitive diagnosis requires diagnostic testing. Venography is the most accurate diagnostic test, but it is invasive, and injection of contrast raises the possibility of allergic reaction. Since venography is relatively expensive and not easily repeatable, it is not generally appropriate for evaluating a subclinical DVT.

Ultrasonography is a reliable, noninvasive, relatively inexpensive test that allows rapid reporting of results. Although not as sensitive as venography, ultrasound is accurate for diagnosing most clinically significant DVTs. In combination with clinical evaluation and serologic D-dimer testing (using a standard blue-top tube), ultrasound provides an accurate clinical diagnosis.[90]

Box 7-1	*Measuring Calf Circumference*

Procedure begins by finding a fixed point on the leg, such as the tibial tuberosity. From the tibial tuberosity, a point is measured approximately 5 cm down the anterior tibia and marked on the skin. At this point the girth of the calf is measured and recorded. This procedure is repeated for the contralateral leg. A discrepancy greater than 1 cm is considered abnormal. A difference of more than 2 cm necessitates emergent evaluation of DVT.

Treatment. Antithrombolytic therapy should be instituted as soon as possible after the diagnosis of a DVT is confirmed. If significant thrombosis is present, hospitalization with full heparinization may be necessary. In some cases, low–molecular weight heparin, fondaparinux, or warfarin therapy may be adequate.[36] Consultation with an internist is appropriate in planning treatment and admitting the patient to the hospital.

Once acute symptoms subside, prophylaxis against future DVTs is started, using an oral anticoagulant such as warfarin or low-dose aspirin. Antiembolic stockings, ambulation, and ankle plantar and dorsiflexion exercises can assist in reducing the risk of a future DVT.

REFERRED PAIN

Irritation of the S1 nerve root can result in calf pain. Referred pain from the lower spine tends to be a deep aching or even a burning pain. Patients with degenerative disk disease are more likely to develop referred pain to the lower extremities. If pain is referred, there is typically no history of local trauma to the leg, although the patient may note some muscle cramping. However, careful questioning can show that leg cramps are not usually associated with activities where the calf muscles are stretched. Additional sensory changes associated with the S1 nerve root distribution, such as tingling over the lateral border of the foot, may be present.

On examination, the calf is usually normal in appearance and nontender to palpation. Painless standing on the tips of the toes helps exclude the calf muscles as the primary site of pain. A brief examination of the lumbosacral spine, including checking reflexes and ROM, should be performed to rule out referred pain.

If there is evidence of nerve root irritation, x-ray studies may be helpful in evaluating degenerative changes in the spine. Treatment is directed at the underlying pathologic condition. PT, therapeutic exercise, NSAIDs, and occasional bracing may be helpful. If there are significant lumbosacral abnormalities, the patient should be referred to an orthopedic surgeon.

DIFFERENTIAL DIAGNOSIS OF KNEE COMPLAINTS

The knee is subject to numerous types of disorders, from trauma to infection to systemic processes. For the most part, any difficulty establishing a differential diagnosis is related to the joint itself. It is not unusual for referred pain from the hip and lumbar nerves to manifest itself as isolated knee pain. Disorders of the foot and ankle, such as excessive pronation or supination, may also be expressed as knee pain.

Hip abnormalities causing knee pain include femoral anteversion, in which the knee and patella, in particular, are subject to unusual forces that result in malalignment, subluxation, and chondromalacia. Arthritis, hamstring atrophy, and even fracture of the hip can be associated with knee complaints. Diffuse anterior knee pain is typical of referred pain from the hip. Nerve root impingement of the lumbar and upper sacral spine may cause weakness of the knee with flexion (L5, S1) or extension (L2, L3). Nerve root irritation or a herniated disk at L5-S1 can produce posterior knee pain.

With a careful history and examination, most potential sites of referred pain can be ruled out. Asking the patient about any joint problems above or below the knee may direct the examination to the true cause of knee pain. Any history of back problems should be carefully evaluated in the patient with knee pain.

DIAGNOSTIC RADIOLOGY

Primary evaluation of bony contours, density, bone lesions, fractures, and other abnormalities is most easily and economically conducted with plain x-ray films. For a basic survey of the knee, AP and lateral views are generally sufficient. A standing AP view of the knees emphasizes narrowing of the joint space (as in OA) that may be easily missed if the patient is supine. For specific concerns, such as patellar malalignment or subluxation, a sunrise view of the knee will provide information on the position of the patella in the trochlear groove of the femur. Additional views, such as notch or oblique projections, are generally left to the discretion of an orthopedic surgeon.

More detailed bony anatomy can be visualized by CT. Evaluating articular margins, medullary canal processes, and bone infection are examples of areas where CT is superior to plain radiographic films. Three-dimensional CT is being used more frequently for the reconstruction of bone, intraarticular fractures, and soft tissue surrounding the bones. This ability is useful for evaluating traumatic or complex fractures or those that are difficult to visualize on plain films. Helical CT reduces the time a patient is in a scanner. Although MRI is preferred for evaluating osteomyelitis, CT remains an excellent diagnostic tool for visualizing sequestra and involvement of cortical bone.[56]

Plain radiographic films and CT both use ionizing radiation, which limits the usefulness of these modalities for patients who are pregnant. CT is also limited if the patient has metal implants near the site of clinical interest. The artifact caused by metallic objects can make interpretation of a CT difficult. Overall, however, both radiography and CT, used judiciously, are simple, accurate, and noninvasive diagnostic tools for evaluating knee complaints.

Because of the significant quantity of soft-tissue structures around and within the knee, MRI has great utility in evaluating pathologic conditions of the knee. MRI is the diagnostic imaging tool of choice for assessing ligaments, tendons, and menisci. MRI best evaluates early changes of OCD, osteomyelitis, osteonecrosis, and soft-tissue tumors.

MRI remains one of the more expensive diagnostic imaging studies but can be cost-effective when used appropriately, because it provides early identification of knee abnormalities. Early diagnosis and definitive treatment can be less expensive than the combined cost of repeated x-ray films, CT, and conservative treatment modalities such as a protracted course of PT. MRI can also distinguish between disorders that will require surgery and those abnormalities that should do well with PT and other conservative measures.

Nuclear medicine imaging studies, such as bone scanning, are helpful for patients who complain of bony knee pain but have an essentially normal physical examination. Bone scans are useful in providing general information about active processes, such as stress fractures, acute arthritic flares, soft-tissue inflammation at the periosteal border, and metabolic processes such as tumor activity. Although sensitive, bone scanning is not specific; nonetheless, it can be an important diagnostic tool to reduce the list of possible diagnoses or to verify a suggested diagnosis. If warranted, more specific studies, such as CT or MRI, can be used to obtain additional information.

INDICATIONS FOR REFERRAL

See the Red Flags box for referral information.

Red Flags *for Knee and Leg Disorders*

Patients with these findings may need to be referred for more extensive work-up.

Signs and Symptoms	Response
Suspected or documented fracture around the knee	Refer immediately to emergency department or orthopedic surgeon
Inability to flex knee; point tenderness over affected portion of patella; trauma, pain, and significant effusion are reported	Possible patellar fracture. Immobilize knee in extended position; refer to orthopedic surgeon for treatment
Difficulty in flexing knee; may have obvious joint deformity; distal femoral tenderness or deformity after trauma	Possible distal femoral fracture; refer to orthopedic surgeon or emergency department.
Knee pain and/or difficulty in walking; swelling and bruising present around knee; knee area tender or painful to palpation; may have bony tenderness at site of injury; ligament pain may be on opposite side of knee; flexion or extension of knee may be uncomfortable or painful; fat globules present in bloody aspirate	Possible tibial plateau fracture. Stabilize knee with splint or immobilizer, keep patient non–weight bearing; refer to orthopedic surgeon for treatment
Ankle pain and weight-bearing activities may not be possible; ankle may be tender on palpation; palpable deformity at site of tenderness may occur	Possible distal fibula fracture. Refer to orthopedic surgeon for evaluation, especially if injury is complicated
Midshaft and fibula fracture	Immediately refer to emergency department or orthopedic surgeon for treatment
Inability to fully extend knee against resistance; may be palpable defect over either quadriceps or patellar tendon, usually adjacent to superior or inferior pole of patella	Possible quadriceps tendon rupture; refer to orthopedic surgeon for immediate surgical correction
No improvement of patellar malalignment after 4 to 6 weeks of consistent exercise	Refer to orthopedic surgeon for possible lateral retinacular release
History of direct trauma to LCL, but may be history of knee "bending out sideways" with fall; pain, stiffness, and localized swelling present; peroneal nerve or muscle damage may be present	Possible LCL injury. Refer to orthopedic surgeon for possible surgical repair
Knee swelling caused by hemarthrosis; pain present to varying degrees; pain and tenderness in posterolateral area of knee or near tibial plateau; positive anterior drawer or Lachman's test	Possible ACL injury. Refer to orthopedic surgeon for further assessment and treatment

Continued

Signs and Symptoms	Response
Vague symptoms of knee instability without significant pain or swelling; pain described as dull aching or stiffness; may be history of trauma to anterior knee; anterior knee lacerations or contusions may be present; positive posterior drawer, Godfrey's, and quadriceps active tests	Possible PCL injury; refer to an orthopedic surgeon for possible surgical intervention
Knee pain after some type of twisting; pain usually well localized to joint line; swelling may be present within 24 hours after injury; locking, catching, giving way of the knee reported; may be pain or feeling of instability when descending stairs; knee may occasionally catch; positive McMurray's and Apley's compression tests	Possible meniscal tear; refer to orthopedic surgeon for possible arthroscopic surgery
Cloudy or purulent aspirate from swollen prepatellar bursa	Possible infected bursa (septic joint); refer patient to orthopedic surgeon or emergency department for definitive treatment
Clear to slightly yellow or pink-tinged serous fluid aspirated from swollen prepatellar bursa	Possible inflammatory bursitis; refer to orthopedic surgeon for corticosteroid injection
Red, painful, swollen knee joint; fever, chills, nausea, and malaise may be present; recent infections may be history; difficulty in bearing weight on the affected extremity; ROM may be limited; pain may be severe	Possible septic joint; refer to orthopedic surgeon or emergency department for in-hospital treatment
Walks with affected leg externally rotated to decrease pain; knee pain may be diffuse; effusion may be present, (usually when there is loose body in joint); may be loss of full extension; knee may be warm to touch	Possible osteochondritis dissecans; refer to orthopedic surgeon for possible arthroscopy or open repair
Symptoms of OA persist after NSAID, physical therapy instituted; ADLs difficult to perform	Refer to a rheumatologist or orthopedic surgeon for discussion of joint replacement therapy
Tense, tender, swollen compartment; passive movement of muscles in involved compartment increases pain; six Ps present—pain, paresis (paralysis), paresthesia, pulses pallor, pressure	Possible compartment syndrome; refer to orthopedic surgeon for surgical decompression (fasciotomy) of leg
Conservative therapy fails for Achilles' tendonitis	Refer to orthopedic surgeon for possible removal of scar tissue from tendon and paratenon
Some calf swelling; pain without weakness during resisted plantar flexion of foot on affected side; positive Thompson's test	Possible complete tear of the Achilles' tendon or calf muscle. Refer to orthopedic surgeon for treatment

ACL, Anterior cruciate ligament; *ADLs,* activities of daily living; *LCL,* lateral collateral ligament; *NSAIDs,* nonsteroidal antiinflammatory drugs; *OA,* osteoarthritis; *PCL,* posterior cruciate ligament; *ROM,* range of motion.

REFERENCES

1. Abramowitz AJ et al: The medial tibial syndrome: the role of surgery, *Orthop Rev* 13:875, 1994.

2. Alfredson H et al: Chronic Achilles tendinitis and calf muscle strength, *Am J Sports Med* 24:829, 1996.

3. Allen CR et al: Posterior cruciate ligament injuries, *Curr Opin Rheumatol* 14:142, 2002.

4. American College of Rheumatology Subcommittee on Osteoarthritis Guidelines: Recommendations for the medical management of osteoarthritis of the hip and knee (2000 update), *Arthritis Rheum* 43:1905, 2000.

5. Baker MM, Juhn MS: Patellofemoral pain syndrome in the female athlete, *Clin Sports Med* 19:315, 2000.

6. Bennett LD, Buckland-Wright JC: Meniscal and articular cartilage changes in knee osteoarthritis: a cross-sectional double-contrast macroradiographic study, *Rheumatology* 41:917, 2002.

7. Bennett JE et al: Factors contributing to the development of medial tibial stress syndrome in high school runners, *J Orthop Sports Med, J Orthop Phys Ther* 31:504, 2001.

8. Reference deleted in proofs.

9. Bharam S et al: Knee fractures in the athlete, *Orthop Clin North Am* 33:565, 2002.

10. Bhattacharyya T et al: The clinical importance of meniscal tears demonstrated by magnetic resonance imaging in osteoarthritis of the knee, *J Bone Joint Surg Am* 85:4, 2003.

11. Boden BP et al: Patellofemoral instability: evaluation and management, *J Am Acad Orthop Surg* 5:47, 1997.

12. Boden BP, Osbahr DC: High-risk stress fractures: evaluation and treatment, *J Am Acad Orthop Surg* 8:344, 2000.

13. Bradley JD et al: Tidal irrigation as treatment for knee osteoarthritis: a sham-controlled, randomized, double-blinded evaluation, *Arthritis Rheum* 46:100, 2002.

14. Brander VA: Osteoarthritis of the knee: pathogenesis, pathophysiology and radiographic progression, *Am J Orthop* 30(8S):6, 2001.

15. Brief AA et al: Use of glucosamine and chondroitin sulfate in the management of osteoarthritis, *J Am Acad Orthop Surg* 9:71, 2001.

16. Butcher JD et al: Lower extremity bursitis, *Am Fam Physician* 53:2317, 1996.

17. Cahill BR: Osteochondritis dessicans of the knee: treatment of juvenile and adult forms, *J Am Acad Orthop Surg* 3:237, 1995.

18. Cahill BR, Ahten SM: The three critical components in the treatment of juvenile osteochondritis dissecans (JOCD), *Clin Sports Med* 20:287, 2001.

19. Calin A: Managing hyperuricemia and gout: challenges and pitfalls, *J Musculoskelet Med* 13:42, 1995.

20. Callahan LR: Stress fractures in women, *Clin Sports Med* 19:303, 2000.

21. Cea-Pereiro JC et al: A comparison between septic bursitis caused by *staphylococcus* and those caused by other organisms, *Clin Rheumatol* 20:10, 2000.

22. Chaisson CE et al: Detecting radiographic knee osteoarthritis: what combination of views is optimal? *Rheumatology* 39:1218, 2000.

23. Cole BJ, Harner CD: Degenerative osteoarthritis of the knee in active patients: evaluation and management, *J Am Acad Orthop Surg* 7:389, 1999.

24. Cook JL et al: Overuse tendinosis, not tendinitis, *Physician Sportsmed* 28:31, 2000.

25. Cosgarea AJ, Jay PR: Posterior cruciate ligament injuries: evaluation and management, *J Am Acad Orthop Surg* 9:297, 2001.

26. Cosagera AJ et al: Evaluation and management of the unstable patella, *Physician Sportsmed* 30:33, 2002.

27. Couture CJ, Karlson: Tibial stress injuries: decisive diagnosis and treatment of "shin splints," *Physician Sportsmed* 30:29, 2002.

28. Curl WW: Popliteal cysts: historical background and current knowledge, *J Am Acad Orthop Surg* 4:129, 1996.

29. Dervin GF et al: Effect of arthroscopic debridement for osteoarthritis of the knee on health-related quality of life, *J Bone Joint Surg Am* 85A:10, 2003.

30. Duri ZAA et al: The immature athlete, *Clin Sports Med* 21:461, 2002.

31. Fithian DC et al: Fate of the anterior cruciate ligament-injured knee, *Orthop Clin North Am* 33:621, 2002.

32. Fleming BD et al: The effect of weightbearing and external loading on anterior cruciate ligament strain, *J Biomech* 34:163, 2001.

33. Fredberg U, Bolvig L: Significance of ultrasonographically detected asymptomatic tendinosis in the patellar and Achilles tendons of elite soccer players: a longitudinal study, *Am J Sports Med* 30:488, 2002.

34. Fredericson M et al: Hip abductor weakness in distance runners with iliotibial band syndrome, *Clin Sports Med* 10:169, 2000.

35. Friedman L et al: Ultrasound of the knee, *Skeletal Radiol* 30:361, 2001.

36. Giangrande PL: Fondaparinux (Arixtra): a new anticoagulant, *Int J Clin Pract* 56:615, 2002.

37. Griffin LY: Noncontact ACL injuries: is prevention possible? *J Musculoskel Med* 18:507, 2001.

38. Griffin LY et al: Appearance of previously injured posterior cruciate ligaments on magnetic resonance imaging, *South Med J* 95:1153, 2002.

39. Handy JR: Popliteal cysts in adults: a review, *Semin Arthritis Rheum* 31:108, 2001.

40. Hewitt TE et al: The effect of neuromuscular training on the incidence of knee injury in female athletes, *Am J Sports Med* 27:699, 1999.

41. Hochberg MC et al: Guidelines for the medical management of osteoarthritis. II. Osteoarthritis of the knee, *Arthritis Rheum* 38:1541, 1995.

42. Hoover TJ, Siefert JA: Soft tissue complications of orthopaedic emergencies, *Emerg Med Clin North Am* 18:115, 2000.

43. Hunt SA et al: Arthroscopic management of osteoarthritis of the knee, *J Am Acad Orthop Surg* 10:356, 2002.

44. Hutchinson MR, Ireland ML: Common compartment syndromes in athletes: treatment and rehabilitation, *Sports Med* 17:200, 1994.

45. Hutchinson MR et al: Chronic exertional compartment syndrome: gauging pressure, *Physician Sportsmed* 27:1999.

46. Ireland ML: The female ACL: why is it more prone to injury? *Orthop Clin North Am* 33:637, 2002.

47. Kellgren JH, Lawrence JS: Radiological assessment of osteoarthritis, *Ann Rheum Dis* 16:494, 1957.

48. Khan KM et al: Histopathologies of common tendinopathies: update and implications for clinical management, *Sports Med* 27:393, 1999.

49. Khan KM et al: Overuse tendinosis, not tendinitis. I. A new paradigm for a different clinical problem, *Physician Sportsmed* 28:38, 2000.

50. Kim SJ et al: Paradoxical phenomena of the McMurray test, *Am J Sports Med* 24:231, 1996.

51. Klimkiewicz JJ, Shaffer B: Meniscal surgery (2002 update): indications and techniques for resection, repair, regeneration, and replacement, *Arthroscopy* 18(Suppl 2):14, 2002.

52. Koski JA et al: Meniscal injury and repair: clinical status, *Orthop Clin North Am* 31:419, 2000.

53. Koval KJ, Helfet DL: Tibial plateau fractures: evaluation and treatment, *J Am Acad Orthop Surg* 3:86, 1995.

54. Lozada CJ, Altman RD: Osteoarthritis. In Robbins L et al, editors: *Clinical care in the rheumatic diseases*, ed 2, Atlanta, 2001, American College of Rheumatology.

55. Mafi N et al: Superior short-term results with eccentric calf muscle training compared to concentric training in a randomized prospective multicenter study on patients with chronic Achilles tendinosis, *Knee Surg Sports Traumatol Arthrosc* 9:42, 2001.

56. Magid D: Computed tomographic imaging of the musculoskeletal system, *Radiol Clin North Am* 32:255, 1994.

57. Malone T et al: Muscular control of the patella, *Clin Sports Med* 21:349, 2002.

58. Margheritini F et al: Posterior cruciate ligament injuries in the athlete: an anatomical, biomechanical and clinical review, *Sports Med* 32:393, 2002.

59. Matava MJ: Patellar tendon ruptures, *J Am Acad Orthop Surg* 4:287, 1996.

60. Matsen FA III: Compartment syndromes. In Barr JS, editor: Instructional course lectures, *Am Acad Orthop Surg* 38:463, 1989.

61. Matsumoto H et al: Roles of the anterior cruciate ligament and medial collateral ligament in preventing valgus instability, *J Orthop Sci* 6:28, 2001.

62. Mazzone MF, McCue T: Common conditions of the Achilles tendon, *Am Fam Phys* 65:1805, 2002.

63. McAlindon TE et al: Glucosamine and chondroitin for treatment of osteoarthritis: a systematic quality assessment and meta-analysis, *J Am Med Assoc* 283:1469, 2000.

64. McConnell J: The physical therapist's approach to patellofemoral disorders, *Clin Sports Med* 21:363, 2002.

65. McQueen MM, Court-Brown CM: Compartment monitoring in tibial fractures: the pressure threshold for decompression, *J Bone Joint Surg* 78B:99, 1996.

66. Merlaragno PG et al: Lower leg compartment syndromes: when to suspect and how to diagnose, *J Musculoskelet Med* 13:14, 1996.

67. Morelli V et al: Alternative therapies for traditional disease states: osteoarthritis, *Am Fam Phys* 67:339, 2003.

68. Moseley JB et al: A controlled trial of arthroscopic surgery for osteoarthritis of the knee, *N Engl J Med* 347:81, 2002.

69. Navarro RA, Soifer TB: Treating the pain of OA, *Orthop Technol Rev* 4:18, 2002.

70. O'Rourke M: Determining the effectiveness of glucosamine and chondroitin for osteoarthritis, *Nurse Pract* 26:44, 2001.

71. Panni AS et al: Overuse injuries of the extensor mechanism in athletes, *Clin Sports Med* 21:483, 2002.

72. Pavelka K et al: Glucosamine sulfate use and delay of progression of knee osteoarthritis: a 3-year, randomized, placebo-controlled, double blind study, *Arch Intern Med* 162:2113, 2002.

73. Peixoto MR et al: Diet and medication in the treatment of hyperuricemia in hypertensive patients, *Arq Bras Cardiol* 76:468, 2001.

74. Perryman JR, Hershman EB: The acute management of soft tissue injuries of the knee, *Orthop Clin North Am* 33:575, 2002.

75. Plancher KD, Tifford CD: Evaluating and managing knee injuries in downhill skiers, *J Musculoskel Med* 19:79, 2002.

76. Post WR et al: Patellofemoral malalignment: looking beyond the viewbox, *Clin Sports Med* 21:521, 2002.

77. Potter HG: Imaging of the multiple-ligament-injured knee, *Clin Sports Med* 19:425, 2000.

78. Reider B: Medial collateral ligament injuries in athletes, *Sports Med* 12:147, 1996.

79. Rosseau I et al: Gout: radiographic findings mimicking infection, *Skeletal Radiol* 30:565, 2001.

80. Sandall W, Aigner T: Articular cartilage and changes in arthritis: cell biology of osteoarthritis, *Arthritis Res* 3:107, 2001.

81. Savio L-Y et al: Biomechanics of knee ligaments, *Am J Sports Med* 27:533, 1999.

82. Savio L-Y et al: Healing and repair of ligament injuries in the knee, *J Am Acad Orthop Surg* 8:364, 2000.

83. Schenck RC, Goodnight JM: Current concepts review: osteochondritis dessicans, *J Bone Joint Surg Am* 78(A):439, 1996.

84. Schlesinger N et al: Local ice therapy during bouts of acute gouty arthritis, *J Rheumatol* 29:331, 2002.

85. Seneviratne A, Rodeo SA: Identifying and managing meniscus tears, *J Musculoskel Med* 17:690, 2000.

86. Sharma L et al: The role of knee alignment in disease progression and functional decline in knee osteoarthritis, *J Am Med Assoc* 286:188, 2001.

87. Shelbourne KD, Klootwyk TE: Low-velocity knee dislocation with sports injuries, *Clin Sports Med* 19:443, 2000.

88. Swan A et al: The value of synovial assays in the diagnosis of joint disease: a literature survey, *Ann Rheum Dis* 61:493, 2002.

89. Swenson TM, Harner CD: Knee ligament and meniscal injuries: current concepts, *Orthop Clin North Am* 26:529, 1995.

90. Tick LW et al: Practical diagnostic management of patients with clinically suspected deep venous thrombosis by clinical probability test, compression ultrasonography, and D-dimer test, *Am J Med* 113:630, 2002.

91. Wang CJ et al: Outcome of surgical reconstruction for posterior cruciate and posterolateral instabilities of the knee, *Injury* 33:815, 2002.

92. Williams P et al: Acute non-traumatic compartment syndrome related to soft tissue injury, *Injury* 27:507, 1996.

93. Wortmann RL: Gout and hyperuricemia, *Curr Opin Rheumatol* 14:281, 2002.

94. Yodlowski ML et al: Surgical treatment of Achilles tendinitis by decompression of the retrocalcaneal bursa and superior calcaneal tuberosity, *Am J Sports Med* 30:318, 2002.

Chapter 8

Ankle

Both chronic and acute ankle complaints are frequently encountered in primary care. Many ankle problems are relatively straightforward in their history and presentation, especially after acute trauma. However, variations in the anatomy of the foot and ankle or a vague history can complicate the presentation, assessment, and treatment of ankle complaints.

Frequently referred to as a hinge joint, the ankle is subject to biomechanical forces that make the joint far more complex than a simple hinge joint. The interaction of the articular surfaces, muscles, ligaments, and joint capsule allows complex combination movement in response to activity and joint loading. Understanding basic ankle anatomy and some joint biomechanics is crucial to be able to assess and treat ankle pathologic conditions accurately.

ANATOMY

Bony Structures

Three bones, the tibia, the fibula, and the talus, make up the ankle joint (Figure 8-1). The tibia is the primary weight-bearing bone of the lower leg. The flattened distal portion of the tibia, the plafond, articulates with the dome of the talus, forming a saddle-shaped joint. A downward-projecting prominence of the medial distal tibia, known as the medial malleolus, articulates with the medial portion of the talus. A complex of ligaments and an interosseous membrane connect the tibia and

fibula. The distal tibia and fibula are also joined by these structures, forming the inferior tibiofibular joint (Figure 8-2). Although often thought of as primarily a muscle attachment for the leg, the fibula receives nearly 20% of the weight-bearing load.[26] The distal portion of the fibula, the lateral malleolus, articulates with the lateral facet of the talus. It is this bony conformity of the ankle mortise that provides a major portion of ankle stability when bearing weight.

The talus, formerly called the astragalus, is the second largest bone in the foot. The dome of the talus receives 80% of load-bearing weight.[28] In addition to articulating with the medial and lateral malleoli, the talar dome also articulates with the calcaneus and navicular bones of the foot. The articulation of the talus and calcaneus is the subtalar joint.

Collectively the articular surfaces of the tibia, fibula, and talar dome make up the square-shaped border of the ankle joint, commonly called the ankle mortise. In carpentry terms, a mortise joint refers to a "square peg in a square hole" arrangement; this type of joint is used where a strong connection is required. In the body the ankle mortise is a strong joint whose stability is affected by the supporting ligaments, the musculotendinous structure, and even the joint position during loading stress. The downward force of weight bearing helps increase the stability of the joint.

Most ankle movements are complex. For example, plantar flexion of the ankle causes internal rotation of the talus. Ankle dorsiflexion causes slight vertical

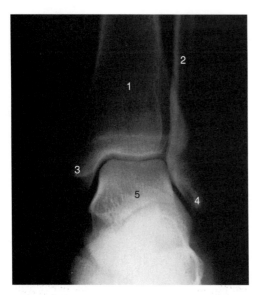

Figure 8-1   The Ankle Joint. Distal tibia (1); distal portion of fibula (2); medial malleolus (3); lateral malleolus (4); talus (5). (From C.L.A.S.S.: *Clinical anatomy principles*, St Louis, 1996, Mosby.)

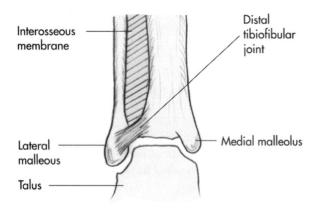

Figure 8-2 The distal or inferior tibiofibular joint is formed by the interosseous membrane and the distal tibiofibular ligament. (From C.L.A.S.S.: *Clinical anatomy principles*, St Louis, 1996, Mosby.)

motion of the fibula, as well as external rotation and posterolateral movement of the talus.[47] Inversion and eversion of the foot actually occur in the subtalar joint, which is stronger than the ankle joint. Recognizing the

complexity of ankle movements will help the practitioner more accurately assess and treat ankle injuries.

Ligaments

Ligamentous structures supply a large proportion of the ankle's stability. In fact, when the ankle is not bearing weight, ligaments provide the majority of the joint's stability. When ligamentous injury occurs, the severity of the damage can range from a minimal effect on weight bearing and joint stability to a dislocation of the ankle.

Clinically the three major ankle ligamentous complexes are those of the medial and lateral ankle and the syndesmosis. Medially, the deltoid ligament is a broad, tough, triangular structure. It extends anteriorly to the navicular bone, inferiorly to the medial calcaneus, and posteriorly to the medial side of the talus. There are two separate parts to the deltoid ligament, the deep and superficial fibers, but in clinical practice the deltoid ligament is usually considered a single unit (Figure 8-3). The deep fibers constitute one of the primary stabilizers of the weight-bearing ankle.[27] The deltoid ligament prevents lateral displacement of the talus, excessive eversion, plantar flexion, and dorsiflexion of the foot.[48] The deltoid ligament is much stronger than the lateral ankle ligaments. Consequently, injury to the medial ankle requires significantly more force than that necessary to damage the lateral ankle ligaments. Medial malleolar injuries, such as avulsion fractures, are often seen in association with deltoid ligament sprains.

Laterally there are three primary ligaments that provide stability to the ankle. All three attach to the distal fibula; each is named for its anatomic location. Moving anteriorly to posteriorly, the ligaments are the anterior talofibular ligament (ATFL), the calcaneofibular ligament (CFL), and the posterior talofibular ligament (TFL) (Figure 8-4). Working together as the lateral collateral ligaments, they prevent excessive anterior and posterior displacement of the foot by stabilizing the lateral malleolus on the talus and calcaneus. Collectively as well as individually, these ligaments are not as strong as the deltoid. As a result, the lateral ligaments are more frequently injured.

The third major ligamentous support of the ankle is the syndesmosis. Consisting of the anterior inferior tibiofibular ligament, the posterior inferior tibiofibular

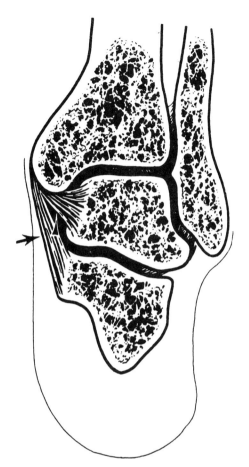

Figure 8-3   The Medial (Deltoid) Ankle Ligament, Shown in a Coronal Section. The superficial fibers *(arrow)* and the deep fibers *(arrowhead)* are indicated. (From Canale ST, editor: *Campbell's operative orthopaedics*, ed 10, vol 3, St Louis, 2003, Mosby.)

ing in a widened ankle mortise. Forced external rotation of the talus within the ankle mortise can have the same result.

Muscles and Tendons

Most of the muscular structures around the ankle are actually the musculotendinous units or tendons of the leg (see Chapter 7). Many of these structures cross the ankle joint and insert into the foot, a fact that further emphasizes the integral relationship of ankle stability and locomotion (Figure 8-5). Medially there are three important tendons at the ankle. The tibialis posterior tendon begins at the posterior side of the interosseous membrane; it passes through a groove behind the medial malleolus and inserts into the navicular and medial cuneiform bones of the foot. Two of the tendon's main functions are maintaining the arch of the foot and allowing inversion of the foot. Lying just behind the tibialis posterior tendon is the flexor digitorum longus tendon, one of the direct flexors of the toes. It also assists the gastrocnemius and soleus muscles in plantar flexing the foot to stand on the tips of the toes. Providing similar action to that of the flexor digitorum longus, the flexor hallucis longus lies on the posterior portion of the ankle rather than medially.

Directly on the posterior aspect of the ankle lies the Achilles' tendon, the thickest and strongest tendon in the body. Immediately medial to it lies the plantaris tendon. Both tendons insert into the posterior aspect of the calcaneus. The Achilles' tendon is responsible for powerful plantar flexion of the foot. In walking, it allows the toe-off phase; the plantaris tendon assists the Achilles' tendon in its action.

Laterally the tendons of the peroneal muscle (i.e., the peroneus longus and peroneus brevis tendons) pass just behind the lateral malleolus before inserting on the foot (Figure 8-6). The peroneus longus crosses under the cuboid bone and runs obliquely across the foot before inserting into the base of the first metatarsal. The peroneus brevis lies in front of the longus, closer to the fibula, and runs through a sheath on the lateral calcaneus, finally inserting into the base of the fifth metatarsal. The peroneal tendons are the primary everters of the foot. They also aid with plantar flexion of the foot.

ligament, and the interosseous membrane that connects the length of the tibia and fibula, the syndesmotic complex plays a role in maintaining the ankle mortise. Its importance in this function is receiving greater clinical attention. Syndesmotic injury resulting in ankle instability most often occurs in combination with a deltoid ligamentous injury or with a fibular fracture that is more than 3 to 4 cm proximal to the ankle joint line.[47] Forced dorsiflexion injuries can force the talus upward between the tibia and fibula, tearing the syndesmosis and result-

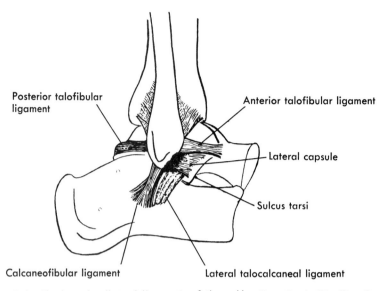

Figure 8-4 The lateral collateral ligaments of the ankle. (From Canale ST, editor: Campbell's operative orthopaedics, ed 10, vol 3, St Louis, 2003, Mosby.)

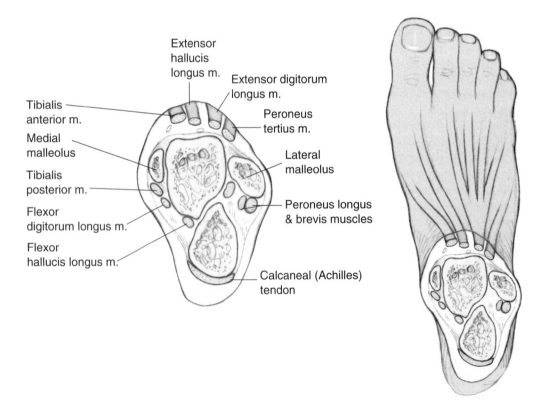

Figure 8-5 Relationship of tendons and osseous structures at the ankle joint. (From C.L.A.S.S.: *Clinical anatomy principles*, St Louis, 1996, Mosby

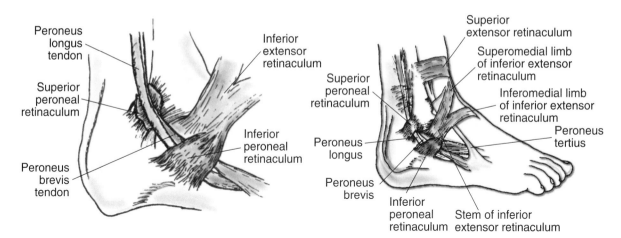

Figure 8-6   Peroneal tendons and their superior and inferior retinaculi. The peroneal tendons are the primary everters of the foot.

Anteriorly the extensor digitorum longus muscle lies just lateral to the tibia. It forms its tendinous attachment above the ankle. After crossing the anterior ankle, the tendon divides into four parts, or slips, that insert into the dorsal base of the second through fifth toes. Medial to the extensor digitorum longus lie the extensor hallucis longus muscle and tendon. The muscle begins at about the middle of the anterior fibula and quickly becomes mostly tendon. It crosses the anterior ankle and inserts into the dorsal base of the distal phalanx of the great toe. The most medial and prominent anterior tendon is the tibialis anterior tendon. It lies on the lateral side of the tibia and is easily visible when the patient dorsiflexes and inverts the foot. The tendon passes along the dorsum of the foot and inserts into the medial aspect of the base of the first metatarsal. Together all three anterior musculotendinous units help fix the bones of the leg in a perpendicular position to the foot while standing. The net effect is increasing overall ankle strength. Table 8-1 summarizes the location and action of several important tendons that cross the ankle joint.

Neurovascular Structures

Nerves of the lower lumbar and upper sacral spine provide innervation to the ankle. Knowledge of the appropriate nerve root that supplies each area of the ankle assists the practitioner in evaluating both local (i.e.,

peripheral) nerve injury and referred pain from the lower back. (Table 8-1 includes a summary of innervation to the ankle.)

Arterial supply to the ankle is primarily through the branches of the anterior tibial and popliteal arteries. The anterior tibial artery follows the anterior surface of the interosseous membrane down to the anterior tibia. At the ankle joint, it lies beneath the extensor hallucis tendon. Beyond the ankle, it becomes the dorsalis pedis. Smaller malleolar arteries, which supply the ankle joint, also arise from the anterior tibial artery. Two main branches of the popliteal artery, the posterior tibial and the peroneal, branch into smaller divisions that supply the tibia and ankle before reaching the foot (Figure 8-7). As indicated by its name, the posterior tibial artery is responsible for the posterior tibial pulse.

Arterial injury to the ankle is usually attributable to significant trauma and therefore is not commonly seen in the primary care setting. Unfortunately, severe soft-tissue trauma to the ankle can occur as the result of low-velocity torquing injuries; the extent of damage may not be readily apparent on initial examination. Soft-tissue swelling can impede both nerve and vascular integrity to some degree. In most cases the damage is temporary and without long-term sequelae, but any obvious loss of pulse or movement should be evaluated by an orthopedic surgeon.

| TABLE 8-1 | Important Tendons That Cross the Ankle Joint | | | |

Location	Tendon	Action	Insertion	Nerve Supply
Medial ankle	Tibialis posterior (palpable just behind medial malleolus)	Prevents excessive inversion of foot; helps maintain normal arch of foot	Navicular and medial cuneiform bones of foot	L5, S1
	Flexor digitorum longus (sometimes palpable just behind tibialis posterior tendon)	Flexes lesser (second through fifth) toes	Base of distal phalanges of second through fifth toes (plantar surface)	L5, S1
Posterior ankle	Flexor hallucis longus (cannot be palpated at ankle)	Flexes great toe	Passes medial calcaneus into base of distal phalanx of great toe (plantar surface)	L5, S1 S1, S2
	Achilles' (easily palpable at posterior ankle)	Plantar flexes foot	Posterior surface of calcaneus	
	Plantaris (may be palpable just medial to Achilles' tendon)	Plantar flexes foot	Posterior surface of calcaneus	L4, L5, S1 (through branch of internal popliteal nerve)
Lateral ankle	Peroneus longus (palpable posterior to lateral malleolus)	Provides foot eversion; assists with plantar flexion; helps maintain transverse arch of foot	Lateral base of first metatarsal	L4, L5, S1 (through branch of external popliteal nerve)
	Peroneous brevis (immediately posterior to lateral malleolus)	Plantar flexes foot; helps evert foot	Base of fifth metatarsal	L4, L5, S1 (through branch of external popliteal nerve)
Anterior ankle	Extensor digitorum longus (palpable when toes are extended)	Extends lesser (second through fifth) toes	Dorsal base of distal phalanges of second through fifth toes	L4, L5, S1 (through anterior tibial nerve)
	Extensor hallucis longus (palpable over anterior ankle when great toe is extended; lies lateral to tibialis anterior)	Extends great toe	Dorsal base of distal phalanx of great toe	L4, L5, S1 (through anterior tibial nerve)
	Tibialis anterior (palpable just medial to anterior tibia; easily palpable with inversion and dorsiflexion of foot)	Dorsiflexes foot; assists with inversion and eversion of foot	Base of medial cuneiform and first metatarsal	L4, L5, S1 (through anterior tibial nerve)

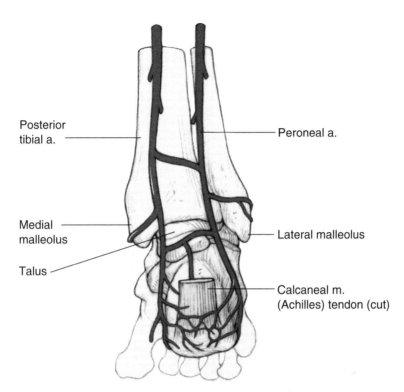

Figure 8-7 Arterial blood supply to the ankle (posterior). Severe ankle trauma can cause significant vascular compromise. (From C.L.A.S.S.: *Clinical anatomy principles*, St Louis, 1996, Mosby.)

EXAMINATION

Evaluation of the ankle begins with inspection of both ankles. Asymmetry, obvious deformity of the joint or soft tissue, discoloration, or difference in active range of motion (ROM) should be noted. The most common cause of ankle asymmetry is soft-tissue swelling. Swelling can cause apparent deformity of the ankle, but true deformity is the result of fracture or dislocation.[49] Varicosities may cause soft-tissue swelling and may be associated with discoloration of the ankle; neither of these findings is necessarily attributable to trauma.

Differences in active range of motion (ROM) are important. When compared with the contralateral joint, decreased dorsiflexion may indicate injury to the tibialis anterior tendons or injury to the talus. Plantar flexion and inversion of the foot are painful and their range diminished with lateral collateral ligament injuries. Inability to evert the foot may indicate injury to the deltoid ligament or to the peroneal tendons.

Obvious deformity over a bone with significant ecchymosis is a cardinal sign of fracture. Dislocation of the ankle can have a similar appearance; swelling can obscure discrete areas of abnormality. Swelling or ecchymosis proximal to the ankle may indicate bony injury of the tibia or fibula.

Observing the ROM of both ankles provides clues to help locate the area of injury. Normal active ROM of the ankle includes dorsiflexion, plantar flexion, eversion, and inversion. The neutral position of the ankle is with the foot nearly perpendicular to the leg. Normal ROM is shown in Table 8-2. Before palpating the ankle, the patient should be asked to point out the most painful site; this area should be examined last.

TABLE 8-2   Degrees of Normal Active Range of Motion of the Ankle

Movement	Degrees	Action
Dorsiflexion	15-20	15 degrees
Plantar flexion	45-50	50 degrees
Eversion (ankle at 90 degrees to leg)	5	5 degrees
Inversion (ankle at 90 degrees to leg)	5	5 degrees

ROM, Range of motion.

Palpation should begin in the area of least tenderness and should include bone, tendons, ligaments, soft tissue, and a check of distal pulses and sensation. Palpation of osseous structures usually begins on the uninjured side of the affected ankle. In most cases this is the medial malleolus. Beginning at the most prominent area of bone, the examiner should palpate both distally and proximally for any pain or tenderness and then continue inferiorly and anteriorly to the deltoid ligament. Just below the medial malleolus and slightly anterior is the head of the talus. The posterior tibial pulse should be checked just behind the medial malleolus. Next, the examiner should palpate the anterior aspect of the joint and dorsum of the proximal foot to evaluate the distal talus. Palpation of the posterior ankle will alert the practitioner to tenderness or a thickening of the Achilles' tendon. Finally, the site of pain, usually the lateral ankle, should be palpated. Again, the lateral malleolus should be located and palpated inferiorly to assess the CFL or the possibility of an avulsion fracture distal to the fibula. Returning to the lateral malleolus, the practitioner should palpate anteriorly to find the anterior TFL. The dorsalis pedis pulse should also be evaluated for its presence and quality.

While palpating the ankle, resisted and passive ROM are assessed. Resisted ROM is relatively easy to evaluate by comparing bilateral strength. The practitioner places his or her hand against the patient's foot, resisting the patient during ROM. Any unilateral weakness is noted. Passive ROM is useful in assessing patient guarding or injury as the cause of diminished ROM. Care should be taken to gently palpate and move the foot to prevent increased pain or inflammation.

Once palpation is completed and ROM evaluated, stability of the ankle joint itself should be tested. Two common tests, the anterior drawer and talar tilt tests, are used to evaluate lateral ankle stability. Although some orthopedic surgeons recommend performing these tests with the patient anesthetized,[4] both have added clinical utility if the patient is able to cooperate. The anterior drawer test evaluates the integrity of the anterior TFL (Figure 8-8). For the anterior drawer test, the patient should sit with the knee flexed to 90 degrees. If the knee is extended, the biomechanics of the talotibial junction are altered and may result in a false negative test.[45] The practitioner stabilizes the tibia with one hand, then grasps the back of the heel with the other, pulling the foot forward. In a classically positive test, a small dimple, known as the suction sign, will appear just anterior to the distal fibula. In acute injury, however, swelling may hide the suction sign; in this case the practitioner notes whether there is a discernible forward glide to the foot. If there is detectable forward motion greater than that shown by the unaffected ankle, the anterior drawer test is positive.

Integrity of the CFL is assessed by the talar tilt test. This test can be performed with the patient either sitting or lying with the affected side up (Figure 8-9). In either position, the patient's knee is flexed to 90 degrees and

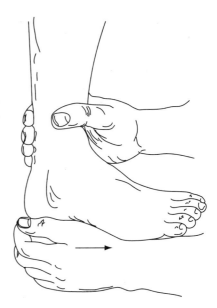

Figure 8-8 The Anterior Drawer Test Evaluates the Anterior Talofibular Ligament. When compared with the uninjured side, asymmetric forward gliding of the foot is indicative of damage to the ligament. (From Rubin A, Sallis R: A study to develop clinical decision rules for the use of radiography in acute ankle injuries, *Ann Emerg Med* 21(1):384-390, 1992, with permission from the American College of Emergency Physicians.)

the foot is perpendicular to the leg (i.e., 0 degrees of dorsiflexion).

If the patient is lying down, the practitioner sits on the examining table and supports the medial side of the patient's leg by placing it on the practitioner's leg. Using one or both of his or her hands, the practitioner attempts to tilt the talus from side to side. The talus is just below the medial and lateral malleoli. Normally talar movement is limited and has a definite end point.

With the patient sitting, the practitioner uses one hand to stabilize the medial aspect of the tibia. Using the other hand, the practitioner holds the patient's heel and forcibly inverts it. In a positive test, the affected ankle will have more palpable movement and there is usually dimpling over the lateral ankle. Ideally, talar tilt testing is performed bilaterally while an AP or mortise x-ray is being taken. Bilateral films make comparison of joint opening (laxity) easier to discern. The use of

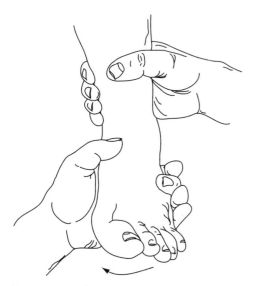

Figure 8-9   Talar Tilt Test. This maneuver is used to test the integrity of the calcaneofibular ligament. (From Rubin A, Sallis R: A study to develop clinical decision rules for the use of radiography in acute ankle injuries, *Ann Emerg Med* 21(1):384-390, 1992, with permission from the American College of Emergency Physicians.)

any talar tilt testing is controversial, with its use still being recommended by orthopedists and discouraged by radiologists.[9]

ABNORMALITIES AND TREATMENT

Sprains and Strains

Ankle sprains are frequently seen in both primary care and orthopedic surgery practices. It is estimated that 85% of ankle injuries are sprains.[48] Most sprains involve the lateral malleolar ligaments, but the medial ligaments and ankle syndesmosis can also be injured. Avulsion fractures of the lateral and medial malleoli are also seen with many ankle sprains.

Several different classification systems have been proposed for grading the severity of ankle sprains. Clinically, a grade I through grade III system is simple, sufficient, and similar to the system of grading sprains of any other joint. Figure 8-10 illustrates the pathology associated with each grade of sprain.

A grade I sprain causes stretching of the involved ligament, but there is no macroscopic tear of the ligament. The ankle is stable, and although the ankle may be painful, the patient has normal function of the joint. Ligamentous injury that results in some macroscopic tearing (i.e., bruising) with moderate swelling and pain, as well as some functional limitation, is classified a grade II injury. A severe injury is classified as a grade III sprain, a complete disruption of the ligament(s) with marked swelling, ecchymosis and joint instability. Table 8-3 summarizes the grading of sprains.

More than one factor is responsible for the high frequency of lateral ankle sprains. The deltoid ligament, on the medial side, is stronger than the lateral ligaments. The two major divisions of the deltoid, the superficial and deep components, stabilize the ankle by preventing excessive eversion of the hindfoot and by preventing external rotation of the talus. Biomechanical studies indicate that ankle instability is most likely with external rotation of the talus.[26] Without the countereffect of the deep deltoid ligament during plantar flexion, the talus would externally rotate. However, the strength of the deltoid ligament pulls the talus into internal rotation.[27]

The lateral malleolus is comprised of three smaller, relatively weaker ligaments, which limit anterior and posterior displacement of the talus and inversion of the ankle.[48] However, when the foot is plantar flexed, the narrow posterior talus is pulled within the mortise, and the talus rotates slightly internally. With the talus in a plantar-flexed, internally rotated position, the anterior TFL is relatively more stressed than the CFL and the posterior TFL. The net result is increased stress on a relatively weak ligament, resulting in injury to the anterior TFL.

Injury to the CFL and posterior TFL occurs with increasing rotational stress. Increased force at the time of injury, common in contact sports, can also result in greater lateral ligamentous injury.

Since the deltoid ligament is broader and stronger than the ligaments on the lateral side, medial ankle sprains require greater force to cause injury, and injury tends to be more severe. Medial, or deltoid, ligamentous sprains are less common than lateral sprains. The usual mechanism of injury for a deltoid sprain is a forced eversion of

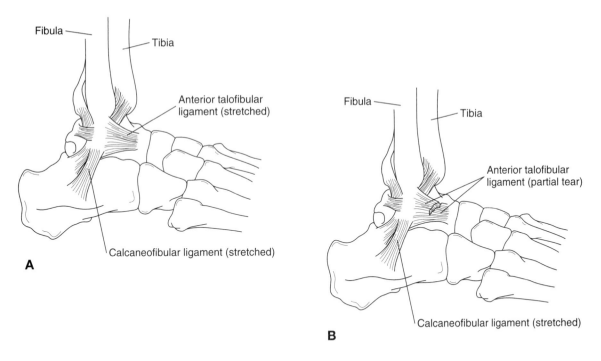

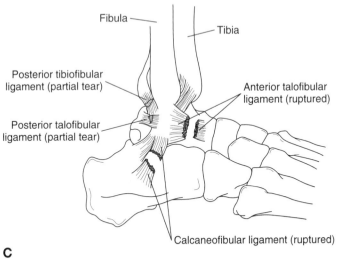

Figure 8-10   Grades of Ankle Sprain. A, Grade I with stretching but not tearing of the ligaments. **B,** Grade II with partial ligament tearing. **C,** Grade III with complete tearing of ligament(s), resulting in joint instability. (Redrawn from Wolfe MW and others: Management of ankle sprains, *Am Fam Physician* 63(1):94, 2001.)

TABLE 8-3	Characteristics of Grades I, II, and III Sprains	
Grade	**Ligamentous Injury**	**Physical Findings**
I	Stretching	Tenderness to palpation
		Mild swelling
		Normal function
II	Partial tearing	Tenderness to palpation
		Moderate swelling and ecchymosis
		Some instability of joint
		Decreased weight bearing and ROM
III	Complete rupture	Pain with palpation
		Marked ecchymosis, and edema
		Gross joint instability
		Inability to bear weight
		Injury to adjacent structures not uncommon

ROM, Range of motion.

the ankle. These injuries are also sometimes associated with the concurrent forced dorsiflexion of the foot.

A third type of sprain, syndesmosis injury, (sometimes called a "high" ankle sprain) tends to occur with severe external rotation. These injuries occur when force is applied to the proximal leg when the foot is held or planted in external rotation.[44] They can also occur when the foot is supinated and everted or pronated with eversion. Syndesmotic sprains are increasingly being recognized as a cause of persistent ankle pain and account for up to 20% of ankle sprains.[44,45] Because the syndesmotic structures connect the lateral tibia and medial fibula, pain is usually lateral to the tibia. As a result, these injuries can be confused with a lateral sprain. Depending on the severity of the syndesmotic sprain, the ankle mortise may be disrupted, leading to posttraumatic degenerative changes of the joint.

Lateral Ankle

The nature of the activity preceding injury to the lateral ankle varies; however, the history almost always involves some type of inversion injury. An acute event such as a fall during a sporting activity may happen so suddenly that the patient can recall little other than the fall. It is important to ask the patient what he or she was doing when the injury occurred to estimate the severity of sprain more accurately. High-impact injury leads to more serious ligamentous damage or associated injury.

Lateral ankle injury associated with significant inversion or plantar flexion, such as falling during a basketball game or twisting the ankle while stepping down a stair or curb, may be associated with another injury. An avulsion fracture of the distal fibula may result from the lower bone density at the distal fibula compared to the bone density of the lateral talar attachment site.[22] Peroneal tendonitis or even fractures to the base of the fifth metatarsal are not unusual in these instances. More often than not, the patient will remember feeling or hearing a pop or crack in or around the ankle. This popping or cracking is more often attributable to ligamentous tearing rather than to a bone fracture.

Swelling over the lateral ankle occurs almost immediately and is often described as ranging in size anywhere from a golf ball to a grapefruit. As a rule, weight bearing on the affected leg is difficult or impossible for a few hours after injury. Inability to bear weight for longer than 2 or 3 hours, significant ecchymosis, or feelings of ankle instability are indicative of a more severe injury.

Many patients will initially treat themselves. The method of rest, ice, compression, and elevation (RICE) is useful in decreasing pain and swelling and is well known to most individuals who participate in athletic events. However, not all patients are aware of RICE; it is therefore important to find out what treatment, if any, the patient has tried. Application of warm compresses or a heating pad will worsen edema in the period immediately after injury.

Numbness and tingling of the toes is not typical; when it does occur, it should be temporary. Numbness or tingling that persists after swelling has begun to resolve should be carefully evaluated to rule out peripheral nerve injury. Previous injuries of a similar nature and prior treatment, if any, should be noted. Repeated or significant injury that has not been properly rehabilitated predisposes the patient to recurrent sprains.

Once the history has been obtained, the practitioner should inspect the ankle for deformity, swelling, and discoloration. Significant bruising occurs rapidly with complete ligamentous disruption or fracture.

Obvious deformity other than that at the site of injury usually indicates an associated problem such as a hematoma, fracture, and preexisting problems (e.g., hallux valgus or excessive pronation or supination). The patient should be asked to point to the most painful area. As a rule, the less time between injury and evaluation, the more specific the site of pain. As time increases between injury and assessment, pain tends to become more generalized. Having noted the area(s) of pain, the practitioner examines the most tender areas last.

After palpating the medial and anterior portions of the ankle, the examiner should locate and palpate the anterior TFL, CFL, and posterior TFL. Most lateral ankle sprains include some component of plantar flexion of the foot at the time of injury. In most cases the lateral malleolar ligaments are injured in an anterior to posterior order. The CFL is the second most frequently injured ligament. Tightening of the CFL occurs with more dorsiflexion of the foot or when the foot is more perpendicular to the leg. When the CFL is injured, it is usually after the anterior TFL is torn. The CFL, like the other lateral ligaments, usually tears toward the middle of the tendon, but it is not unusual for it to avulse a fragment of bone from the distal fibula or lateral calcaneus. If there is a rotational component to the inversion, the PTFL is injured.

Complete tearing of the anterior TFL or CFL causes ankle instability. An anterior drawer test should be performed to evaluate the anterior TFL, and a talar tilt test should be conducted to evaluate the CFL. Figure 8-11 shows a positive anterior drawer test. Radiographic verification of anterior movement of the talus is shown in Figure 8-12. (Both tests are discussed in this chapter under "Examination.") Pain is common with the anterior drawer test when the patient has a partial tear of the anterior TFL; if the ligament is completely torn there may be very little pain. Performing either the anterior drawer test or talar tilt test can be extremely difficult

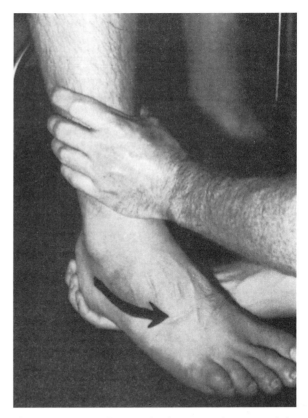

Figure 8-11 Positive anterior drawer test for a tear of the anterior talofibular ligament. The arrow indicates the direction of force applied to the posterior calcaneus. (From Canale ST, editor: *Campbell's operative orthopaedics*, ed 10, vol 3, St Louis, 2003, Mosby.)

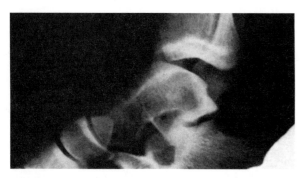

Figure 8-12 Radiographic appearance of a positive anterior drawer test at the ankle. Note the asymmetry of the joint as the talus moves anteriorly. (From Canale ST, editor: *Campbell's operative orthopaedics*, ed 10, vol 3, St Louis, 2003, Mosby.)

when the patient is experiencing acute pain and cannot relax the ankle.

It is not uncommon to have associated injuries with lateral ankle sprains.[14] The CFL is confluent with a portion of the peroneal tendon sheath; as the peroneal tendons begin their course to the fifth metatarsal, the tendons also glide over part of the superficial CFL. As a result, injury to the peroneal tendons or a fracture of the base of the fifth metatarsal is not unusual with a grade II or grade III calcaneofibular sprain. Ankle instability, suggested fracture, or associated tendon injury are reasons to refer the patient to an orthopedic surgeon.[11]

Testing the strength of the peroneal tendons begins by asking the patient to sit on the edge of the examining table with his or her legs dangling over the side. The practitioner uses one hand to stabilize the patient's tibia and then places the other hand with the palm against the lateral border of the patient's foot. The patient is asked to evert the foot against the resistance provided by the practitioner's hand. The uninjured and injured sides are compared. Pain or weakness with resisted eversion may indicate peroneal tendonitis or a partial tear of the peroneus brevis tendon.

Neurovascular status of the ankle and foot should also be assessed. Both the dorsalis pedis and posterior tibial pulses should be palpated and assessed for quality. Vascular injury is rare with an isolated lateral ligament sprain; however, if there is significant swelling, venous and capillary flow may be temporarily reduced. Damage

to the peroneal nerve can be indicated by decreased ankle ROM and difficulty extending the toes.

Medial Ankle

History. Eversion injuries of the ankle tend to result in deltoid ligamentous damage. Forced dorsiflexion of the foot, in combination with eversion, is common. Although comprising only approximately 5% of all ankle sprains, injuries to the deltoid ligament tend to be more severe. Injuries such as running into a fence while chasing a fly ball, falling during contact sports, slipping on an inclined surface, or tripping while climbing stairs are fairly common ways of injuring the deltoid ligament.

Important questions to ask the patient with a suggested deltoid sprain include those concerned with the patient's ability to bear weight, the rapidity of swelling, and the presence of any obvious deformity. Immediate inability to bear weight should raise the possibility of fracture, as should the patient's report of an immediate deformity. Less severe injury is likely if the patient is able to stand or continue activity after the injury. With ligamentous rupture, swelling is almost instantaneous, weight bearing is difficult but not necessarily impossible, and bruising occurs within hours.

Physical Examination and Diagnosis. As usual, the examiner should ask the patient to point to the most painful area and examine this area last. The examiner must first assess movements that are least likely to cause pain, such as inversion and plantar flexion, looking for associated lateral ankle injury. The lateral, anterior, and posterior portions of the ankle should be palpated, checking for tenderness or palpable deformity. The practitioner should gently palpate the medial malleolus and note any bony tenderness. If the malleolus is painful, caution should be used in performing ROM.

After evaluating the rest of the ankle, the patient should actively evert and dorsiflex the foot. The contralateral ROM should be compared and any discrepancies noted. If the injured ankle has decreased active ROM, the practitioner should passively evert and dorsiflex the foot and note any improvement in ROM or complaints of pain. If the patient is able to actively move the ankle without significant pain, the practitioner can use his or her hand to provide resistance to active ROM. Weakness on the affected side may be attributable to pain; however, significant weakness may indicate fracture or injury to associated structures.

Neurovascular status should also be assessed. The dorsalis pedis artery passes along the anteromedial portion of the ankle, becoming the dorsalis pedis pulse. The posterior tibial artery and pulse is palpable just posterior to the medial malleolus; fracture in this area may interrupt the artery. Congenital absence of a palpable pulse in the dorsalis pedis or posterior tibialis is normal in a percentage of the population. The absence of a unilateral pedal or dorsalis pedis pulse is only clinically significant if it was previously known to be present.

Tenderness over the medial malleolus, gross deformity, significant weakness, or neurovascular compromise are four criteria that necessitate referral to an orthopedic surgeon.

Syndesmosis

History. Injury to the syndesmosis is most frequently associated with a forceful external rotational force and medial ligament sprain. In fact, complete disruption of the syndesmosis does not affect the biomechanics of the ankle unless there is also a significant deltoid ligamentous injury.[26,29] This injury is often overlooked but can result in prolonged rehabilitation and, if untreated, chronic ankle pain and arthritis.[50] The history is essentially the same for an injury to the syndesmosis as it is for a sprain of the deltoid ligament, but the forced eversion component of the injury may be more prominent than the dorsiflexion.

Physical Examination. While evaluating the ankle for lateral and medial ligamentous injury, the practitioner can perform a squeeze test to obtain some rudimentary information about the syndesmosis. To conduct the squeeze test, the practitioner manually squeezes the distal tibia and fibula together (Figure 8-13). Usually the practitioner can exert this manual lateral-medial compression with one hand. The presence of ankle pain is a positive test. In acute injury, however, findings may not be reliable. Another clinical tool is the external rotation test. With the patient's knee flexed to 90 degrees, the foot is externally rotated. Pain occurs with a positive test.[44,49] If a syndesmotic injury is suggested, x-ray films are more useful in evaluating the injury. A widened or asymmetric mortise joint may necessitate surgical

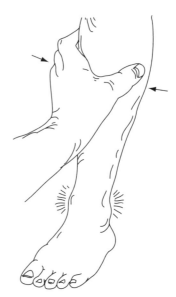

Figure 8-13 The Squeeze Test for Evaluating a Syndesmotic Injury. A positive test is ankle pain with bilateral compression of the tibia and fibula. (From Rubin A, Sallis R: A study to develop clinical decision rules for the use of radiography in acute ankle injuries, *Ann Emerg Med* 21(1):384-390, 1992, with permission from the American College of Emergency Physicians.)

repair. The patient should be splinted and referred to an orthopedic surgeon.

Diagnosis. For the most part, history and physical examination are all that are required to diagnose an ankle sprain accurately. Most patients with mild-to-moderate (grades I to II) injuries do not need x-ray evaluation.

Exceptions to that caveat have been defined by what are known as the Ottawa rules[40] (Figure 8-14). Under these guidelines, x-ray films are necessary for the patient who:

- Is unable to bear weight initially after injury or when examined.
- Has tenderness over the posterior edge of the distal 6 cm or distal tip of the medial or lateral malleolus.
- Has tenderness over the fifth metatarsal or tarsal navicular.

Radiographic Studies. Radiographic evaluation of the ankle should be considered if there is point tenderness over a bone, if the patient has a history of previous ankle injury, if there is obvious deformity, or if the

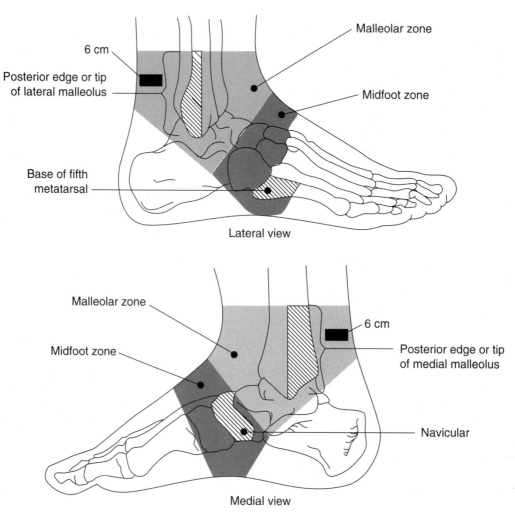

Figure 8-14 Ottawa Ankle Rules; Guidelines for Obtaining X-ray Films after Injury.
Tenderness over any bony area in the shaded regions or an inability to bear weight immediately after injury or during the physical examination meets the guidelines for ankle x-ray films. (From Rubin A, Sallis R: A study to develop clinical decision rules for the use of radiography in acute ankle injuries, *Ann Emerg Med* 21(1):384-390, 1992, with permission from the American College of Emergency Physicians.)

patient complains of grossly diffuse pain. X-ray stress views are best performed in a hospital, a sports medicine clinic, or an orthopedic surgical practice where proper positioning and stressing of the ankle joint are easily accomplished. In an ankle with stable ligaments, external forces will not significantly alter the radiographic appearance of the ankle mortise. A normal ankle will not usually show mortise widening greater than approximately 10 degrees.[4] If there is lateral ligamentous disruption, forced inversion of the ankle will show a widening of the lateral malleolus (Figure 8-15). Significant widening may be an indication for surgical intervention; however, an orthopedic surgeon should make this decision.

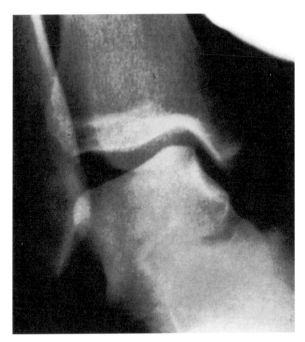

Figure 8-15 A Positive Stress View of the Ankle.
Complete disruption of the lateral collateral ligaments is indicated. Note the widened lateral ankle mortise as the talus tilts when valgus stress is applied to the ankle joint. (From Canale ST, editor: *Campbell's operative orthopaedics*, ed 10, vol 3, St Louis, 2003, Mosby.)

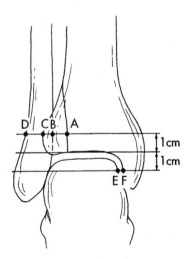

A = Lateral border of posterior tibial malleolus
B = Medial border of fibula
C = Lateral border of anterior tibial prominence
D = Lateral border of fibula
E = Medial border of talus
F = Lateral border of medial malleolus
AB = Tibiofibular clear space
BC = Tibiofibular overlap
EF = Medial clear space

Figure 8-16 Evaluation of Ankle Joint Clear Space.
Normal tibiofibular overlap (BC) should be more than 1 mm, tibiofibular clear space (AB) less than 6 mm, and a medial clear space (EF) less than 4 mm. (From Coughlin MJ, Mann RA: *Surgery of the foot and ankle*, ed 7, vol 2, St Louis, 1999, Mosby.)

Radiographic evaluation of a suggested syndesmotic injury is based on knowledge of normal anatomic relationships of the ankle bones. A widened syndesmosis is present if there is less than 6 mm of space visualized on a mortise view between the distal tibia and fibula. The syndesmotic space is measured by using an AP view of the ankle and measuring 1 cm above the tibial plafond. A perpendicular line is then drawn across the ankle joint. Normally there is more than 1 mm of overlap between the tibia and fibula.[1] This area is known as the clear space. Figure 8-16 illustrates evaluation of clear space on plain x-ray.

The basic x-ray projections are AP, lateral, and mortise (Figures 8-17 and 8-18).[8] Some orthopedic surgeons delete the AP view because it does not always offer more information than that visualized in the lateral and mortise views. However, deleting the AP view remains an orthopedic decision. If ankle instability is suggested or noted on clinical examination, stress views of the ankle may be indicated.

Of the three projections, the mortise view is probably the most important. Normally the saddle-shaped tibiotalar joint is highly congruent. Functionally this means that there is a very small margin for maintaining this congruity. During normal walking the ankle bears four to five times the person's body weight; a shift of the joint more than a couple of millimeters will cause uneven wearing of the articular cartilage and may accelerate degenerative changes.

The mortise projection is similar to an AP film, but a mortise view requires the foot to be in 15 degrees of internal rotation. When viewed, the lateral, superior, and

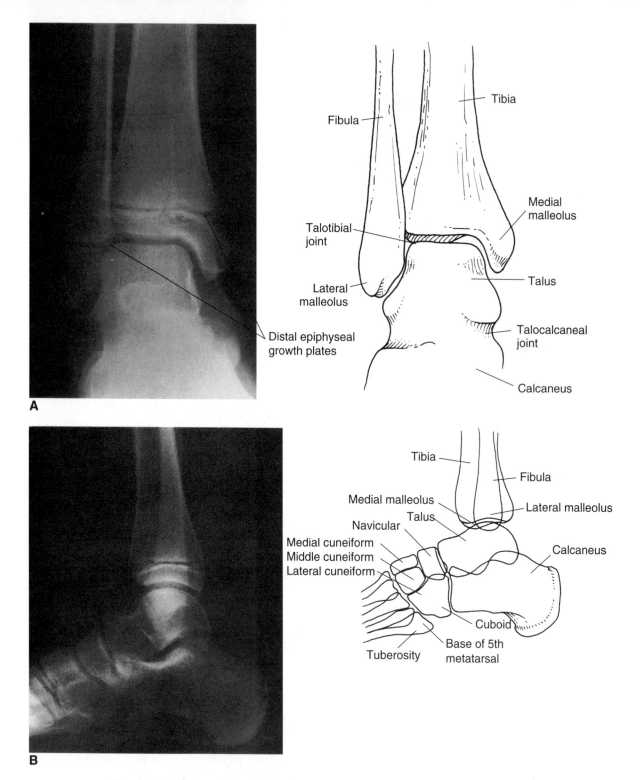

Figure 8-17 Radiographic evaluation of the normal ankle. **A,** Anteroposterior view. **B,** Lateral view. (From Coughlin MJ, Mann RA: *Surgery of the foot and ankle*, ed 7, vol 1, St Louis, 1999, Mosby.)

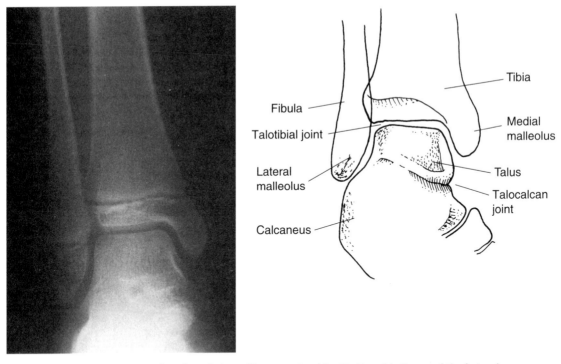

Figure 8-18 Mortise view of the ankle. (From Coughlin MJ, Mann RA: *Surgery of the foot and ankle*, ed 7, vol 1, St Louis, 1999, Mosby.)

medial joint spaces should be equally distanced. Unequal widening of the joint space indicates more severe ligamentous injury, and the patient should be referred to an orthopedic surgeon for further evaluation.

Computed tomography (CT) and magnetic resonance imaging (MRI) are generally not appropriate for acute evaluation of the ankle in an outpatient setting. Ankle pain, swelling, and instability that persists beyond 4 to 6 weeks may require these tests to evaluate the ankle for fracture, osteochondritis, or other occult pathologic conditions. Other causes of chronic ankle pain or instability include impingement attributable to synovial scarring, osteochondral lesions, cartilage damage, congenital abnormalities, or tumor.[15,41] In any case, persistent symptoms after appropriate treatment necessitate a referral to an orthopedic surgeon.

Treatment. RICE is the initial treatment for an ankle injury. Rest does not mean immobilization unless a fracture is suggested; rather, decreased weight bearing and stabilization with a splint are indicated. A rigid splint

or crutches will lessen strain on the injured ankle. Applications of ice or a cold pack for 10 to 20 minutes every 1 to 2 hours help relieve swelling and pain. Icing the ankle should generally continue for the first 24 to 48 hours after injury. Compression can be accomplished with an elastic bandage. Care must be taken not to apply the bandage too tightly, since continued swelling can occur, causing circulatory problems. The elastic bandage should be applied in a distal to proximal direction to improve lymphatic and vascular drainage. Elevation of the ankle above the level of the heart for the first 24 to 48 hours after injury will lessen dependent edema. Once swelling begins to diminish (usually 48 to 72 hours after injury), the patient should be encouraged to begin bearing weight if there is no joint instability. The practitioner should emphasize that although there may be some pain initially, weight bearing with the splint will not cause further ligamentous damage.

Nonsteroidal antiinflammatory drugs (NSAIDs) are the primary medications of choice for ankle sprains.

Acetaminophen can be added for its analgesic effect. Except in significant ligamentous injuries, narcotics are not usually needed to control pain. If narcotic analgesia is required, it is generally necessary only for a few days.

When discussing treatment with the patient, the prolonged recovery time of an ankle sprain should be emphasized. Although great improvement in symptoms usually occurs in 3 to 4 weeks, it can easily be 6 to 8 weeks before most symptoms have resolved. Intermittent swelling of the joint for 4 to 6 months after injury is not uncommon.

Rehabilitation of the ankle joint varies, to some degree, on the individual and his or her lifestyle. The athletic individual may require more aggressive rehabilitation than the older, sedentary, or bedridden patient. Regardless of patient lifestyle, the goal of rehabilitation is to promote the healing of the ligaments with as little residual scar tissue as possible, allowing the return of a stable, functional ankle. Early physical therapy (PT), emphasizing ROM, a reduction of pain and swelling, and an improvement in strength, is appropriate for grades I and II sprains. Treatment of grade III sprains is controversial with regard to surgical intervention versus functional rehabilitation.[31,35]

Rehabilitation is directed at restoring function and strengthening the ankle. Active ROM, gait training, and resistive exercises are often used. The return to weight-bearing status assists in decreasing pain and swelling. Most patients require only a short course of PT. Once a patient is able to demonstrate satisfactory compliance with an exercise program, rehabilitation can continue at home.

If the practitioner is concerned about the severity of ligamentous injury, referral to an orthopedic surgeon within 48 to 72 hours of injury is reasonable in most instances. For the first 48 hours after injury, acute swelling may make accurate clinical evaluation difficult. Immediate referral to an orthopedic surgeon is appropriate if there is pain over bony areas (especially over the medial or lateral malleolus), obvious deformity of the ankle, neurovascular compromise, or significant weakness or instability of the joint. If immediate referral to an orthopedic surgeon is indicated, x-ray films of the ankle should also be provided.

Ankle Fractures

Perhaps surprisingly, ankle fractures occur in a greater percentage in nonathletes than in athletic individuals. Not surprisingly, ankle fractures are among the most frequent fractures treated by orthopedic surgeons. Fractures of the lateral malleolus are often seen in conjunction with lateral ankle ligamentous injuries. Some fractures, such as those of the dome of the talus, can be subtle in their physical and radiographic presentation. In a skeletally immature patient (i.e., the epiphyseal plates are still open), ligaments are relatively stronger than bone and an ankle inversion "sprain" may result in a Salter-Harris grade II injury to the distal epiphysis. (Table 8-4 summarizes the Salter-Harris classification system.) When the epiphyseal plates have fused, there is

---

TABLE 8-4   Salter-Harris Classification of Epiphyseal Fractures

Grade	Characteristics of Injury
I	Separation of epiphysis; rarely affects growth
	Often missed on plain x-ray film; mistaken for sprain on clinical examination
II	Fracture through epiphysis; fracture line extends toward metaphysis (shaft) of bone
III	Fracture through epiphysis; fracture line extends distally toward joint
	May affect growth if not properly reduced
IV	Fracture of epiphysis with fracture line extending both proximally toward shaft and distally into joint
	High risk for premature closure of epiphyseal plate
V	Crush injury to epiphyseal plate; can be mistaken for Salter-Harris grade I on plain films
	Arrest of epiphyseal growth plate can occur

no need to worry about damage to the epiphyseal growth plates. When treating fractures near a joint in adolescents whose epiphyseal plates have not yet closed, it is prudent to refer them to an orthopedic surgeon.

The majority of ankle fractures are the result of acute trauma, whether from a sporting activity, fall, or direct blow. These types of injury generally involve the lateral or the medial malleolus, or both malleoli. Stress fractures of the ankle can also occur, but these tend to involve the anteromedial aspect of the distal tibia.

Ankle fractures are primarily classified using one of two systems. The Lauge-Hansen system is based on the position of the foot and the direction of the injuring force at the time of injury. The second system, the Danis-Weber, is based on the level of the fibular fracture in relationship to the ankle joint. Some orthopedic surgeons use a modification of the Danis-Weber system, the AO classification. This system includes the variables of posterior or medial malleolar injury.[47] Regardless of which system is used, the more proximal (i.e., higher) the fibular fracture, the more unstable the joint and the more likely the need for surgical stabilization. Figure 8-19 shows a widened ankle mortise caused by a fibular fracture above the joint.

Fractures at or above the level of the talar dome should always be referred to an orthopedic surgeon. Small, nondisplaced avulsion fractures from the distal tip of either the lateral or medial malleolus can often be managed with a rigid ankle brace for 4 to 6 weeks. Fractures near the level of the talar dome must be carefully evaluated with consideration given to the ankle mortise. Because of the high congruity of the ankle joint, a talar shift of even 1 mm can decrease joint contact area by as much as 40%.[43]

High-impact axial loading of the ankle joint, such as those that occur in motor vehicle accidents or from a fall from a height, may involve the distal tibial articular surface or plafond. Energy from this type of impact is transmitted up the tibia and causes a comminuted fracture known as a pilon fracture. Tibial pilon fractures (Figure 8-20) result in immediate severe pain and swelling, as well as an inability to bear weight on the ankle. These serious injuries generally require surgical stabilization.

In a primary care setting, a patient who has a history of ankle trauma and tenderness over a bony prominence,

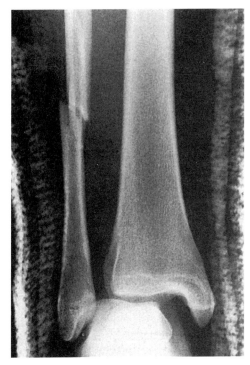

Figure 8-19 Widened lateral ankle joint caused by a fracture of the fibula proximal to the mortise and with disruption of the syndesmosis. (From Donatto KC: Ankle fractures and syndesmosis injuries, *Orthop Clin North Am* 32(1):79-90, 2001.)

an inability to bear weight on an injured ankle, or an obvious ankle deformity should be splinted and referred to an emergency department or orthopedic surgeon. X-ray films are always appropriate in this situation.

History. Acute ankle fractures are the result of direct or indirect trauma. As a rule, the greater the impact, the more complex the fracture with more fragments, greater displacement, and more extensive soft-tissue damage. Patients may not recall the presence of a rotational component to their injury, but they can generally remember how they fell, which side of the ankle sustained a blow, and what activity produced the injury.

Hearing a crack or pop may indicate a fracture, but these sounds are also frequently associated with ligamentous injury. Immediate or rapid onset of ecchymosis and swelling may indicate either ligamentous tearing or bone injury. Inability to bear weight on the injured ankle

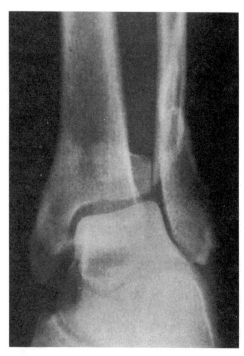

Figure 8-20   Tibial Pilon Fracture. This injury is the result of significant axial loading of the ankle. (From Coughlin MJ, Mann RA: *Surgery of the foot and ankle*, ed 7, vol 2, St Louis, 1999, Mosby.)

is typical with a fracture, but this finding can also occur with a sprain.

Point tenderness is a classic finding in fracture, but the high association of ligamentous injuries with ankle fractures may obscure a well-localized feeling of pain. Patient self-treatment should be explored to determine the relative probability of further, post-insult injury having occurred. A stable spiral fracture of the fibula may become impacted or displaced by the patient who has spent 1 or 2 days "trying to walk out the pain." The use and efficacy of medication and the presence or absence of associated symptoms, such as numbness, tingling, and cyanosis, can indicate the presence of associated neurologic or vascular injury.

Physical Examination. As with other ankle injuries, the practitioner must first look for obvious deformity or discoloration. The presence and location of fracture blisters should be noted. The areas of least pain

are gently palpated, progressing to more tender soft-tissue and bony prominences. The vascular status is evaluated by checking both the dorsalis pedis and posterior tibial pulses, and comparing contralateral pulses. The presence and type of edema is noted, as well as the briskness of capillary refill in the toes. (Normal capillary refill time is less than 2 to 3 seconds.) Sensation to light touch and proprioception should also be evaluated.

Asking the patient to wiggle his or her toes can test motor function. In the presence of acute injury, most patients will be unable or unwilling to move the affected ankle. Passive movement of the ankle should be approached cautiously, if at all. If a fracture is suggested, x-ray films should be obtained after immobilizing the joint.

Radiographic Studies. At a minimum, lateral and mortise views of the ankle should be obtained.[6,8] If radiographic facilities are not readily available, the ankle should be splinted and the patient referred to an emergency department or orthopedic surgeon. A pre-formed splint, loosely secured with an elastic bandage, is appropriate. If no splinting material is available, the patient should maintain a non–weight-bearing status and be referred to an appropriate facility.

Although most fractures can be seen on plain x-ray films, bony overlap, degenerative changes, or poor positioning during the x-ray procedure can obscure details, including some fractures. Evaluation of the ankle mortise is at least as important as searching for a fracture.

A lateral x-ray view shows anterior or posterior distal tibial fractures, posterior or spiral fibular fractures, and some fractures of the talar dome. Anterior or posterior displacement of the talus can also be evaluated.

The mortise film is essentially an AP view of the ankle, but the foot is internally rotated 15 degrees. This position makes evaluation of the mortise easier by reducing the apparent overlap of the fibula on the tibia. Several parameters are evaluated to determine stability of the joint. Of these measurements, most are subject to controversy[47] and are not essential to primary care management.

CT is useful in evaluating the joint itself, providing information on displacement of comminuted fractures and determining bone position. CT evaluation of the ankle is generally not necessary in an acute primary care setting.

Pilon Fractures

Direct axial loading of the ankle can cause an impaction fracture involving the distal tibial articular surface (Figure 8-21). Though uncommon, representing only 1% to 10% of lower extremity fractures, pilon fractures usually result in significant joint surface damage. The articular surface of the tibia (the plafond) is disrupted, and the fracture is comminuted. Fractures of this type are the result of a significant force, such as a motor vehicle accident or fall from a great height but can also result from a low-energy injury.[38]

Other than significant swelling and pain, there may be no obvious deformity of the ankle. These fractures should be treated surgically. In spite of surgical repair, functional return is often poor. Impaction and comminution of fracture fragments disrupt the articular surface of the distal tibia, often resulting in posttraumatic arthritis. These patients should be stabilized, placed on non–weight-bearing status, and urgently referred to an emergency department or orthopedic surgeon.

Maisonneuve Fracture

When a fracture of the medial malleolus occurs in combination with a fractured fibula above the joint line, it creates an unstable ankle (Figure 8-22). This type of injury, called a Maisonneuve fracture, occurs when there is pronation of the foot combined with external rotation of the talus. The force of the injury is transmitted up the fibular shaft. The deltoid ligament is frequently torn, and a widening of the medial malleolus is visualized on x-ray (see Figure 8-19). The deltoid ligament may flip into the widened medial joint, making nonsurgical reduction impossible. These patients should be splinted, placed on non–weight-bearing status, and urgently referred.

Achilles' Tendinopathy

A paratenon, rather than a synovial sheath, covers the Achilles' tendon. Lying beneath the paratenon, the epitenon surrounds the Achilles tendon. A multitude of terms, including tendinosis, tenopathy, paratenonitis, tenosynovitis, and achillodynia are used to describe pain in the Achilles tendon.[37] As with other forms of tendinopathy, histopathologic studies are necessary to differentiate tendon degradation from inflammation. Tendonitis does not involve intrinsic changes of sub-

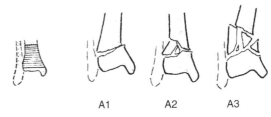

43-A Tibia distal, extra-articular fracture

A1 .... metaphyseal simple
A2 .... metaphyseal Wedge
A3 .... metaphyseal complex

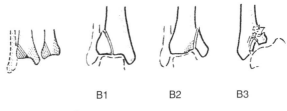

43-B Tibia distal, partial articular fracture

B1 .... pure split
B2 .... split-depression
B3 .... depression multifragmentary

43-C Tibia distal, complete articular fracture

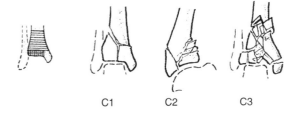

C1 .... articular simple, metaphyseal simple
C2 .... articular simple, metaphyseal multifragmentary
C3 .... multifragmentary

Figure 8-21 Diagrammatic representation of various types of tibial pilon fractures. (From Borrelli J Jr, Ellis E: Pilon fractures: assessment and treatment, *Orthop Clin North Am* 33(1):231-245, 2002.)

stance of the tendon. The term tendinosis is becoming more commonly used to describe Achilles tendon pain since most studies show degeneration of the tendon

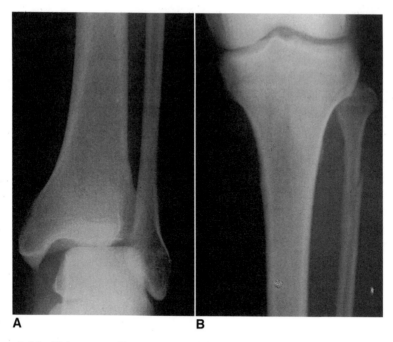

A   **B**

Figure 8-22   Maisonneuve Fracture. A, Initial x-ray showed widening of the medial ankle mortise due to lateral displacement of the talus. **B,** X-ray of the proximal fibula shows spiral fracture. (From Browner BD et al, editors: *Skeletal trauma,* ed 3, vol 2, Philadelphia, 2003, WB Saunders.)

rather than inflammation.[21] Tendinosis may or may not be associated with tendonitis. The most common site of Achilles tendinopathy is 2 to 6 cm proximal to its insertion on the calcaneus, where the tendon is relatively avascular.[2]

History. As with other forms of tendinopathy, Achilles' tendinopathy is generally the result of overuse or overstretching, or of a combination of the two. Runners and joggers, particularly men older than age 40, are prone to developing pain in the Achilles' tendon. Symptoms of pain, stiffness at the beginning of a run, and swelling over the tendon can be acute or chronic. If symptoms persist longer than 6 months, Achilles' tendinopathy can be considered chronic.

During running, the Achilles' tendon is subject to forces equivalent to ten times the individual's body weight.[6] As the foot strikes the ground and during the toe-off, additional rotational forces are placed on the tendon. The tendons of patients with flat feet (especially with hyperpronation of the feet), forefoot varus deformity, or unusually high arches are also subject to additional stresses. Training errors, such as a sudden increase in distance or intensity or running, poorly fitted shoes, or a dramatic change in running surfaces can compound the already significant stresses placed on the tendon.

Initially the paratenon that surrounds the tendon becomes inflamed and adheres to the tendon, further aggravating the inflammatory process. At this stage, rest, ice, and antiinflammatory medication will usually resolve symptoms. Continued stressing of the tendon can lead to degenerative changes of the tendon that can progress to actual tears.[10]

In runners, stiffness in the morning (or at the start of a run) is typical, followed by a period of increased mobility with gradually increasing pain. As the tendon becomes more inflamed and adhesions develop between the tendon and paratenon, pain may occur with normal walking. It is important that the patient be asked to

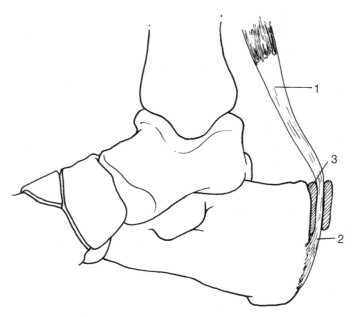

Figure 8-23 Site of Achilles' Tendon Pain. Area is relatively avascular and is a common site for tendonitis and tendinosis *(1)*. Pain can also occur at the tendon insertion *(2)*, or in conjunction with retrocalcaneal bursitis *(3)*.

relate the onset of symptoms, self-treatment and results, and any changes in activity level.

Physical Examination and Diagnosis. The presenting symptom is typically pain, 1 to 2 inches (2 to 6 cm) proximal to the insertion of the Achilles' tendon on the superior aspect of the posterior calcaneus (Figure 8-23). The tendon is frequently thickened and warmer to the touch when compared with the unaffected side. Crepitus is sometimes present. Resisted plantar flexion of the foot tends to increase pain, and the patient may complain of weakness.

Swelling at the posterolateral border of the superior calcaneus may be present with insertional Achilles' tendinosis. The retrocalcaneal bursa may become inflamed, causing pain and swelling anterior to the Achilles' tendon insertion. As long as the tendon is intact, the patient will be able to actively plantar flex the foot. "Pushing down on the gas pedal" or standing on the tips of the toes can be used to evaluate strength.

Clinically, tendinosis is somewhat different than tendonitis. With tendinosis, the tendon is thickened several centimeters. The tendon may be nontender or quite painful with compression, but it may not have any increased temperature when palpated. Tendinosis is more likely to limit the patient's ability to stand on the tips of the toes or perform toe raises. Nodules, attributable to calcifications in the tendon, may occasionally be palpable.[42]

Treatment. Conservative treatment with rest, ice, and NSAIDs will reduce local inflammation. Rest may involve decreasing running distance or, in severe cases, may include using crutches on the affected side to maintain nonweight bearing during activities for 1 to 2 weeks. Intermittent application of ice will also reduce swelling and generally increase comfort. Regular administration of NSAIDs for 1 or 2 weeks will generally relieve pain and inflammation. If abnormal biomechanics of the foot are noted, corrective orthotics may alleviate symptoms. Many physical therapists can fabricate orthotics, or they can be purchased at some specialty footwear stores. Most podiatrists will also fabricate custom orthotics, but usually at a higher cost than the other two sources. In some cases, cast immobilization may be appropriate.[42] Injection of steroids is not indicated.

Rehabilitation exercises for mild cases can be performed at home. The patient stands approximately 18 to 24 inches away from a wall and, keeping his or her knees straight, leans forward toward the wall. Once the upper torso is against the wall, the patient holds this position for 5 to 10 seconds and repeats this maneuver ten times, working up to three sets of ten. These wall leans should also be repeated with the knees flexed to 45 degrees. This exercise isolates the gastrocnemius and soleus muscles.

Further strengthening of the Achilles' tendon can be accomplished by using elastic bands, or even a bicycle tire inner tube. The patient sits with his or her legs extended and loops the band over the ball of the ipsilateral foot, then actively plantar flexes the foot, holding the position for 5 seconds. Initially, this exercise should be repeated ten times. As the patient becomes able to perform this stretch, repetitions can gradually increase to three sets of ten performed twice a day.

Formal PT is beneficial in many cases. Ultrasound can make stretching less painful. Electric muscle stimulation and massage may help release adhesions that develop in chronic tendonitis. Orthotics can help correct excessive pronation of the foot.

Improvement in symptoms usually occurs within 2 to 3 weeks. Once the patient is pain-free with equal plantar flexion strength, resumption of running or sports is appropriate. In selected recalcitrant cases, surgical reconstruction of the Achilles' tendon may be indicated.[30] After surgical repair, more than 6 months of rehabilitation may be necessary to achieve normal plantar flexion.[3]

Achilles' Tendon Rupture

History and Physical Examination. Rupture of the Achilles' tendon can be caused by an acute injury or by untreated chronic tendonitis. An acute rupture is typically described as a sudden sharp pain, often feeling like, "I was hit with a baseball bat." Immediate swelling almost always occurs, and attempts to continue activity are extremely difficult. Any activity requiring forceful contraction of the Achilles' tendon, such as running from a stationary position (i.e., starting a sprint or running bases) or pushing a stalled car, can lead to acute tearing.

Rupture attributable to chronic tendonitis is associated with little pain. The patient may not recall a specific event, but he or she may report difficulty climbing stairs and weakness in the ankle. Achilles' tendon rupture is associated with men over the age of 30 years, often the "weekend warrior" type of athlete. Usually there is no significant predisposing medical history, although the administration of fluoroquinolone antibiotics has recently, though rarely, been associated with spontaneous rupture.[13]

Diagnosis. A palpable gap in the Achilles' tendon or a positive Thompson's test is almost pathognomonic for rupture of the Achilles' tendon. Rapid diagnosis is important to decrease complications associated with delayed treatment. A significant gap may not always be palpable, but if the Achilles' tendon is ruptured, it is always more difficult to palpate distinctly than the contralateral structure.

Thompson's test is the most useful clinical tool for diagnosing a complete rupture of the Achilles' tendon. To perform the test, the examiner asks the patient to lie prone on the exam table, with his or her feet hanging over the edge to relax the calves.[25] The practitioner then squeezes the patient's calf; a normal reaction is plantar flexion of the foot (Figure 8-24). A positive test is absence of plantar flexion and is highly suggestive of a ruptured tendon. The Copeland test can be used to better quantify an equivocal Thompson's test.[7] To perform this test, a sphygmomanometer is placed on the patient's affected calf and inflated to 100 mm Hg. The ipsilateral foot is then dorsiflexed. Normally, the pressure will rise to about 140 mm Hg. If the Achilles' tendon is ruptured, there will be minimal change in pressure.

Additional testing such as ultrasound is rarely necessary in cases of acute Achilles' tendon rupture. It may be appropriate, however, if there is any question of tendon integrity.

Even with appropriate clinical evaluation, if there is any suggestion of tendon rupture, the patient should be referred to an orthopedic surgeon. It has been reported that up to 25% of Achilles' tendon tears are misdiagnosed.[17,25]

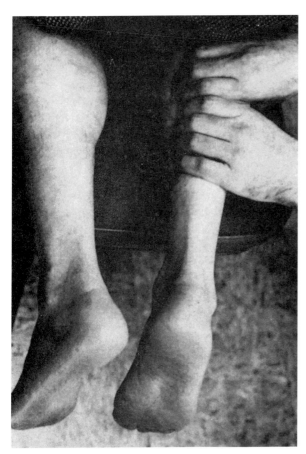

Figure 8-24 Positive Thompson's Test on the Right. When the calf is squeezed, a normal response is plantar flexion of the foot. In this example the foot remains in a neutral position. (From Mercier LR: *Practical orthopedics*, ed 5, St Louis, 2000, Mosby.)

Treatment. Both surgical and nonsurgical approaches have been used to treat acute ruptures of the Achilles' tendon. For active or athletic individuals, surgical repair is generally indicated. Surgical repair offers the advantages of an earlier return to activity, restoration of Achilles' tendon length, and the recovery of greater strength compared to patients treated nonoperatively.[44]

Nonoperative treatment consists of immobilization in either a cast or a cast boot for 8 to 12 weeks, followed by PT. A cast boot should have a locking hinge to allow 15 degrees of plantar flexion. When casted, the foot is placed in the same 15 degrees of plantar flexion to allow the ends of the tendon to fibrose with scar tissue. Disadvantages of casting include muscle atrophy, joint stiffness, and disuse osteopenia. Nonoperative treatment has been shown to have a higher rate of re-rupture.[5,28] Casting remains a viable alternative for the sedentary, older person or for those who have risk factors that make them poor candidates for surgical treatment.

Other Causes of Ankle Pain

Ankle pain, especially of a chronic nature, can be attributable to many factors. Chronic pain after trauma such as a sprain or a fracture is most often caused by incomplete rehabilitation.[32] The location of pain is the first clue in deciphering its cause.

Lateral ankle pain may be the result of a poorly rehabilitated sprain, more significant ligamentous injury than originally diagnosed, an occult fracture, or peroneal tendon instability. Anterior ankle pain can indicate the presence of a syndesmotic injury, osteophytes, or impingement. Osteochondral fractures of the talus attributable to vascular, cartilage, or bony injury may develop weeks to months after an ankle injury. Pain from an osteochondral injury may come from anywhere in the ankle joint. Posterior ankle pain may be a symptom of os trigonum, or posterior impingement, syndrome.[46]

A patient with persistent pain after an ankle sprain who has not undergone any rehabilitation program is a good candidate for a formal PT program. Therapy should include ROM, stretching, and muscle-strengthening exercises. Activities designed to improve proprioception are also important.

Persistent pain or instability after a sprain may also indicate more severe ligamentous damage than first diagnosed. Complete rupture of one or more ligaments can cause a "giving way" of the ankle, a difficulty navigating uneven surfaces, or positive anterior drawer or talar tilt testing. Patients with these symptoms should be referred to an orthopedic surgeon. MRI evaluation may be helpful in determining the extent of ligamentous damage.

Peroneal Tendon Problems

Lateral ankle pain should be evaluated for possible peroneal tendon abnormality if pain persists after a sprain has had adequate time to heal.[36] Chronic pain from a sprain tends to be localized to the injured area. Pain from peroneal tendonitis tends to be more proximal and usually runs along the posterior fibula. Unlike the pain with most lateral ankle sprains, peroneal tendon pain is exacerbated by eversion of the foot. Weakness of eversion is not uncommon.

Injury to the superior peroneal retinaculum (SPR) can cause peroneal tendon instability. Located along the posterior fibula approximately 2 cm proximal to the tip of the bone, the SPR is a fibrous band of tissue whose primary function is to keep the peroneal tendons in the retromalleolar sulcus (Figure 8-25). Most often the SPR is not torn, but pulled away from the lateral malleolus.[24] When the tendons are no longer held in place, they tend to subluxate with certain ankle movements. As they move out of the sulcus, the patient may feel or hear a snapping or popping over the lateral ankle. The tendon movement usually causes a sharp, burning pain that extends proximally over the lateral ankle and calf. Occasionally, the subluxating tendon is visible as it pops out of its normal sulcus.

Conditions associated with peroneal tendonitis or instability include lateral ankle sprain (especially from

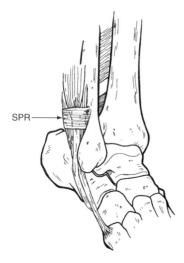

Figure 8-25   The superior peroneal retinaculum (SPR) helps stabilize the peroneal tendons in the sulcus at the distal end of the fibula.

forced dorsiflexion attributable to sudden deceleration), cerebral palsy and other neuromuscular diseases, avulsion fracture of the posterior distal fibula, and even congenital dislocation.[24]

Treatment of peroneal tendonitis is usually rest, ice, and NSAIDs. PT is often useful in regaining strength, and stretching exercises will often prevent recurrence.

Acute tendon instability should be initially treated with immobilization, followed by PT to improve strength and proprioception.[39] If there is no improvement after 4 to 6 weeks, most orthopedic surgeons will proceed with surgical repair.

Osteochondritis Dissecans (Osteonecrosis)

Osteochondral damage of the talar dome, including fractures, can be the result of forceful ankle inversion or eversion that "jams" the talus into the medial or lateral malleolus, damaging the bone and articular cartilage. Over time, these damaged areas may necrose and separate from the talus (Figure 8-26). Repeated ankle sprains can cause cumulative trauma to the talus, also causing osteochondral lesions.

Osteonecrotic changes in the talus are often not evident on x-ray films for 6 weeks or more after injury (Figure 8-27). When present, osseous changes are often subtle. CT and MRI are sensitive tools used for evaluating these lesions (Figure 8-28). A bone scan, though sensitive, is less specific and may not show changes as early as an MRI.

Although some lesions will heal without specific treatment, the area of defect may separate and become a loose body within the joint. In addition to joint pain, locking or catching, and instability, posttraumatic arthritis can develop. Surgical treatment is indicated if healing does not occur after a 6-week course of immobilization. Arthroscopic surgical drilling of the lesion and removal of any loose fragments is usually successful in allowing the bone to heal.

Ideally a patient with any prolonged ankle pain will be referred to an orthopedic surgeon before significant joint symptoms develop. If symptoms have been present for 1 month or longer after appropriate rehabilitation, repeat x-ray studies are appropriate.

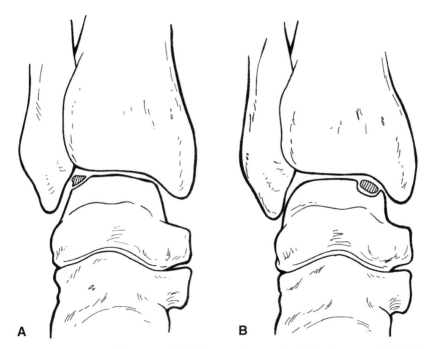

Figure 8-26 Lateral **(A)** and medial **(B)** areas of osteochondritis dissecans of the talus. Lateral injuries often follow acute trauma. The injured areas of bone and cartilage may separate from the talus.

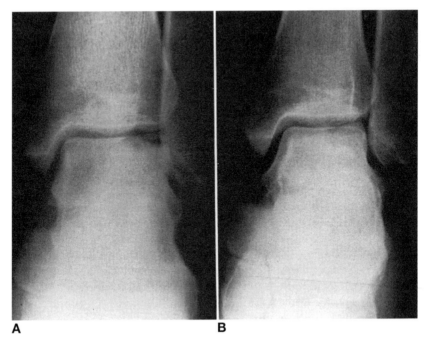

Figure 8-27 **A,** Plain x-ray film showing osteonecrotic lesion of the lateral talar dome. Pain persisted for 8 months before the area was surgically excised. **B,** X-ray film showing appearance of osteonecrotic lesion 3 years after surgery. At this time, the ankle was still painless. (From Canale ST, editor: *Campbell's operative orthopaedics*, ed 10, vol 3, St Louis, 2003, Mosby.)

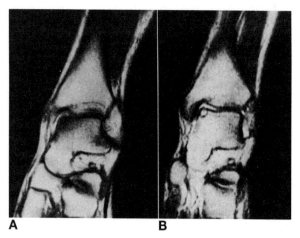

A   **B**

Figure 8-28   Magnetic Resonance Image of the Talus Showing Osteonecrotic Lesions of the Talus. A, Lateral view of the talus indicates osteonecrotic area. **B,** Coronal view of detached talar fragment. (From Firooznia H et al, editors: *MRI and CT of the musculoskeletal system*, St Louis, 1992, Mosby.)

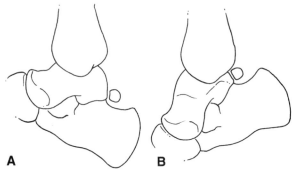

A   **B**

Figure 8-29   Posterior Impingement Test. A, When the foot is dorsiflexed, the os trigonum is relatively free of surrounding bone. **B,** Plantar flexing the foot and pushing upward on the heel will compress the bone and posterior ankle soft tissues, causing pain in a symptomatic ankle. (From Bucholz RW: *Orthopaedic decision making*, ed 2, St Louis, 1996, Mosby.)

Posterior Impingement Syndrome

Chronic posterior ankle pain can be a symptom of os trigonum syndrome, also known as posterior impingement syndrome. This entity is more common in dancers, especially ballet dancers, than in other populations. In patients who have an accessory ossicle known as the os trigonum (see Chapter 9), an acute ankle sprain may cause loosening of the soft-tissue attachments of the bone, resulting in its instability. The basic pathologic condition is impingement of the soft tissues in the posterior ankle when the foot is plantar flexed. This condition can also occur with an enlarged posterior talar tubercle. Posterior impingement syndrome is a clinical diagnosis. Posterior ankle pain that occurs with forcible plantar flexion of the foot is the primary test used to diagnose this entity (Figure 8-29). Lateral ankle x-ray films may confirm the presence of an os trigonum or a prominent posterior talar tubercle, but their absence does not exclude the diagnosis. Further imaging studies are rarely indicated.[12]

Treatment is usually conservative with rest, ice, PT, and antiinflammatory medications. If symptoms do not resolve with conservative therapy, the patient should be referred to an orthopedic surgeon.

IMAGING STUDIES

X-Ray Films

The American College of Radiology has developed specific criteria for the appropriateness of imaging studies used to evaluate ankle fractures and chronic ankle pain.[6,9] These guidelines are useful to help the practitioner in deciding what imaging studies are suitable for specific conditions.

X-ray films are the primary initial diagnostic imaging study for evaluating the ankle. Bony contour, alignment, density, and joint integrity can be quickly and inexpensively evaluated. Although not all ankle injuries are appropriate for x-ray evaluation, plain radiographic films should initially be used to evaluate any area of bony tenderness or deformity.

When used appropriately, ultrasound (US), scintography, CT, and MRI provide additional and specific information about ankle abnormalities.

Ultrasound

US is most often used for evaluating tendons. In the case of Achilles' tendon rupture, US is a rapid, safe, and relatively inexpensive tool to localize and assess the extent of injury. Another use for US of the ankle is with suggested transient peroneal tendon instability. A tear in the retinaculum covering the peroneal tendons may result in intermittent subluxation of the tendons. Since subluxation is most likely to occur during dorsiflexion and inversion, the real-time imaging of US offers an advantage and may allow better visualization of the problem than either MRI or CT.[18] The primary limitation of US is the expertise of the ultrasonographer.

Magnetic Resonance Imaging

MRI of the ankle is useful in evaluating tendons, cartilage, synovial lesions, tumors, and bone injury. MRI can distinguish subtle differences in the tendon substance such as a longitudinal split, degenerative change, partial tears, or tenosynovitis. Examining soft-tissue structural integrity is useful in evaluating chronic ankle pain that may be attributable to a partial rupture or to scar tissue, as well as in evaluating chronic inflammation of a tendon or a ligament. MRI readily evaluates bone marrow edema, an early change associated with trauma. Other osseous lesions that can be detected by MRI include bone contusion, osteochondral lesions, stress fracture, occult fracture, and osteonecrosis (ON). One of the earliest changes associated with ON is marrow edema. MRI is excellent for identifying marrow edema and can therefore identify ON before inflammatory changes show on bone scan.

Evaluation of hyaline (articular) cartilage is appropriate for MRI, but this scanning choice is not perfect. Gadolinium-enhanced MRI is beneficial for earlier detection of cartilaginous defects.[16]

Differences in the MRI appearance of fat, synovial fluid, and soft tissue make MRI the preferred tool for evaluating most soft-tissue masses. Although MRI can determine basic composition of a mass, malignant tumors cannot be differentiated from those that are benign either by signal intensity of the tumor border or by its margin.[23]

Magnetic resonance arthrography is useful for evaluating chronic ankle instability since it is much more accurate than stress radiography in identifying chronic ligament tears.

Computed Tomography

Evaluation of osseous structures is the primary use of CT. One of the greatest benefits of CT is its capability of visualizing occult or unusual fractures. CT provides more detailed information on fracture extent, healing, and alignment than other imaging studies. Alignment of normal osseous structures, accessory ossicles, and osseous tumors are best visualized by CT. Like MRI, CT is useful in evaluating osteochondritis dissecans. Unlike MRI, CT provides information about tumor histology, mineralization, and cortical integrity of bone.[20]

Other imaging procedures include CT arthrography, tenography, and joint arthrography. Tenography can be used to identify abnormalities of the tendon sheath and to inject medication (usually local anesthetics or steroids) into the site of pathology.[19]

INDICATIONS FOR REFERRAL

See the following Red Flags Box for referral information.

Red Flags *for Ankle Disorders*

Patients with these findings may need to be referred for more extensive work-up.

Signs and Symptoms	Response
Ankle instability (positive anterior drawer and talar tilt tests); suggested fracture or associated tendon injury with grade II or grade III calcaneofibular lateral ankle sprain	Refer to orthopedic surgeon
Medial ankle sprain with tenderness over medial malleolus; gross deformity, significant weakness, or neurovascular compromise	Possible fracture; refer to orthopedic surgeon
Positive squeeze test for lateral or medial ligamentous injury	Possible syndesmotic injury; refer to orthopedic surgeon
Pain over bony areas (especially medial or lateral malleolus), obvious deformity of the ankle, neurovascular compromise, or significant weakness or instability of joint	Possible severe ligamentous injury or fracture; refer to orthopedic surgeon
Fracture is near joint in adolescent whose epiphyseal plates have not yet closed	High risk for premature epiphyseal plate closure or growth arrest; refer to orthopedic surgeon for further examination and work-up
Fracture is at or above level of talar dome	Risk for decreased joint contact area; always refer to orthopedic surgeon for further treatment
Immediate severe pain and swelling; inability to bear weight on ankle	Possible tibial pilon fracture; immediately refer to emergency department or orthopedic surgeon for surgical stabilization
Fracture of medial malleolus occurs in combination with fractured fibula above the joint line, creating an unstable ankle	Possible Maisonneuve fracture; immediately refer to emergency department or orthopedic surgeon for surgical reduction
Palpable gap in Achilles' tendon or positive Thompson's test	Possible Achilles' tendon rupture; refer to orthopedic surgeon for possible surgical repair
Ankle gives way; difficulty in navigating uneven surfaces; positive anterior drawer or talar tilt tests after treatment for sprain	Possible severe ligamentous damage; refer to orthopedic surgeon for further evaluation
No improvement in peroneal tendon instability after 4 to 6 weeks of casting	Refer to orthopedic surgeon for surgical repair
No improvement of symptoms of osteochondritis dissecans after 6 weeks of immobilization and nonweight–bearing status	Refer to orthopedic surgeon for possible surgical drilling of lesion and removal of any loose fragments
No improvement of symptoms of posterior impingement syndrome after conservative treatment	Refer to orthopedic surgeon for possible surgical management

REFERENCES

1. Adelaar RS et al: Ankle and foot trauma. In Kasser JR, editor: *Orthopaedic knowledge update 5*, Rosemont, IL, 1996, American Academy of Orthopaedic Surgeons.
2. Ahmed IM et al: Blood supply of the Achilles tendon, *J Orthop Res* 16:591, 1998.
3. Angerman P, Hovgaard D: Chronic Achilles tendinopathy in athletic individuals: results of nonsurgical treatment, *Foot Ankle Int* 20:304, 1999.
4. Bennett WF: Lateral ankle sprains. Part I: anatomy, biomechanics, diagnosis and natural history, *Orthop Rev* 23:381, 1994.
5. Bhandari M et al: Treatment of acute Achilles tendon ruptures: a systematic overview and metaanalysis, *Clin Orthop* 400:190, 2002.
6. Brage ME et al: Ankle fracture classification: a comparison of reliability of three x-ray views versus two, *Foot Ankle Int* 19(12):555, 1996.
7. Copeland SA: Rupture of the Achilles tendon: a new clinical test, *Ann R Coll Surg Engl* 72:270, 1990.
8. Dalinka MK et al: *Imaging of suspected ankle fractures,* Expert Panel on Musculoskeletal Imaging, American College of Radiology, ACR Appropriateness Criteria, Reston, Va, 1999, American College of Radiology, accessed 02/20/03, website: www.acr.org.
9. DeSmet AA: *Chronic ankle pain,* Expert Panel on Musculoskeletal Imaging, American College of Radiology, ACR Appropriateness Criteria, Reston, Va, 2002, American College of Radiology, accessed 02/22/03, website: www.acr.org.
10. Fredericson M: Common injuries in runners, *Sports Med* (1):49, 1996.
11. Gray JM, Alpar EK: Peroneal tenosynovitis following ankle sprain, *Injury* 32:487, 2001.
12. Hamilton WG et al: Pain in the posterior aspect of the ankle in dancers, *J Bone Joint Surg Am* 78A(10):1491, 1996.
13. Harrell RM: Fluoroquinolone-induced tendinopathy: what do we know? *South Med J* 92:622, 1999.
14. Hertel J: Functional instability following lateral ankle sprain, *Sports Med* 29:361, 2000.
15. Hintermann B et al: Arthroscopic findings in patients with chronic ankle instability, *Am J Sports Med* 30:402, 2002.
16. Hochman MG et al: MR imaging of the symptomatic ankle and foot, *Orthop Clin North Am* 28(4):659, 1997.
17. Inglis AE et al: Ruptures of the tendo Achilles—an objective assessment of surgical and nonsurgical treatment, *J Bone Joint Surg Am* 58A(7):990, 1976.
18. Jacobson JA, van Holsbeeck MT: Musculoskeletal ultrasonography, *Orthop Clin North Am* 29(1):135, 1998.
19. Jaffee NW et al: Diagnostic and therapeutic ankle tenography: outcomes and complications, *Am J Radiol* 176:365, 2001.
20. Javoshida S et al: An integrated approach to the evaluation of osseous tumors, *Orthop Clin North Am* 29(1):19, 1998.
21. Kader D et al: Achilles tendinopathy: some aspects of basic science and clinical management, *Br J Sports Med* 36:239, 2002.
22. Kumai T et al: The functional anatomy of the human talofibular ligament in relation to ankle sprain, *J Anat* 200:457, 2002.
23. Marcantonio DR et al: Practical considerations in the imaging of soft tissue tumors, *Orthop Clin North Am* 29(1):1, 1998.
24. Mason RB, Henderson IJP: Traumatic peroneal instability, *Am J Sports Med* 24(5):652, 1996.
25. Mazzone MF, McCue T: Common conditions of the Achilles tendon, *Am Fam Physician* 65:1805, 2002.
26. Michelson JD: Fractures about the ankle, *J Bone Joint Surg Am* 77A:142, 1995.
27. Michelson JD et al: Motion of the ankle in a simulated supination-external rotation fracture model, *J Bone Joint Surg Am* 78A:1024, 1996.
28. Moller M and others: Acute rupture of tendon Achillis: a prospective randomized study of comparison between surgical and non-surgical treatment, *J Bone Joint Surg Br* 83(6):843, 2001.
29. Nussbaum ED et al: Prospective evaluation of syndesmotic ankle sprain without diastasis, *Am J Sports Med* 29:31, 2001.
30. Paavola M et al: Surgical treatment of chronic Achilles tendinopathy: a prospective seven month follow up study, *Br J Sports Med* 36:178, 2002.
31. Pijnenburg CM et al: Treatment of ruptures of the lateral ankle ligaments: a meta-analysis, *J Bone Joint Surg Am* 82:761, 2000.
32. Renstrom PA: Persistently painful ankle, *J Am Acad Orthop Surg* 2:270, 1994.
33. Reference deleted on proofs.
34. Reference deleted on proofs.

35. Safran MR et al: Lateral ankle sprains: a comprehensive review. Part 2: treatment and rehabilitation with an emphasis on the athlete, *Med Sci Sports Exerc* 31:S438, 1999.

36. Scanlan RL, Gehl RS: Peroneal tendon injuries, *Clin Podiatr Med Surg* 19:419, 2002.

37. Schepsis AA et al: Achilles tendon disorders in athletes, *Am J Sports Med* 30:287, 2002.

38. Sirkin M, Sanders R: The treatment of pilon fractures, *Orthop Clin North Am* 32:91, 2000.

39. Smith AM, Teasdall R: Managing tendon disorders of the foot and ankle, *J Musculoskel Med* 19:196, 2002.

40. Stiell IG et al: A study to develop clinical decision rules for the use of radiography in acute ankle injuries, *Ann Emerg Med* 21:384, 1992.

41. Stokes W, Western GB: Persistent ankle pain after a 'simple sprain,' *Phys Sportsmed* 29:49, 2001.

42. Teitz CC et al: Tendon problems in athletic individuals, *J Bone Joint Surg Am* 79A:138, 1997.

43. Thordarson DB: Detecting and treating common foot and ankle fractures, *Phys Sportsmed* 24:29, 1996.

44. Title C, Katchis SD: Traumatic foot and ankle injuries in the athlete, *Orthop Clin North Am* 33:587, 2002.

45. Trevino SG et al: Management of acute and chronic lateral ligament injuries of the ankle, *Orthop Clin North Am* 25:1, 1994.

46. Umans H: Ankle impingement syndromes, *Semin Musculoskel Radiol* 6:133, 2002.

47. Vander Griend R et al: Fractures of the ankle and distal part of the tibia, *J Bone Joint Surg Am* 78A:1772, 1996.

48. Veenema KR: Ankle sprain: primary care evaluation and rehabilitation, *J Musculoskel Med* 17:563, 2000.

49. Wolfe MW et al: Management of ankle sprains, *Am Fam Phys* 63:93, 2003.

50. Zwipp H et al: Ligamentous injuries about the ankle and subtalar joints, *Clin Podiatr Med* 19:195, 2002.

Chapter 9

Foot

Trauma, infection, overuse, and developmental and degenerative processes all affect the foot. Any of these, in turn, can affect other areas of the lower extremity by altering the normal biomechanics of gait. A basic understanding of the structure and biomechanics of the foot will aid the practitioner in identifying, diagnosing, and treating many problems of the foot.

ANATOMY

Under normal conditions the feet are subject to numerous forces. When standing, forces exerted on the foot are equivalent to those of four times a person's body weight. These forces are even greater with walking and running.

Normal gait and locomotion depend a great deal on a normally functioning foot. When walking, jogging, or running, the foot must remain flexible enough to accommodate uneven terrain, yet stable enough to level the body and allow forward movement. The correct interplay between bones, muscles, ligaments, tendons, and neurovascular structures allows both the necessary flexibility and stability.

A basic review of normal gait will aid the practitioner in localizing and diagnosing a number of foot problems. Usually, normal gait is divided into two phases: swing and stance. The swing phase is the shorter of the two, accounting for 38% to 40% of the entire cycle. It begins with a toe-off and ends at the next foot strike. (Once called "heel strike," this phase of gait is more correctly termed "foot strike," since the latter also encompasses pathologic gaits where the heel may not make contact with the ground.[7]) During the normal swing phase, the foot clears the ground; the opposite tibia becomes vertical, and then there is foot strike of the opposite foot. The remaining 60% to 62% of the cycle, the stance phase, begins with a foot strike and ends at toe-off. The stance phase is often further divided into intervals of foot strike to opposite toe-off, reversal of fore shear to aft shear, and opposite foot strike. Figure 9-1 illustrates the normal gait cycle.

Around the ankle and foot the tibialis anterior muscle is responsible for the swing phase. The remainder of the foot muscles are used during the stance phase. Muscular weakness of the tibialis anterior causes what is known as a "slip gait" (i.e., the affected foot "slips" out of dorsiflexion during the swing phase). Complete loss of tibialis anterior function results in a "step gait" in which there is no dorsiflexion of the foot. Clinically the patient's foot remains in passive plantar flexion, and a slipping of the foot occurs when it makes contact with the ground.

As the foot strikes the ground to initiate the stance phase, the foot muscles are fairly relaxed to accommodate the terrain and absorb the body's impact. The foot pronates and the area of weight bearing moves medial to the talus. As gait progresses, the tibia rotates externally while the subtalar joint rotates internally. Internal rotation of the subtalar joints "locks" the transverse metatarsal joint so that the heel can rise against a firm lever. As the ankle passively plantar flexes, the subtalar joint everts while the tibia rotates internally. During this

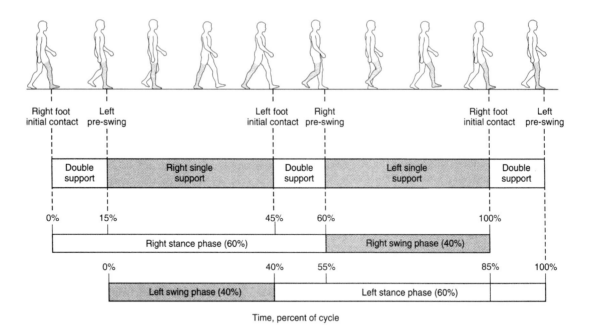

Figure 9-1 Normal gait pattern showing stance and swing phases. (Adapted from Inman VT, Ralston HJ, Todd F: *Human walking,* Baltimore, 1981, Williams & Wilkins, p 26.)

time (formerly called the "foot flat" phase) there is opposite toe-off and reversal of fore shear to aft shear.[7] As the heel rises, the foot actively plantar flexes and body weight is transferred from the calcaneus to the metatarsal heads and to the toes. The intrinsic muscles of the foot help maintain foot stability at this point. During toe-off, the calf muscles are quiet, whereas the anterior tibialis causes active dorsiflexion of the ankle, allowing the toes to clear the ground. At this time the foot remains fairly rigid as it rotates internally and the tibia rotates externally.

During the swing phase, the tibialis anterior muscle supinates the unloaded foot, increasing its stability in preparation for the next foot strike. Excessive supination, such as in pes cavus, causes poor shock absorption as the foot fails to adequately pronate; stress fractures tend to be more common.[47]

BONY STRUCTURES

Traditionally, bony structures of the foot are divided into three sections. The forefoot includes the metatarsals and

phalanges. The midfoot is composed of the tarsal bones, which are the navicular, the three cuneiform bones, and the cuboid. Finally, the talus and calcaneus make up the hindfoot. In all, there are twenty-six bones in the foot, which, when combined with their articulations, are critical to human locomotion (Figure 9-2).

In addition to the five metatarsals and fourteen phalanges of the forefoot, two sesamoid bones are present on the plantar surface of the foot joint just proximal to the metatarsophalangeal (MTP) joint of the great toe. As with other sesamoid bones, these two are located within the substance of a tendon; in this case, it is the flexor hallucis brevis tendon. Sesamoids have an articular surface covered with hyaline cartilage. They function to alter the direction of the tendon's pull as it crosses the joint. In the foot these sesamoids decrease pressure on the first MTP joint and provide additional power to the great toe when pushing off during walking, running, or jumping.

Sesamoid bones are commonly found along the MTP joints and at the interphalangeal (IP) joints of the first and second toes (Figure 9-3). Sesamoids may be bipartite and on x-ray films are occasionally mistaken

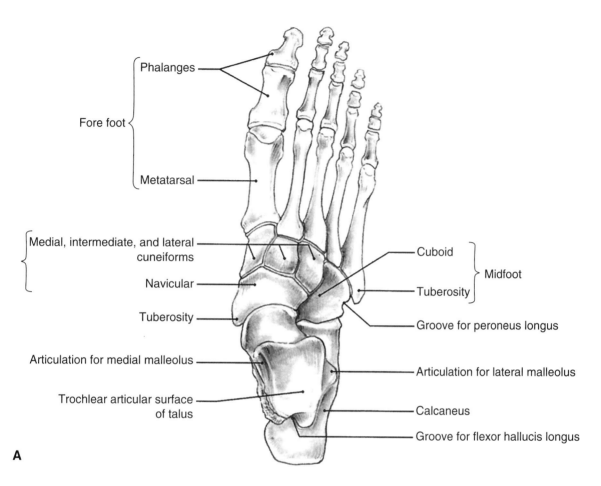

A

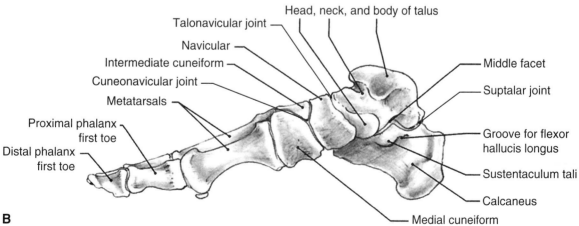

B

Figure 9-2   Bony anatomy of the foot. **A,** Dorsal view. **B,** Medial view.

Continued

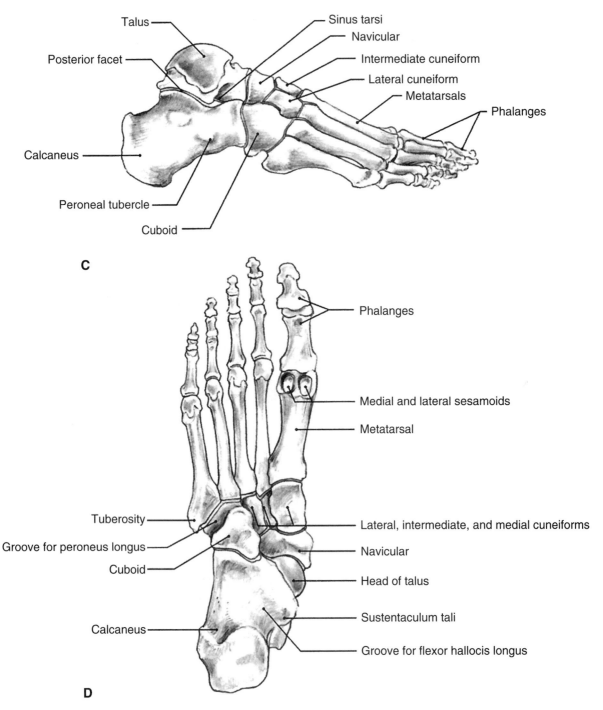

Talus

Posterior facet

Calcaneus

Peroneal tubercle

Cuboid

Sinus tarsi

Navicular

Intermediate cuneiform

Lateral cuneiform

Metatarsals

Phalanges

C

Phalanges

Medial and lateral sesamoids

Metatarsal

Tuberosity

Groove for peroneus longus

Cuboid

Calcaneus

Lateral, intermediate, and medial cuneiforms

Navicular

Head of talus

Sustentaculum tali

Groove for flexor hallocis longus

D

Figure 9-2, cont'd C, Lateral view. **D,** Plantar view. (From Noble J: *Textbook of primary care medicine,* ed 2, St Louis, 1996, Mosby.)

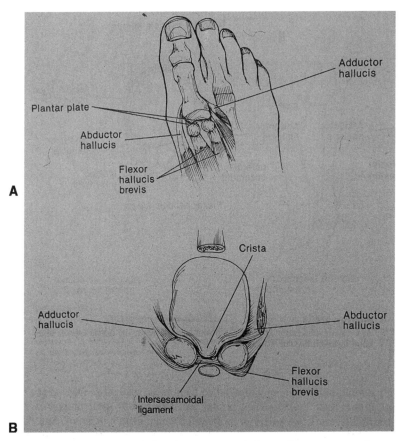

Figure 9-3   **Sesamoid Bones of the First Metatarsal.** Sesamoids serve as tendon attachments and help strengthen the force of the great toe when it is hyperextended. **A,** Dorsal view. **B,** Coronal view. (From Wargon C: Common foot injuries. In Sallis RE, Massimino F, editors: *ACSM's essentials of sports medicine*, St Louis, 1997, Mosby.)

for a fracture. Bipartite sesamoids are usually present bilaterally.

Separating the forefoot and the midfoot is the tarsometatarsal (TMT), or Lisfranc's, joint. Normally there is little movement at this joint. It functions primarily as a stabilizer of the longitudinal and transverse metatarsal arches.[25] It also allows the foot to support the body's weight at midstance and toe-off.

The midfoot contains the first, second, and third (or medial, middle, and lateral) cuneiforms, the tarsal navicular, and the cuboid bones. Proximally, the wedge-shaped cuneiforms all articulate with the distal ends of their corresponding metatarsals. The fourth and fifth metatarsals articulate proximally with the cuboid, which, in turn, also articulates with the calcaneus.

Between the cuneiform and the talus bones is the tarsal navicular, located on the medial side of the foot. Occasionally the navicular bone may be unusually prominent, or an accessory navicular may be present, causing localized pain. Clinically this is often easily visible as a bony protrusion on the medial aspect of the foot.

Chopart's joint is the transverse tarsal joint, made up of the talonavicular and calcaneocuboid joints that separate the midfoot and the hindfoot. Depending on the position of the subtalar joint, Chopart's joint becomes relatively flexible, allowing the foot to adjust to an uneven surface. During toe-off, the joint becomes more stable, enabling the foot to act as a lever to support the body's weight during push-off.

The two largest bones in the foot, the calcaneus and the talus, make up the hindfoot. The calcaneus, the larger of the two, is critical to supporting the body's weight when standing and to withstanding the impact of the foot-strike phase of gait. Roughly box-shaped, the calcaneus, or os calcis, also forms a strong lever for the muscles of the calf. Several tendons involved in ankle movement and walking attach to the various surfaces of this bone. A horizontal ridge of bone called the sustentaculum tali projects from the upper medial surface of the calcaneus. The top of the sustentaculum tali is convex and serves to support the anterior articular surface of the talus. The flexor hallucis longus tendon passes through a groove on the underside of the sustentaculum tali, and part of the posterior tibial tendon (PTT) also attaches to the ridge. Both the Achilles' and plantaris tendons attach to the posterior surface of the calcaneus. The calcaneus articulates with the talus and the cuboid bones.

The talocalcaneal joint, commonly known as the subtalar joint, is a complex articulation that permits rotation around an oblique axis, allowing a triplanar motion of the foot (Figure 9-4). Clinically, when heel strike occurs, the subtalar joint everts while the tibia rotates internally. This combined motion absorbs some of the force of foot strike and allows walking on uneven surfaces. As gait progresses to toe-off, the subtalar joint actively inverts while the tibia rotates externally. In this position the subtalar and transverse tarsal joints are nonparallel and the foot is relatively more stable. Forceful, excessive inversion or eversion of the subtalar joint can cause its dislocation.

The uppermost bone of the foot, the talus, supports the weight of the body at the ankle. In combination with the medial and lateral malleoli it forms the ankle joint, also known as the talocrural joint. The uppermost portion of the talus, the trochlea or dome, is wider anteriorly than posteriorly.[2] As a result, when the foot is dorsiflexed the talus becomes more tightly wedged between the malleoli, stabilizing the ankle against inversion and eversion.

Approximately 60% to 70% of the talus is covered with articular cartilage.[2] Distally the head of the talus articulates with the navicular bone, forming part of the

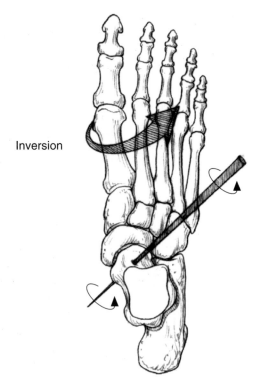

Inversion

Figure 9-4   Representation of complex movement of the subtalar joint. The movements of the foot involve more than one axis of motion. (From Mathers LH, editor: C.L.A.S.S.: *Clinical anatomy principles*, St Louis, 1996, Mosby.)

transverse tarsal joint. Inferiorly the talus articulates with the calcaneus bone along the middle calcaneal articular surface. The medial side of the inferior talus features a deep groove called the talar sulcus, which forms the roof of the tarsal sinus.

In addition to the normal twenty-six bones of the foot, accessory ossicles have been identified in numerous areas of the foot (Figure 9-5). Accessory ossicles differ from sesamoid bones in that the former do not usually have an articular surface and are not necessarily found within a tendon. These accessory ossicles can be mistaken for fractures on x-ray films.

The two most common accessory ossicles in the foot are the accessory navicular (discussed earlier) and the os trigonum. The os trigonum is the ununited lateral tuberosity of the posterior talus. As a rule the os trigonum is asymptomatic, but impingement of the bone between the posterior tibia and calcaneus can

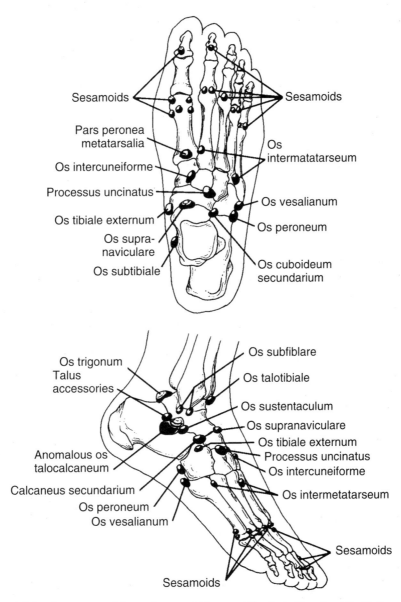

Figure 9-5   Accessory ossicles and sesamoid bones of the foot. (From Coughlin MJ, Mann RA, editors: *Surgery of the foot and ankle*, ed 7, vol 1, St Louis, 1999, Mosby.)

occur in individuals who frequently or forcefully plantar flex the foot. Ballet dancers and rock climbers may complain of posterior foot or ankle pain if there is impingement of the os trigonum and posterior foot and ankle soft tissues.

SOFT-TISSUE STRUCTURES

Ligaments

The balance of stability and flexibility in the foot is maintained thanks to the proper interplay of osseous structures, ligaments, tendons, and muscles. As in the hand, there are multiple ligaments in the foot. In addition to providing stability to the bones of the foot, its ligaments also help form and stabilize joint capsules.

In the forefoot, IP ligaments stabilize the medial and lateral joints and allow only plantar flexion and dorsiflexion of the toes. Plantar ligaments along each toe join these collateral ligaments. These ligaments limit extension of the toes, but a considerable degree of flexion is allowed.

Metatarsal ligaments are divided into dorsal, plantar, and interosseous regions. These ligaments form the bases of the second through fourth metatarsals. Similar to the thumb, at its base the first metatarsal is not connected to the second metatarsal by any ligaments. Both the dorsal and plantar ligaments run transversely between adjacent metatarsals two through four. The interosseous ligaments lie between the lateral shafts of the bones.

In the midfoot region, ligaments follow the same pattern of dorsal, plantar, and interosseous attachment. The dorsal ligaments connect the proximal metatarsals with their adjoining cuneiform bones. The plantar ligaments of the first and second metatarsals are stronger than their dorsal counterparts. Three interosseous ligaments connect the second and third metatarsals to the first and third cuneiforms. Along the proximal metatarsals, the strength of the dorsal, plantar, and interosseous ligaments also helps maintain the transverse arch of the foot.

There are three major ligaments that connect the tarsals and metatarsals. The first of these, the plantar calcaneonavicular ligament, begins at the distal surface and medial bony ridge of the calcaneus (i.e., the sustentaculum tali). From there the ligament covers the entire inferior surface of the navicular. Medially the ligament joins with the deltoid ligament. A portion of the plantar calcaneonavicular ligament forms part of the socket for the head of the talus. Because of its dense, fibroelastic structure, this ligament is commonly referred to as the spring ligament. One of its major functions is support of the longitudinal arch of the foot.

The bifurcate ligament is made up of the calcaneocuboid and calcaneonavicular ligaments, but not the plantar calcaneonavicular ligament. A portion of the calcaneocuboid ligament forms a primary connection between the first and second rows of the tarsals. The calcaneonavicular portion of the bifurcate ligament is more dorsal and lateral than the plantar calcaneonavicular ligament.

The long plantar ligament extends from the inferior surface of the calcaneus to the undersurface of the cuboid and then to the bases of the second, third, and fourth metatarsals. Like the spring ligament, the long plantar ligament is quite strong and important in the support of the bones of the foot. Maintenance of the longitudinal arch of the foot is largely a function of the long plantar ligament.

Fascia

A strong, dense fibrous membrane extends along the plantar surface of the foot from the calcaneus to each of the metatarsal heads (Figure 9-6). Known as the plantar fascia, it has both superficial and deep layers. The deep

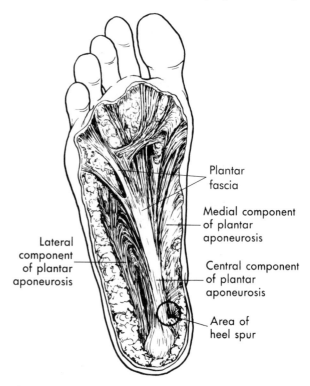

Figure 9-6   Drawing of the plantar fascia and the adjoining plantar aponeuroses. (Redrawn after Sarrafian SK: *Anatomy of the foot and ankle: descriptive, topographic, functional,* Philadelphia, 1983, JB Lippincott.)

layer helps hold the flexor tendons of the toes. Laterally the plantar fascia blends with the transverse metatarsal ligament. Two intermuscular septa extend upward into the foot and separate the internal, middle, and external muscle groups of the foot. The upper surface of the fascia helps attach the flexor brevis digitorum muscle.

Tendons

Stability and flexibility of the foot are enhanced by the presence of a large number of tendons and muscles. Of all the muscles and tendons of the foot, only the posterior tibial, or a slip from it, attaches to each of the tarsal and metatarsal bones. The PTT is the primary inverter of the foot, and its other functions include assisting the foot with plantar flexion and maintaining the medial longitudinal arch.

Other important tendons of the foot are the tibialis anterior, the peroneus longus and brevis, the flexor and extensor hallucis, and the extensor and flexor longus and brevis digitorum tendons. Dorsiflexion of the foot at the ankle is a primary function of the tibialis anterior; it also helps maintain the longitudinal arch. The peroneal muscles and tendons are primary everters of the foot. Flexion and extension of the toes are the responsibility of the corresponding hallucis (great toe) and digitorum (lesser toes) tendons. Table 9-1 shows

TABLE 9-1	Tendinous Attachment Sites on Bones of the Foot	
Bony Attachment	**Number of Muscles**	**Muscle and Tendon Attachments**
Calcaneus	8	Posterior tibial
		Achilles'
		Abductor hallucis
		Abductor minimi digiti
		Flexor brevis digitorum
		Extensor brevis digitorum
		Flexor accessorius (quadratus plantae)
Talus		Primarily a site of ligamentous attachment; several tendons cross the bone
Cuboid	2	Part of flexor brevis hallucis; slip of posterior tibial
Navicular	1	Slip of posterior tibial
First cuneiform	3	Tibialis posterior and anterior peroneus longus
Second (middle) cuneiform	1	Slip of posterior tibial
Third (lateral) cuneiform	2	Slip of posterior tibial
		Flexor brevis hallucis
First metatarsal	3	Part of tibialis anterior
		Peroneus longus
		First dorsal interosseous
Second metatarsal	4	Adductor obliquus hallucis
		First and second dorsal interosseous
		Slip from posterior tibial
Third metatarsal	5	Adductor obliquus hallucis
		Second and third dorsal interosseous
		First plantar interosseous
		Slip of posterior tibial tendon
Fourth metatarsal	5	Adductor obliquus hallucis
		Third and fourth dorsal interosseous
		Plantar interosseous
		Slip of posterior tibial

Continued

TABLE 9-1   Tendinous Attachment Sites on Bones of the Foot—cont'd

Bony Attachment	Number of Muscles	Muscle and Tendon Attachments
Fifth metatarsal	6	Peroneus brevis Peroneus tertius Flexor brevis minimi digiti Adductor transversus hallucis Fourth dorsal Third plantar
Great toe	7	Innermost tendon of extensor brevis digitorum Abductor hallucis Adductor obliquus hallucis Flexor brevis hallucis Adductor transversus hallucis Extensor longus hallucis Flexor longus hallucis
Lesser toes (2-5)		Note: The common tendon of the extensor longus and extensor brevis tendons insert in the middle and distal phalanges of each of the lesser toes
Second toe	3	First and second dorsal interosseous First lumbrical
Third toe	3	Third dorsal and first plantar interosseous Second lumbrical
Fourth toe	3	Fourth dorsal and second plantar interosseous Third lumbrical
Fifth toe	4	Flexor brevis minimi digiti Abductor minimi digiti Third plantar interosseous Fourth lumbrical

the numerous muscles and their tendon attachments on the foot.

Muscles

The muscles of the foot have been classified in various ways. Perhaps the easiest division is into either extrinsic or intrinsic muscles. Extrinsic muscles lie in the leg, but their tendons function in the foot. These include most of the muscles attached to the tendons previously discussed. The peroneal, tibialis anterior, soleus, gastrocnemius, plantaris, tibialis posterior, and flexor digitorum and hallucis muscles are included in this group.

Muscles that are entirely within the foot are known as intrinsic muscles, most of which lie on the plantar surface of the foot. In fact, the dorsum of the foot has only one muscle, the extensor brevis digitorum. As the name implies, this muscle's function is to extend the toes. The lateral edges of the muscle blend with the lateral portions of the plantar fascia. The extensor brevis digitorum has five tendinous attachments, one to each of the phalanges. A portion, or slip, of the extensor brevis hallucis muscle attaches to the great toe and is sometimes considered a separate muscle.

On the plantar surface of the foot, there are four layers of intrinsic muscles. The names, attachments, and innervations are shown in Table 9-2.

TABLE 9-2	Plantar Muscles of the Foot

Muscle	Attachments	Innervation	Actions
First Layer			
Abductor hallucis	Calcaneus to base of proximal phalanx of great toe	Medial plantar (S2-S3)	Abducts great toe
Flexor digitorum brevis	Calcaneus to sides of middle phalanges of toes 2-5	Medial plantar (S2-S3)	Flexes toes 2-5
Abductor digiti minimi	Calcaneus to proximal phalanx of fifth toe	Lateral plantar (S2-S3)	Abducts fifth toe
Second Layer			
Quadratus plantae	Calcaneus to tendons of FDL	Lateral plantar (S2-S3)	Stabilizes long flexor Flexes toes
Lumbricals	Tendons of FDL to extensor hood and middle toes 2-5	Lateral plantar (except hood and middle toes 2-5)	Flexes PIP Extends DIP joints
Third Layer			
Flexor hallucis brevis	Cuneiform/cuboid to base of proximal phalanx of first toe	Medial plantar (S2-S3)	Flexes great toe
Adductor hallucis (two heads—oblique and transverse)	Oblique head: bases of metatarsals 2-4 to base of proximal phalanx of first toe Transverse head: MTP joints of toes 3-5 to base of proximal phalanx of first toe	Lateral plantar	Abducts first toe
Flexor digiti minimi (flexor digiti minimi brevis)	Base of fifth metatarsal to proximal phalanx of fifth toe	Lateral plantar	Flexes fifth toe
Fourth Layer			
Interossei (dorsal)	Adjacent sides of metatarsals to proximal phalanges and extensor sheaths of toes	Lateral plantar (S2-S3)	*Ab*ducts
Interossei (plantar)	Adjacent sides of metatarsals to proximal phalanges and extensor sheaths of toes Tendons of peroneus longus and tibialis posterior	Lateral plantar (S2-S3)	*Ad*ducts

From Mathers LH, editor: C.L.A.S.S.: *Clinical anatomy principles*, St Louis, 1996, Mosby.
DIP, Distal interphalangeal; *FDL,* flexor digitorum longus; *MTP,* metatarsophalangeal; *PIP,* proximal interphalangeal.

NEUROVASCULAR STRUCTURES

Nerves

Nerve root function from L4 to S2 supplies sensation to the foot (Figure 9-7). The L4 dermatome covers the medial side of the ankle and foot. Sensation along the dorsum of the foot is primarily a function of L5. The lateral side of the foot and the Achilles' reflex are supplied by S1.

Branches of the sciatic nerve provide motor function of the foot. One of these branches, the common peroneal (i.e., lateral popliteal) nerve, allows dorsiflexion of the foot at the ankle. Injury to the lateral popliteal nerve results in a foot-slap type of gait and prevents the foot from dorsiflexing during the swing phase of locomotion. This nerve wraps around the head of the fibula and can be easily injured secondary to a proximal fibular fracture or from a direct blow to this area.

The superficial peroneal (i.e., musculocutaneous) nerve supplies the medial side of the great toe, the lateral side of the second, and both the medial and lateral sides of the third and fourth toes. This nerve also communicates with part of the saphenous nerve.

Anteriorly the deep peroneal (i.e., anterior tibial) nerve supplies the extensor muscles of the foot, including the tibialis anterior. A lateral branch supplies the extensor digitorum brevis muscle. Injury to this nerve results in weakness or an inability to extend the toes.

The tibial (i.e., medial popliteal) nerve runs posteriorly behind the medial malleolus and through the tarsal tunnel. From there it divides into the medial and lateral plantar nerves. With the exception of the extensor digitorum brevis muscle, all the intrinsic muscles of the foot receive their motor innervation from the tibial nerve. Branches of this nerve can become trapped within the tarsal tunnel, giving rise to tarsal tunnel syndrome.

The medial and lateral plantar nerves divide into the digital nerves of the toes. The two branches join in the third web space; this anastomosis may help explain the frequency of neuromas at this location. The lateral plantar nerve supplies part of the sole of the foot. Entrapment of the nerve is thought to play a role in painful heel syndrome.

Vascular Supply

The anterior and posterior tibial arteries, along with the peroneal artery, supply the foot. All three arteries are branches of the popliteal artery. As the anterior tibial artery descends into the foot and divides, it gives rise to the dorsalis pedis artery and pulse (Figure 9-8). The dor-

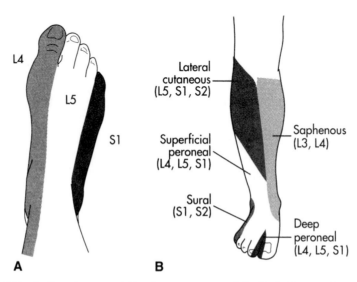

Figure 9-7 **A,** Dermatomes and **B,** cutaneous nerves of the foot. (From Hartley A: *Practical joint assessment: lower quadrant,* ed 2, St Louis, 1995, Mosby.)

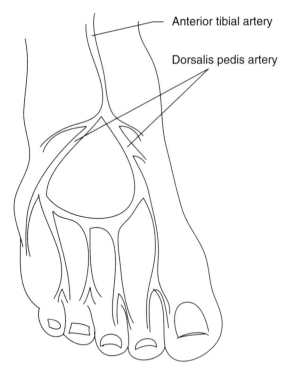

Figure 9-8   Arterial blood supply to the dorsum of the foot. (From Mathers LH, editor: C.L.A.S.S.: *Clinical anatomy principles*, St Louis, 1996, Mosby.)

sal metatarsal arteries branch off the dorsalis pedis artery.[30]

The posterior tibial artery lies medial to the posterior tibial nerve. In the foot the artery forms part of the neurovascular bundle in the tarsal tunnel. From the tarsal tunnel it further divides into the plantar metatarsal arteries and the medial and lateral plantar arteries. These divisions supply the metatarsal heads and web spaces of the toes. In some people the posterior tibial artery may be congenitally absent and replaced by a large peroneal artery. Branches of the peroneal artery supply the calcaneus and lateral malleolus.

EXAMINATION

Alterations in normal biomechanics of the foot are often the cause of lower extremity complaints. The complex interplay of muscles, bones, ligaments, and tendons allows adequate shock absorption and stability during walking, jumping, and running.

Evaluation of normal walking and standing, as well as an examination of foot structure, is important in discerning the causes of numerous foot complaints.[7] Variations in anatomy can predispose a patient to certain problems.

As with other anatomic areas, the examiner compares contralateral structures. Normally the appearance of both feet should be similar, though most individuals have one foot slightly larger than the other.

The practitioner begins with the patient comfortably seated and barefoot. Any obvious abnormalities, such as swelling, discoloration, bumps, scars, or other signs of trauma are noted. The examiner should ask the patient to actively flex and extend the toes, plantar flex and dorsiflex the foot, and internally and externally rotate the foot.

Normally the toes can flex at each of the joints. Flexion at the MTP joints is approximately 45 degrees. Active extension of the toes beyond 0 degrees occurs only at the MTP joints. Extension of approximately 40 degrees at the MTP joints is required for the normal toe-off phase during locomotion.

The bones of the foot are palpated, leaving any tender areas for last. Most of the bones are easy to palpate along the dorsum of the foot. Beginning with the great toe, the practitioner palpates back toward the foot. The lesser toes can be palpated in a similar manner. The MTP joints are normally nontender. The first metatarsal becomes larger at its base; its articulation with the first cuneiform is usually easy to feel. Continuing proximally along the medial aspect of the foot, the navicular forms a rounded, palpable, and occasionally visible prominence on the medial midfoot. Immediately behind the navicular process is the talus. With the foot everted and dorsiflexed, the rounded head of the talus is easily visible on the medial aspect of the dorsum of the foot, just in front of the ankle.

The practitioner palpates the medial malleolus and then moves approximately 1 cm downward toward the ground. The small calcaneal ridge of bone, known as the sustentaculum tali, is sometimes palpable.

Returning to the lesser toes, the examiner palpates proximally along the metatarsals of the lesser toes. The second and third metatarsals articulate with the second and third cuneiforms. The fourth and fifth metatarsals share an articulation with the cuboid. The base of the fifth metatarsal forms an easily palpable bony prominence on the lateral border of the midfoot; just behind this prominence lies the cuboid. The cuboid articulates with the calcaneus, which is easily palpable.

The metatarsal heads, plantar fascia, and plantar surface are palpable along the sole of the foot. Painful nodules between the metatarsal heads may indicate the presence of a neuroma.

Next the patient is asked to stand normally, facing the practitioner. Any asymmetry of the foot (i.e., bunions, dislocations, fractures, synovitis, toe deformities, corns, calluses, and contractures) should be noted. An assessment of the patient's weight-bearing stance is made. Do the patient's ankles appear symmetric? Is there any unusual pronation or supination? The patient is asked to make a one-quarter (90 degrees) turn to more easily assess the arch of the foot. After a second one-quarter turn (the patient is now facing away from the practi-

tioner), pronation and supination are assessed again. Soft-tissue prominence around the medial malleolus in combination with an apparent asymmetry of the Achilles' tendon is typical of excessive foot pronation. The practitioner should note how many of the lesser toes are visible laterally. Normally only the fifth and sometimes the fourth toes are visible to the lateral side of the foot when viewed from the back of the heel (Figure 9-9). Excessive pronation causes valgus abnormality of the calcaneus, and most of the toes are visible (i.e., the "too many toes" sign).

Asking the patient to walk, the practitioner can assess basic neuromuscular function. (Detailed biomechanical gait analysis requires referral to a motion analysis laboratory.) Toe walking requires the gastrocnemius-soleus muscle complex and the Achilles' tendon to be functioning normally. Toe walking also requires integrity of the S1 nerve root.

An inability to walk on the heels can indicate an injury to the tibialis anterior muscle or to the deep peroneal nerve. Extension of the toes is also a function of the deep peroneal nerve.

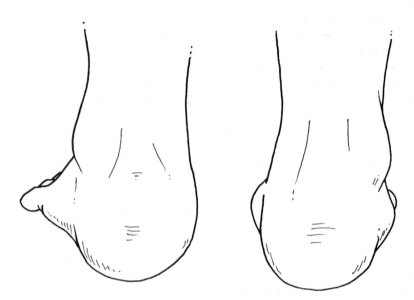

Figure 9-9   Right foot demonstrates normal weight-bearing stance, which is compared with pronated, everted forefoot on left. (From Bucholz RW: *Orthopaedic decision making*, ed 2, St Louis, 1996, Mosby.)

PATHOLOGIC CONDITIONS AND TREATMENT

FRACTURES

Phalanges

Toe fractures are among the most frequent fractures of the foot and are often seen in the primary care setting. The great toe and little toe seem to take the brunt of these injuries. As a rule a patient will have a clear recollection of a specific event that caused the injury. Striking a hard or immovable object while walking barefoot is a common history for lesser toe fractures. Fractures of the great toe tend to involve greater force or a heavy object dropped on the digit.

Examination usually reveals a swollen, sometimes ecchymotic digit. Point tenderness indicates the site of the fracture. Care must be taken to ascertain that there is no rotational deformity of the digit. This is most easily done by assessing the planar orientation of the nail beds and comparing the contralateral foot. Plain anteroposterior (AP) and lateral x-ray films will confirm the diagnosis (Figure 9-10). An oblique x-ray view can help determine whether there is any displacement of the fracture.

Regardless of which toe is involved, nondisplaced fractures of the distal or middle phalanges are fairly easily treated. With padding between the injured toe and its adjoining digit, the two toes are taped together. Referred to as "buddy taping," the uninjured toe serves as a splint to support the fractured digit. Wearing a supportive or postoperative shoe may increase the patient's comfort.

Both the tape and padding should be changed if either becomes wet or dirty. Treatment of a fracture of the proximal phalanx should include the use of a postoperative shoe to prevent displacement of the fracture during walking. Approximately 2 to 3 weeks is usually sufficient for healing; immobilization can then be discontinued, but the patient should be advised to wear the shoe for another 1 to 2 weeks.

Displaced or rotated fractures (Figure 9-11) require reduction before immobilization. When either problem is present, the practitioner should gently buddy tape the digits for stabilization and refer the patient to an orthopedic surgeon.

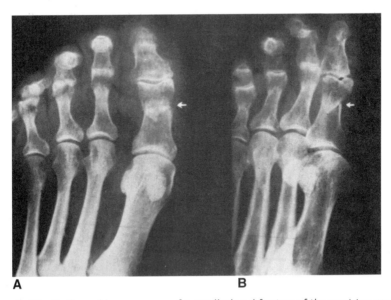

Figure 9-10   Radiographic appearance of a nondisplaced fracture of the great toe proximal phalanx. **A,** Anteroposterior view. **B,** Oblique view. (From Mann RA, Coughlin MJ, editors: *Surgery of the foot and ankle,* ed 6, vol 2, St Louis, 1993, Mosby.)

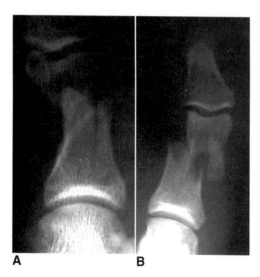

Figure 9-11 Displaced fractures of the great toe proximal phalanx. **A,** Mildly displaced fracture, **B,** comminuted, displaced fracture. (From Coughlin MJ, Mann RA, editors: *Surgery of the foot and ankle,* ed 7, vol 2, St Louis, 1999, Mosby.)

Metatarsals

Either acute injury or repetitive microtrauma can cause metatarsal fractures. Fractures of the lesser toe metatarsals occur more commonly than fractures of the first metatarsal. (Fractures of the fifth metatarsal are discussed separately.)

A direct blow to the dorsum of the foot is a common cause of a second, third, fourth, or fifth metatarsal fracture. As a rule the patient can easily remember the specific insult.

Pain and swelling occur almost immediately with discoloration developing hours to days later. Weight bearing is painful, and movement of the toes may increase discomfort. Initial numbness of the foot or toes is not unusual, but it generally resolves within the first day.

On examination, swelling usually extends to the dorsum and sometimes the sole of the foot. Point tenderness at the site of a metatarsal injury is a hallmark of the fracture. Pain is often described as deep aching or even burning that becomes sharp when the site is palpated or with weight bearing.

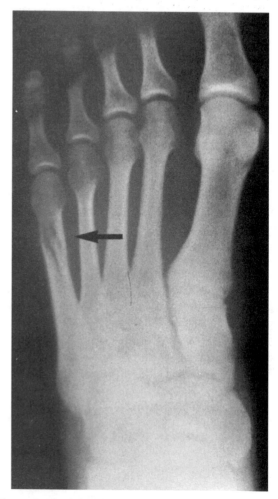

Figure 9-12 Spiral fracture of the fifth metatarsal shaft. (From Coughlin MJ, Mann RA, editors: *Surgery of the foot and ankle,* ed 7, vol 2, St Louis, 1999, Mosby.)

Plain x-ray films will confirm the diagnosis. AP, lateral, and oblique views should be ordered to evaluate the fracture for any displacement (Figure 9-12).

A patient with a known or suggested acute metatarsal fracture should be nonweight-bearing on the affected foot until appropriate immobilization can be used. Wrapping the foot with an elastic bandage may increase patient comfort, but the practitioner must use care to avoid wrapping the foot too tightly. If the fracture is not displaced, treatment generally consists of a short leg walking cast or fracture boot. The foot usually remains immobilized for 3 to 4 weeks; then the patient can begin using a supportive shoe.[25] Referral to an orthopedic surgeon is always appropriate.

Metatarsal Stress Fracture

Metatarsal stress fractures can be attributable to a number of factors. Whether the result of training errors, overuse, alteration of the foot's biomechanics, metabolic disorders, or some other cause, the basic pathophysiology is the body's inability to maintain a balance of bone repair and breakdown. The high incidence of these fractures in military recruits has led to the term "march fracture" to describe metatarsal stress fractures.

Athletes who participate in running or jumping activities are more likely to sustain stress fractures. Often, increasing distance, starting to run on inclines, or wearing poorly fitting footwear are identified as new stressors that lead to stress fractures.[24]

Patient history may reveal a change in activity level, but the most consistent history is localized pain and tenderness in the forefoot. For a number of reasons, including the biomechanics of the foot, the third metatarsal is most often affected; the second, fourth, first, and fifth are, in order, the next most commonly involved.[48] Pain often begins insidiously, but it tends to intensify with running, jogging, and sometimes walking. It is not unusual for a patient to have pain for 2 to 3 weeks (or more) before seeking treatment.[29]

Careful attention should be paid to the patient's history of activity level, footwear, and, in the case of runners, types of running surfaces. Prevention of recurrent fracture is an important goal of therapy. Running shoes should be replaced every 300 to 400 miles or 3 to 6 months to ensure adequate shock absorption.[15] Abnormal foot biomechanics, such as pes cavus or planus, excessive pronation, or a heavy heel strike, should be evaluated and corrected with therapy, gait training, or orthotics.

Examination rarely reveals any significant discoloration, although there may be mild erythema in conjunction with some localized warmth and diffuse swelling over the dorsum of the foot. Point tenderness over the affected metatarsal shaft is common. If the entire metatarsal is tender, placing a vibrating tuning fork over the shaft of the bone can help localize pain.

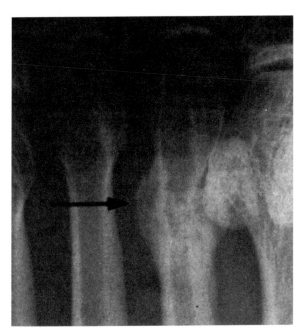

Figure 9-13 Healing stress fracture of the second metatarsal showing abundant callus formation. (From Mercier LR: *Practical orthopedics*, ed 5, St Louis, 2000, Mosby.)

Plain x-ray films are rarely useful for initial diagnosis during the first 1 or 2 weeks of symptoms. Evidence of a fracture may not be evident until 3 to 4 weeks after the onset of pain, when callus formation becomes visible (Figure 9-13). Plain x-ray films can be useful in identifying underlying disease processes, such as rheumatoid arthritis (RA) or osteoporosis, that can complicate a stress fracture. For evaluating the presence of a stress fracture, bone scanning with technetium 99m is the standard because its great sensitivity shows nearly all stress fractures.[24] Magnetic resonance imaging (MRI) is highly specific and accurate, but its expense makes it impractical for routine diagnosis of stress fractures.

Treatment consists of limiting the patient's activity for 3 to 4 weeks. Casting is rarely necessary because most fractures will heal once the source of stress is removed. The underlying biomechanical, hormonal, hematologic, or nutritional problems should also be addressed to prevent recurrence. Nonsteroidal antiinflammatory drugs (NSAIDs) can decrease pain by reducing inflammation. An elastic bandage used with a postoperative shoe or even a well-cushioned running shoe will provide adequate stability for bone healing. Most patients can resume normal activities in 6 to 8 weeks.[47]

Metatarsal Fractures

Left untreated, metatarsal stress fractures can progress to cortical fractures that are visible on x-ray films. Most metatarsal fractures, however, are the result of direct trauma. Indirect trauma, such as forced plantar flexion of the foot, can also result in metatarsal fractures.

The history for most metatarsal fractures is fairly straightforward. Patients can usually recount an acute event such as a fall, a heavy object falling on the foot, or slamming on the brakes in a motor vehicle accident.

Pain is usually well localized over the metatarsal fracture. Bruising usually develops within a few days of injury. Weight bearing exacerbates pain. Numbness or tingling of the toes can occur, but usually resolves within a day or so.

Examination reveals localized tenderness to palpation over the fracture site. Tenderness may be more acute over either the dorsal or plantar surface of the bone. There may be palpable deformity if the fracture is displaced. Depending on the location of the fracture, the patient will have a varying degree of difficulty moving the toe. The more distal the metatarsal fracture, the more likely the patient will report more significant pain or difficulty moving the associated toe.

An x-ray study is the most cost-effective diagnostic tool for evaluating fractures. Plain films should include AP, lateral, and oblique views to evaluate the fracture for any displacement.

Displaced fractures should be referred to an orthopedic surgeon for reduction or for internal fixation. Without reduction, displaced fractures will alter the normal weight-bearing biomechanics of the foot. As a result, deformity and postfracture metatarsalgia may occur.[39]

Treatment of a nondisplaced metatarsal fracture consists of 3 to 4 weeks of immobilization, usually with a short leg walking cast or a fracture boot. Multiple metatarsal fractures, displaced fractures, or fractures of the first or fifth metatarsals should always be referred to an orthopedic surgeon for treatment.

Fifth Metatarsal Fractures

One of the most frequently fractured metatarsals is the fifth. In addition to direct trauma, a patient often reports indirect injury, such as a severe ankle sprain or a misstep down a step or off a curb, as the cause of the fracture.

Controversy exists surrounding the best method of treatment for fifth metatarsal fractures. Part of the reason for this controversy is the relatively high incidence of delayed healing, fibrous union, and nonunion associated with fractures of proximal portion of the bone.

Proximal fifth metatarsal fractures are often incorrectly lumped together under the term "Jones fracture." A true Jones fracture is a transverse break through the junction of the proximal diaphysis (i.e., shaft) and metaphysis within a 1.5-cm area distal to the proximal tuberosity, or the base, of the bone.[10] A true Jones fracture does not extend into the fourth to fifth intermetatarsal articulation.[36]

Healing of proximal fifth metatarsal fractures largely depends on the anatomy and vascular supply of the affected area. The proximal tuberosity is primarily cortical bone and has an excellent blood supply. Fractures in this area, which are classified as zone 1, are most often avulsion injuries. These occur as the result of extreme stress at the site of soft-tissue attachment. When stress is great enough, a portion of bone will "pull off," resulting in a fracture. Although they often extend into the metatarsocuboid joint, they usually heal well and without surgery.[10,50]

Moving toward the more distal part of the tuberosity, zone 2 is the area where a true Jones fracture occurs (Figure 9-14). This area is immediately distal to the articulation between the fourth and fifth metatarsals. This type of fracture most often occurs when the foot is plantar flexed and adducted. Running or field sports, as well as missteps off a curb, can cause this type of injury. This area lies between the rich metaphyseal blood supply at each end of the bone and the main branches of the intramedullary nutrient artery that generally enters the middle third of the bone. As a result, healing in this area can be prolonged and nonunion can occur.[10]

Treatment of a Jones fracture remains controversial; disagreements arise over the length of immobilization, weight-bearing versus nonweight-bearing status while casted, surgical fixation, and use of postsurgical protec-

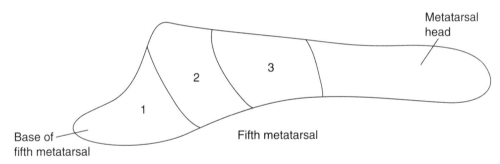

Figure 9-14 Approximate locations of the three anatomic zones of the proximal fifth metatarsal. Fractures in zone 1 usually heal very well. Jones fractures occur in zone 2. Zone 2 and 3 fractures may have a prolonged healing time.

tion.[10,35,50] A nondisplaced Jones fracture usually heals when the foot is placed in a nonweight-bearing cast for 6 to 8 weeks.[36] Surgical fixation with an intramedullary screw allows an earlier return to sports than does casting alone.

The proximal branch of the nutrient artery supplies the most distal part of the proximal third of the metatarsal, considered zone 3. Bone injury in this area often damages this same arterial branch, resulting in delayed healing. Fractures in zone 3 tend to be stress fractures.[10,35] As is typical of stress fractures, initial x-ray films may be negative. A visible fracture line may not become apparent for several days to 2 and 3 weeks after injury. Once again there is controversy among orthopedic surgeons regarding optimal treatment.

Fractures of the midshaft and neck of the fifth metatarsal are similar to fractures of the other lesser metatarsals. Blood supply to the diaphysis is good, and healing almost universally occurs without surgery or prolonged immobilization.

History. In addition to some traumatic event, the patient typically reports the sudden onset of acute pain over the lateral portion of the midfoot. Bruising usually occurs within 24 hours and may be noted over the dorsum of the foot before settling into more dependent areas. Walking may vary from feeling uncomfortable to being impossible. Movement of the toes often increases pain. An associated lateral ankle injury is not uncommon. In fact, the patient may report foot pain only after the ankle has been immobilized.

Physical Examination. Swelling over the lateral dorsum of the foot, with or without discoloration, is typical. If it has been longer than 24 hours since the injury, bruising is usually apparent over the inferior lateral border of the foot. If there is associated lateral ankle ligamentous damage, edema and ecchymosis may extend from the ankle to the lateral toes.

Pain increases with plantar flexion and inversion of the foot. As with other fractures, the cardinal sign is point tenderness over the fracture. Numbness and tingling of the toes, if present, usually resolve spontaneously in the first 1 or 2 days.

Diagnosis. Plain x-ray films are used to confirm the practitioner's clinical diagnosis. AP, lateral, and oblique x-ray views should be ordered. An oblique view is particularly important in evaluating proximal fifth metatarsal fractures, since some fracture lines are apparent only on this view (Figure 9-15).

Treatment. Small, nondisplaced avulsion fractures of the proximal tuberosity can be treated with a soft dressing, such as cast padding and an elastic bandage with the use of a supportive postoperative shoe. Weight bearing as tolerated is usually allowed. Some patients may initially be more comfortable using crutches. Most of these fractures will heal within 3 to 6 weeks, even if radiographic evidence of callus is not evident.[10,35,36] Jones or displaced fractures should be referred to an orthopedic surgeon. The same is true if x-ray facilities are unavailable or the practitioner is uncertain of how to determine the type of fracture. Using an elastic bandage and crutches for nonweight-bearing activities is a safe,

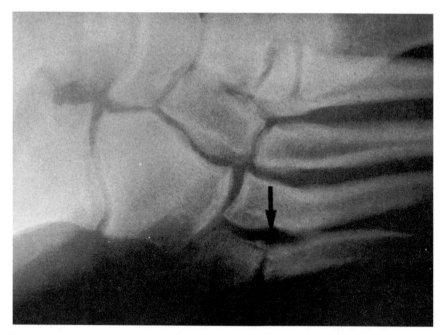

Figure 9-15   True Jones Fracture of the Fifth Metatarsal. Note some widening of the fracture line. (From Coughlin MJ, Mann RA, editors: *Surgery of the foot and ankle*, ed 7, vol 2, St Louis, 1999, Mosby.)

practical measure until the patient is referred for orthopedic evaluation.

Tarsometatarsal Fracture

Fracture of the proximal metatarsal bones is sometimes called a Lisfranc's fracture. A true Lisfranc's injury is a fracture-dislocation of the TMT joint. Injury to this area can occur as the result of direct trauma, such as a heavy object falling on the foot, or indirect trauma from a significant forefoot twisting injury.[44]

These injuries are frequently missed on initial examination; failure to treat them can result in the loss of the transverse arch's stability and the eventual development of posttraumatic arthritis.[42] The transverse arch is crucial in stabilizing the foot at the end of the stance phase of gait, as it allows a rigid platform for pushing off.

Midfoot instability can result from instability between the first and second metatarsals. As noted earlier in this chapter, there is no intermetatarsal ligament between the first and second metatarsals; longitudinal and oblique plantar ligaments join them. The joint itself is made up of the base of the second metatarsal and its articulation with the medial and lateral cuneiforms (Figure 9-16). Lisfranc's ligament passes from the second metatarsal to the medial cuneiform, bypassing the first metatarsal; it also runs along the plantar aspect of the foot. Any disruption of this ligament will cause midfoot instability.

Pain with weight-bearing activities, difficulty with walking, and excessive midfoot swelling after trauma may indicate an injury to the TMT area. A simple clinical stress test can assist in identifying proximal TMT instability (Figure 9-17). To perform this test, the practitioner grasps the patient's first metatarsal in one hand, the second metatarsal in the other, and then both plantar flexes and dorsiflexes the bones. Pain with these movements is a positive test.[45]

Radiographic films of the area can be difficult to interpret, since findings may be subtle. Assessment of several radiographic features can assist in determining abnormalities of alignment.[32] First, the medial aspect of the second metatarsal normally aligns with the medial

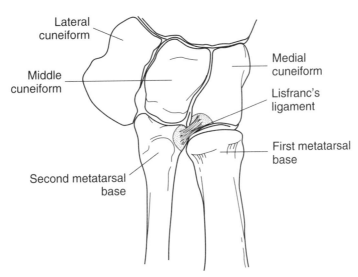

Figure 9-16 Anatomic Drawing of Lisfranc's Ligament and Joint. This ligament is important in stabilizing the midfoot. (From Coughlin MJ, Mann RA, editors: *Surgery of the foot and ankle*, ed 7, vol 2, St Louis, 1999, Mosby.)

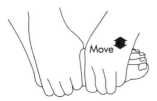

Figure 9-17 Clinical Stress Test for Tarsometatarsal Instability. While grasping the foot at the tarsometatarsal joint, the forefoot is moved in a dorsal and a plantar direction. (From Hartley A: *Practical joint assessment: lower quadrant*, ed 2, 1995, Mosby.)

border of the second, or middle, cuneiform on an AP x-ray film. On an oblique view, the lateral border of the third metatarsal should line up with the lateral border of the lateral cuneiform, and the medial border of the fourth metatarsal should be aligned with the medial border of the cuboid. On the lateral view, a metatarsal should line up with its respective tarsal bone.

Any midfoot injury resulting from a significant force can be appropriately referred to an orthopedic surgeon. It is advisable to refer the patient soon after such an injury, because early stabilization has a higher success rate than delayed intervention.[45] Surgical repair performed more than 6 weeks after injury has a higher incidence of complications and a worse outcome overall.

Tarsals

Any of the tarsal bones can be broken. Of the seven tarsals, perhaps fractures of the calcaneus and talus are the most serious. When standing normally an individual's body weight is evenly distributed between the calcaneus and metatarsal heads. Injury to the calcaneus not only affects weight bearing, it frequently alters the biomechanics of the calcaneus-talus (i.e., subtalar) joint. In turn, subtalar joint disruption alters the mobility of the foot. Talus fractures are associated with a high incidence of secondary osteonecrosis (ON) of the bone.[2] Fractures of the other tarsal bones tend to be associated with other injuries to the foot.

Calcaneus

In addition to being the largest bone in the foot, the calcaneus has a unique anatomy that influences the subtalar joint and, indirectly, the ankle joint. A calcaneal fracture that extends to the subtalar joint—and most fractures do—will affect motion of the foot.

Calcaneal fractures are generally the result of a high-energy force, such as a motor vehicle accident or a direct axial load from a fall or a jump from a height.[4] Stress fractures, primarily among military recruits, have also been reported.[21]

Generally calcaneal fractures are classified as either intraarticular or extraarticular. About 75% of calcaneal fractures are intraarticular.[26] Extraarticular fractures are usually avulsion types of injuries from ligament or tendon insertion areas. The Achilles' tendon can avulse the posterior tuberosity of the calcaneus; the bifurcate ligament has also been shown to cause avulsions of the anterior process. If the avulsed fragments are small, treatment is essentially the same as that for an ankle sprain. Large fragments tend to require surgical reattachment.

Fractures caused by axial loading tend to be more serious, since they are more often intraarticular and more frequently have displaced fragments. Intraarticular fractures generally have a worse outcome than extraarticular fractures.[4] A fracture line that extends into either the calcaneocuboid or subtalar joints will affect the person's gait.

Clinically the patient has heel pain that increases with weight bearing. Walking may be impossible because of pain. On examination, the heel may appear widened or shortened when compared with that of the uninjured foot. The arch of the foot may be flattened. Fracture blisters are frequently present.

Initial diagnosis is made by history, examination, and plain x-ray films. Three basic x-ray views should be ordered:

1. Lateral view of the foot
2. Harris axial heel view (sometimes called an os calcis view)
3. Broden's view

The lateral view allows visualization of any loss in calcaneal height and assessment of the calcaneocuboid joint. The Harris view reveals varus-valgus alignment of the calcaneus, as well as any injury to the medial or lateral walls of the bone. Broden's view is similar to a mortise view of the ankle, but Broden's view requires 45 degrees of internal rotation (Figure 9-18). Fractures into the posterior facet are best seen on Broden's view.[32] If any displacement is noted, or if there is the suggestion of

an intraarticular injury, a computed tomography (CT) study should be ordered.

Initial treatment of any calcaneus fracture is immobilization in a bulky dressing and splint, nonweight-bearing status, ice, and elevation. If fracture blisters are present, further treatment should generally wait until the blisters have resolved,[38] but CT scanning and a referral to an orthopedic surgeon can be done soon after injury. Referral to an orthopedic surgeon is essential for any calcaneal fracture.

If the patient's foot can be adequately padded and splinted, CT can be obtained before referral to an orthopedic surgeon. Definitive treatment of a displaced calcaneal fracture is usually surgery, performed within the first 3 weeks of injury. Patients with underlying disease processes, such as diabetes or peripheral vascular disease, may not be surgical candidates and will be treated more conservatively with splinting that allows removal and ankle range of motion (ROM) exercises.

Talus

Talus fractures can range from tiny avulsion fractures attributable to ankle sprains to fractures of the talar body with associated dislocations of the subtalar joint or other talar articulations. Axial loading with hyperdorsiflexion of the ankle is a more serious injury. Osteochondral fractures of the talar dome can occur with an inversion type of ankle sprain. One of the major difficulties associated with talar fractures is that the surface area is primarily articular cartilage. As a result, there is a limited amount of space for blood vessel penetration to the bone and a relatively poor blood supply. Damage to the blood vessels is common at the time of fracture, and delayed healing or ON can result.

History and clinical examination may not distinguish an ankle sprain from a talus fracture.[23] X-ray evaluation of a possible talus fracture is the same as that used for evaluating an ankle sprain. The critical feature in evaluating the x-ray films is actually looking at the talus (Figure 9-19).

Talar fractures have a high incidence of complications. The injured foot should be splinted; the patient should be kept on a nonweight-bearing status with crutches and referred to an orthopedic surgeon as soon

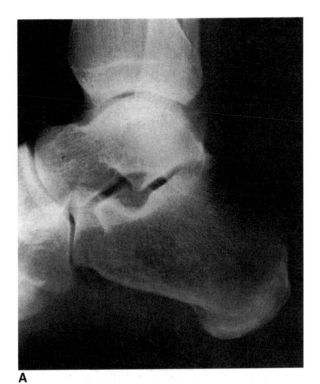

A

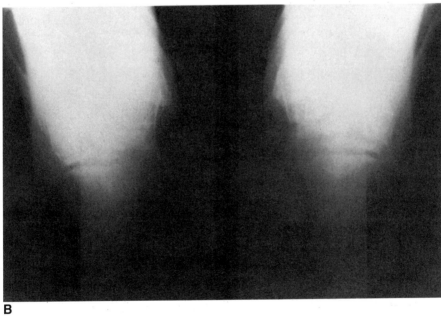

B

Figure 9-18 Basic X-Ray Views of the Calcaneus to Evaluate for Fracture. A, Lateral
view; **B,** Harris axial (or os calcis) view. (Note the fracture lines seen on the Harris view.)

Continued

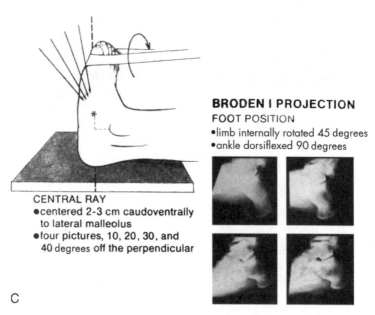

BRODEN I PROJECTION
FOOT POSITION
• limb internally rotated 45 degrees
• ankle dorsiflexed 90 degrees

CENTRAL RAY
• centered 2-3 cm caudoventrally to lateral malleolus
• four pictures, 10, 20, 30, and 40 degrees off the perpendicular

C

Figure 9-18, cont'd   C, Broden's view. (From Mann RA, Coughlin MJ, editors: *Surgery of the foot and ankle*, ed 6, vol 2, St Louis, 1993, Mosby.)

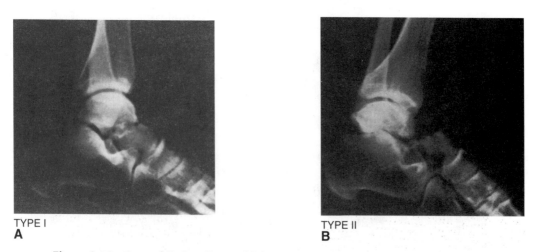

TYPE I
A

TYPE II
B

Figure 9-19   X-ray of Various Types of Talus Fractures. These injuries require immediate referral to an orthopedic surgeon. **A,** Type I fractures are nondisplaced. **B,** Type II fractures are displaced with some subluxation or dislocation of the talocalcaneal joint.

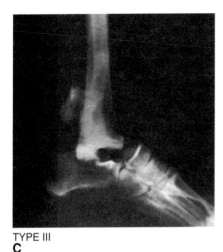

TYPE III
C

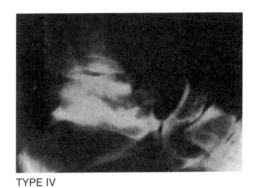

TYPE IV
D

Figure 9-19, cont'd   C, Type III fractures are displaced with a talocalcaneal and talotibial dislocation. **D,** Type IV is a type III fracture with dislocation of the talus from the talonavicular joint. (From Mann RA, Coughlin MJ, editors: *Surgery of the foot and ankle*, ed 6, vol 2, St Louis, 1993, Mosby.)

as possible. Treatment of talar neck or body fractures is usually open reduction and internal fixation. Nondisplaced avulsion fractures can be treated with immobilization.

Tarsal Navicular

Indirect or direct trauma and repetitive microtrauma can cause fractures of the navicular bone. Overall, navicular fractures are encountered relatively infrequently in the primary care setting. A fracture of the navicular body can occur if the talus is forced against the navicular, splitting it. This is an unusual injury. Avulsion fractures from the dorsal aspect of the bone can be seen on a lateral radiograph of the foot. Avulsion fractures are rarely displaced and can be managed symptomatically or, if necessary, with a cast.

Stress fractures typically occur in runners or others who engage in repetitive impact loading. These fractures usually occur in the middle third of the navicular. On examination, there is usually point tenderness at the fracture site; these fractures are difficult to see on plain x-ray films. As a result, there is often a delay of weeks to months before diagnosing these injuries.[48]

Bone scan with confirmatory CT—if the bone scan is positive—is recommended to diagnose a navicular stress fracture.[32,48] Nondisplaced fractures can be treated in a nonweight-bearing cast; displaced fractures require surgery followed by a nonweight-bearing cast.

Cuboid and Cuneiform Bones

Fractures of the cuneiform and the cuboid bones usually occur in combination with other foot injuries. A Lisfranc's injury is suspected if x-ray films reveal small fractures of the second (or middle) cuneiform, the cuboid, or the navicular bones. Lisfranc's injuries require immediate referral to an orthopedic surgeon.

SPRAINS, STRAINS, AND DISLOCATIONS

Toes

Patients with simple IP sprains of the toes rarely seek treatment. A notable contrast is a ligamentous injury to the MTP joint of the great toe, also known as "turf toe." A hyperextended great toe typically causes this injury during a pivot or a forceful push-off. Field sports that involve running, pivoting, and cutting often predispose a patient to this injury.

The patient usually complains of pain and swelling around the base of the great toe. Pain is worse with movement of the digit, especially extension. The MTP joint is usually quite tender to palpation.

On x-ray examination, small calcifications may be seen in the collateral ligamentous area (Figure 9-20). Occasionally a small defect can be seen on the dorsal aspect of the metatarsal head (Figure 9-21).

Treatment consists of buddy taping the great and second toes and wearing a postoperative or other hard-soled shoe for 2 to 3 weeks. Ice and NSAIDs may be useful in decreasing inflammation and pain.

Dislocation of a toe most often involves the fifth (or little) toe. The mechanism of injury is usually the collision of a bare foot with a relatively immovable object, such as a chair, a table leg, or a doorframe. The patient reports immediate onset of pain at the moment of

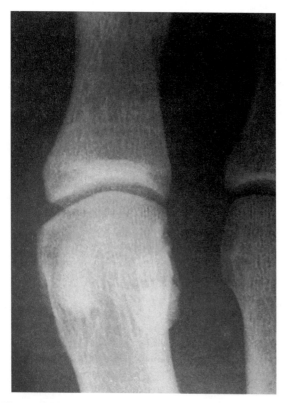

Figure 9-20   Turf Toe Injury. Subtle radiographic findings include calcifications in the collateral ligament(s) with avulsion on the fibular side. (From Coughlin MJ, Mann RA, editors: *Surgery of the foot and ankle*, ed 7, vol 2, St Louis, 1999, Mosby.)

impact and may note hearing or feeling a pop or crack. On inspecting the digit, angulation or some other deviation is noted. Perhaps because of surprise or a mild state of shock, the patient may pull on and relocate the toe.

Continued pain or swelling after such an event is sometimes the patient's initial reason for seeking medical attention. On examination, the digit is swollen and often discolored. There may be some rotation or asymmetry to the digit. Neurovascular compromise is unusual. Careful inspection and comparison of the plane of the contralateral digit's nail should be performed to rule out any rotational deformity.

Diagnosis is based on history, examination, and radiographic films. Plain x-ray projections should include AP, lateral, and oblique views to assess the presence and direction of any persistent dislocation or fracture. Small fractures of the articular surface of the bone are not uncommon.

If dislocation of the joint persists, closed reduction can usually be accomplished in the office. After performing a digital nerve block using plain 1% or 2% lidocaine hydrochloride, the distal phalanx is grasped and gentle traction applied with one hand.[39] Forceful pulling can further traumatize the soft tissue of the digit and turn a simple dislocation into a complex one. However, unless the practitioner has experience in reducing dislocations, the patient should be referred to an orthopedic surgeon.

Once reduced, the affected toe is buddy taped to its adjoining digit for 2 to 3 weeks. Pain control may initially require the use of oral narcotic analgesics. Within the first several days after injury, NSAIDs usually provide adequate relief.

Metatarsophalangeal and Tarsometatarsal Ligaments

Ligamentous injury of the foot can occur in association with ankle sprains, overuse, or acute injury. Many injuries involve forced plantar flexion or dorsiflexion or abnormal rotation of the foot. These traumas can result in stretching or tearing of any of the numerous ligaments that stabilize the foot. In severe injury, dislocation of the foot can occur. Dislocations are dramatic in clinical appearance (Figure 9-22) and are rarely seen in a primary care setting. Although usually easy to reduce, liga-

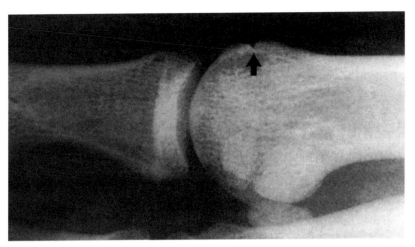

Figure 9-21 A divot on the dorsum of first metatarsal head *(arrow)* is sometimes seen with a turf toe injury.

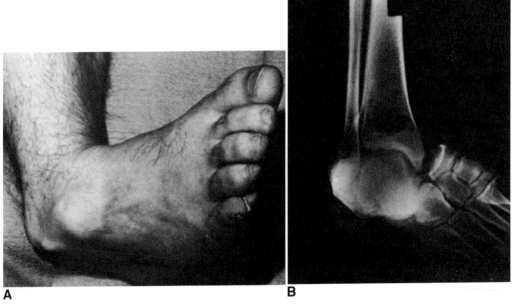

A   **B**

Figure 9-22 Clinical **(A)** and radiographic **(B)** appearance of a medial subtalar dislocation. (From DeLee JC, Curtis R: Subtalar dislocation of the foot. *J Bone Joint Surg Am* 64:433, 1982.)

mentous injuries require follow-up evaluation by an orthopedic surgeon.

The presenting symptoms of milder sprains usually include diffuse pain or tenderness and swelling over the dorsum of the foot. Pain is most pronounced over the area of ligamentous injury. Walking, weight bearing, and running tend to exacerbate pain. Sometimes the patient will feel the need to "stretch out" the foot. Point tenderness is difficult to elicit. Repositioning the foot in the position where the injury occurred can increase pain.

As with other sprains, rest, ice, compression, and elevation are the basic principles of initial treatment. Within the first 48 hours after the injury, the patient should resume some weight-bearing activities. The use of an elastic bandage may improve the patient's sense of security. NSAIDs can help reduce inflammation and its secondary pain. Usually the use of NSAIDs on a regular basis is not indicated for longer than 1 to 2 weeks.

Progressive increases in activity should begin within the first few days after injury. A full return to sports is normal in 4 to 8 weeks, depending on the severity of the sprain. A lace-up splint may improve patient comfort.

NERVE PROBLEMS

Tarsal Tunnel Syndrome

As the posterior tibial nerve courses along the medial aspect of the ankle and foot, it passes through an osteofibrous canal known as the tarsal tunnel. The tarsal tunnel is bordered by the medial malleolus, the medial aspect of the talus and the calcaneus, and the flexor retinaculum (Figure 9-23). Compression or entrapment of the nerve within this tunnel results in burning pain, numbness, and tingling in the plantar aspect of the foot and toes.

Any of the three branches of the posterior tibial nerve (Figure 9-24) can be affected—the medial plantar nerve, the lateral plantar nerve, or the calcaneal nerve.[28] Any process that decreases the size of the tarsal tunnel can cause nerve entrapment. Scar tissue, crush injury, postfracture callus formation, space-occupying lesion, tendon sheath inflammation, and deformity of the foot and heel can alter the normal tunnel and compress the nerve. Even excessive pronation of the foot can cause symptoms.

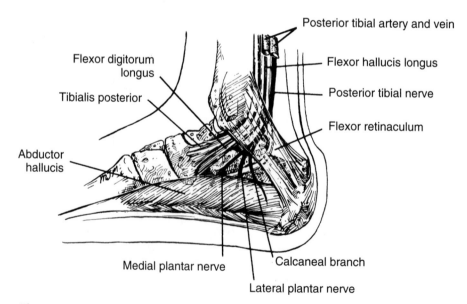

Figure 9-23 Landmarks of the Tarsal Tunnel. The medial malleolus, medial talus, medial calcaneus, and flexor retinaculum make up the borders of the tunnel through which the posterior tibial nerve passes. (From Coughlin MJ, Mann RA, editors: *Surgery of the foot and ankle*, ed 7, vol 1, St Louis, 1999, Mosby.)

Symptoms of pain, burning, and numbness are frequently worse with weight-bearing activities. Occasionally symptoms will radiate to the calf. Rest and elevation of the affected foot may reduce symptoms.

On examination there is diffuse medial foot or ankle pain. Forced plantar flexion and inversion of the foot may reproduce symptoms. Tapping the nerve within the tarsal tunnel can reproduce or cause symptoms; this is a positive Tinel's sign.

A tentative diagnosis can be made on the basis of history and physical examination. Electromyography (EMG) and nerve conduction studies (NCS) provide a more definitive diagnosis if symptoms have been present for at least 6 weeks. EMG and NCS offer little benefit, however, for evaluating acute nerve injury.

Surgical release of the entrapped nerve is the treatment of choice. Once a diagnosis of tarsal tunnel syndrome is made, the patient should be referred to an orthopedic surgeon for definitive treatment. Analgesics and NSAIDs may decrease symptoms but will rarely resolve them.

Morton's Neuroma

Forefoot pain that radiates from the forefoot to the toes and is exacerbated by walking may indicate the presence of Morton's neuroma. Pain is caused by the presence of a lesion, also called an interdigital perineural neuroma, on the interdigital nerve—most commonly on the third and usually between the third and fourth metatarsal heads (Figure 9-25). It is thought that repetitive trauma causes fibrosis and swelling of the nerve. Although the third interdigital nerve is most frequently affected, this neuroma can develop on any interdigital nerve.

Morton's neuroma affects women more often than men, possibly in part because of the relatively tighter shoes women wear. Repetitive dorsiflexion of the toes at the MTP joint (as occurs when wearing high heels) is also associated with development of interdigital perineural fibromas.[37] A common history is a sharp, burning pain in the forefoot while walking. After stopping, removing the shoe, and massaging the area, pain decreases or resolves.

Examination is usually remarkable only for pain between the third and fourth metatarsal heads with direct palpation. Sometimes a practitioner can elicit pain by transversely compressing all the metatarsal heads by grasping the forefoot and squeezing. This is performed with the thumb over the first MTP joint and the fingers around the fifth MTP joint. Occasionally, a firm nodule can be palpated between the metatarsal heads, which may range in size from a large grain of sand to a pea-sized bump.

Treatment should begin with metatarsal pads, more accommodative footwear, or a small pad between the affected toes. Injection of the neuroma with a local anesthetic and a corticosteroid will relieve symptoms in some patients, but most eventually require surgical excision of the lesion.

Metatarsalgia

Pain beneath the metatarsal heads is called *metatarsalgia*. It is often seen in combination with other forefoot abnormalities and is more of a symptom than a diagnosis. Metatarsalgia can affect one, several, or all of the metatarsal heads. Pes cavus, a tight Achilles' tendon, degenerative joint disease of the foot, hammertoe, claw toe, and hallux valgus deformities are some of the conditions with which metatarsalgia is associated.

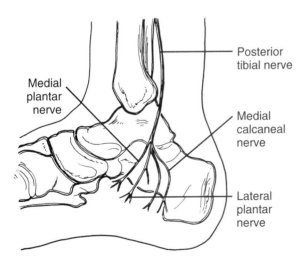

Figure 9-24 Branches of the posterior tibial nerve that may become entrapped at the medial malleolus, causing tarsal tunnel syndrome.

Posterior tibial nerve

Medial plantar nerve

Medial calcaneal nerve

Lateral plantar nerve

Patients typically complain of pain over the ball of the foot. Pain is often described as cramping, but it may also be a burning sensation. Symptoms are worse with walking and tend to improve with rest.

On examination, there may be diffuse tenderness over the ball of the foot. Calluses may be present under the metatarsal heads. Unlike with Morton's neuroma, transverse compression of the metatarsal heads does not usually reproduce or increase pain.

Diagnosis is based primarily on history and examination, but plain x-ray films can help rule out a fracture or joint disease. Weight-bearing lateral and AP views, as well as an oblique x-ray projection, will reveal osteo-phytes, a healing stress fracture, or a shortened first metatarsal. Any of these conditions will cause localized pain at the affected site.

Treatment is directed at readjusting the weight-bearing surface from the metatarsal heads to the shafts of the bones. The use of a metatarsal bar fabricated especially for the patient is useful for changing the weight-bearing area of the foot. The bar is placed proximal to the metatarsal heads so that they are no longer in direct contact with the ground. Symptomatic care with NSAIDs and warm soaks is also prescribed. If these measures do not alleviate symptoms, the patient should be referred to an orthopedic surgeon.

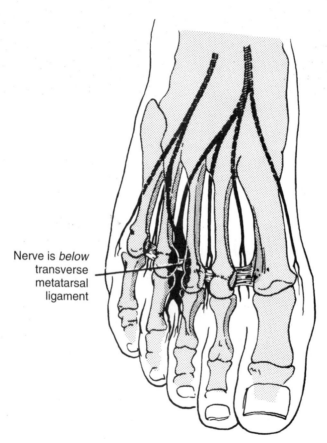

Nerve is *below* transverse metatarsal ligament

Figure 9-25 Diagram showing the most common location of an interdigital perineural fibroma (often called Morton's neuroma). The lesion is occasionally palpable. (From Coughlin MJ, Mann RA, editors: *Surgery of the foot and ankle*, ed 7, vol 1, St Louis, 1999, Mosby.)

DEVELOPMENTAL DISORDERS

Bunions and Bunionettes

One of the most common causes of pain and deformity in the forefoot is the presence of a bunion (Figure 9-26). There is a strong familial tendency in the occurrence of bunions, although footwear can exacerbate or cause bunion deformity.[9] The term bunion is typically used to describe a deformity over the first MTP joint secondary to hallux valgus, or lateral deviation of the great toe (i.e., hallux) and medial deviation of the first metatarsal. When a bunion is present on the lateral side of the foot (i.e., at the fifth MTP joint), it is often termed a bunionette or tailor's bunion.

Structurally there are three main problems when a bunion is present. First, the metatarsal head is quite prominent. As a result, wearing shoes, especially those with a narrow toe box, can be quite painful. Second, the intermetatarsal angle is increased. This alters the pull of the muscles that stabilize the hallux and sesamoid bones. Finally, as a result of the altered muscle pull, the great toe abducts and pronates, frequently overlapping the second toe. The sesamoid bones become displaced, altering the biomechanics of the great toe.[8]

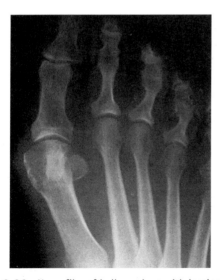

Figure 9-26   X-ray film of hallux valgus with bunion (exostosis) of the first metatarsal. (From Mercier LR: *Practical orthopedics*, ed 5, St Louis, 2000, Mosby.)

Bunionette deformity results in lateral deviation of the fifth metatarsal with medial deviation of the little toe. The toe may be rotated or overlap the adjacent digit.

Subluxation of the MTP joint can occur with either bunion or bunionette deformities. Subluxation can cause an incongruent joint, which can predispose the MTP joint to degenerative changes.

Pain at the site of deformity is the cardinal symptom of a bunion. Weight-bearing activities and wearing shoes typically increase pain, but sharp, shooting pain at night when the patient is barefoot is not uncommon. Numbness and tingling are not associated with bunions unless there is some concomitant process.

Examination should be conducted with the patient standing and sitting, since weight bearing can exaggerate the deformity.[8] Both active and passive ROM of the great toe should be evaluated. Crepitus or pain may indicate degenerative changes in the joint.

Weight-bearing AP and lateral views should be obtained. A special sesamoid or axial view should also be ordered to evaluate any subluxation of the sesamoids, but interpretation of this view is best left for the orthopedic surgeon.

Even though surgery offers definitive correction of the deformity, treatment should begin with conservative measures. Many patients will have relief of symptoms with simple measures such as padding over the bunion, wearing wider shoes, and avoiding high heels. NSAIDs may offer relief of acute symptoms. If symptoms persist, the patient should be referred to an orthopedic surgeon.

Hammertoe Deformity

A flexion deformity of the proximal interphalangeal (PIP) joint of the toe can result in the distal phalanx "pointing down." This deformity, called a hammertoe, also causes hyperextension of the MTP joint of the digit (Figure 9-27). In many individuals the second toe is longer than the others; it is also the one most often affected by a hammertoe deformity.

Caucasian women between the ages of 30 and 60 are most often afflicted. Variations of hammertoe deformity include claw toe and mallet toe deformities. A claw toe deformity results in flexion of the PIP joint and hyperextension of the distal interphalangeal (DIP) joint.

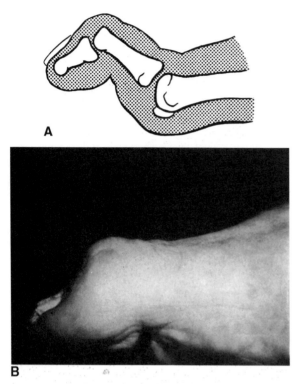

A

B

Figure 9-27   Hammertoe Deformity of the Great Toe.
A, The MTP joint is hyperextended with flexion of the interphalangeal joint. **B,** Clinical appearance of the hammertoe
deformity. (From Coughlin MJ, Mann RA, editors: *Surgery of the foot
and ankle*, ed 7, vol 1, St Louis, 1999, Mosby.)

A flexion deformity of the DIP joint results in a mallet
toe. Figure 9-28 illustrates these variations.

There is a distinct correlation between the types of
shoes worn and the development of this problem. Tight,
ill-fitting shoes are often a major contributor to the
development of hammertoe deformities. Deformity
and pain with certain footwear are often the presenting
complaints.

On examination the deformity is evident. Calluses are
often present from constant rubbing on the tip of the distal phalanx and on the dorsum of the PIP joint. Usually
the callus is painful. Hallux valgus is often present.

If the practitioner can manually straighten the deformity, it is considered a flexible deformity. At this stage,
extension and flexion exercises of the toe may reduce
deformity. Wearing shoes that have a larger toe box and

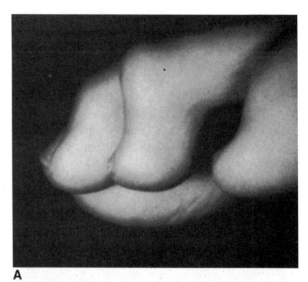

A

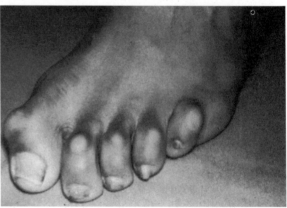

B

Figure 9-28   A, Mallet toe deformity. **B,** Claw toe deformity.
Note the multiple calluses over the dorsum of the interphalangeal and proximal interphangeal joints caused by chronic
irritation of ill-fitting shoes. (**A** from Coughlin MJ, Mann RA, editors: *Surgery of the foot and ankle*, ed 7, vol 1, St Louis, 1999,
Mosby.)

adequate room to allow full extension for the second toe
is also important.[9] Finally, taping the toe in an "over-
and-under" pattern (Figure 9-29) can help correct a flexible hammertoe deformity. A hammertoe that has been
present for some time usually becomes rigid and cannot
be manually reduced. A rigid deformity requires surgical correction.

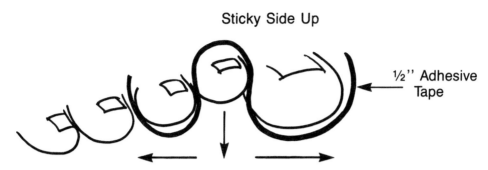

Figure 9-29   The "over-and-under" method of taping a flexible hammertoe deformity of the second toe. (From Mercier LR: *Practical orthopedics*, ed 5, St Louis, 2000, Mosby.)

Freiberg's Disease

One of the more overlooked causes of forefoot pain is an ischemic epiphyseal necrosis of the second (or sometimes third) metatarsal head. This condition is known as Freiberg's disease, necrosis, infraction, or osteochondrosis.

Freiberg's disease occurs primarily in adolescence, but it may not become symptomatic until adulthood. Repetitive trauma, such as marching or running, may exacerbate symptoms. Sometimes the patient may have spontaneous onset of localized pain and stiffness at the second MTP joint.

On examination mild swelling around the joint (i.e., synovitis) and localized tenderness may be the only clinical findings. As the disease progresses, the MTP joint may have decreased flexion and extension.

Radiographic changes may not become visible for a month or more after the onset of symptoms. The most characteristic x-ray finding is a flattening of the second (or third) metatarsal head. Sclerosis at the MTP joint may be evident before flattening occurs. Over time, osteoarthritic changes of the MTP joint can develop (Figure 9-30). MRI may help differentiate Freiberg's from a stress fracture, but MRI is expensive and not usually necessary.

Treatment soon after the onset of symptoms may delay progression of the disease. Although spontaneous resolution can occur, there is no definitive evidence that early treatment can prevent progression. Resolution of symptoms may take up to 1 year.

Metatarsal bars or pads are used to relieve pressure on the metatarsal head. Decreasing the intensity of activity will allow healing to occur. Sometimes custom orthotics are used in an extra-depth shoe to relieve pressure points. Once the metatarsal head has collapsed, symptoms may need to be treated surgically.

Calluses

Repeated irritation over a bony prominence can result in the development of localized hyperkeratosis. This condition, commonly called a callus, is frequently seen under the great toe sesamoids on the plantar surface of the other metatarsal heads. They are sometimes called plantar corns and can be confused with plantar warts. Calluses can be differentiated from plantar warts by the latter being tender to lateral compression; also, plantar warts often contain small central black dots that represent thrombosed small blood vessels.

Pain or even discomfort from the hyperkeratotic skin may prompt the patient to seek care. Unless the patient has tried self-excision, calluses do not usually become infected. Pain is often worse with the wearing of ill-fitting shoes that cause local irritation.

Diagnosis is based on history and the clinical appearance of the lesion. Trimming away the horny layer of skin around the callus will reveal more layers of heaped-up keratin and may reveal a keratin plug.[13]

Treatment centers on removing the source of irritation. Reducing the pressure on the callus can be accomplished by wearing low-heeled shoes with a wide enough toe box to prevent crowding of the toes. Metatarsal pads may also help. Warm soaks followed by use of a pumice stone can help remove the callus layers. Use of keratolytic

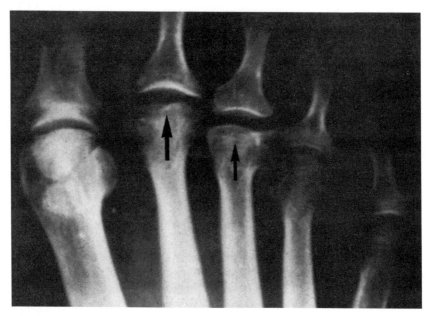

Figure 9-30   X-ray Appearance of Freiberg's Disease. Note flattening of the second and third metatarsal heads (*arrows*). (From Coughlin MJ, Mann RA, editors: *Surgery of the foot and ankle*, ed 7, vol 2, St Louis, 1999, Mosby.)

agents such as salicylic acid should not be used in patients with neuropathy or who may be immunocompromised.[13] Referral to an orthopedic surgeon is rarely necessary.

Corns

Like calluses, corns develop in response to undue pressure over a particular area of the foot. Corns may be either hard or soft. Soft corns tend to develop in areas where there is moisture, such as the area between two toes (Figure 9-31). Hard corns are typically painful and often occur over the fifth MTP joint, especially when there is an underlying bunionette deformity (Figure 9-32).

Pain is more common with a corn than a callus. Breakdown of the skin may occur where the corn rubs against the shoe. When the horny layer of corn is trimmed, a well-defined translucent core can be seen. Treatment with corn pads, moleskin, and better-fitting shoes can help relieve symptoms. Keratolytic agents can be used, after which the layers of the corn can be shaved down. Patients with a tendency to develop corns may require referral to a podiatrist for regular

trimming. As a rule, deep excision of a corn should be avoided because of a tendency for infected ulcers to develop.

Hallux Rigidus

Trauma to or osteoarthritis (OA) of the MTP joint of the great toe can result in pain and limited movement of the joint. This condition is termed hallux rigidus. Although it can occur at any age, it is most common among patients in their 30s and 40s.

Pain and stiffness of the great toe are the patient's primary complaints. Pain is worsened by any activity where the great toe is dorsiflexed (i.e., the toe-off phase of walking). Swelling and mild erythema may also occur.

Examination reveals a swollen, tender joint. Some bony hypertrophy may be palpable. Flexion and extension are limited. Neurovascular status to the toe is usually normal. On x-ray examination, there is usually joint space narrowing and osteophytes are often present (Figure 9-33).

Treatment with nonnarcotic analgesics, NSAIDs, moist heat, and a supportive shoe can decrease symp-

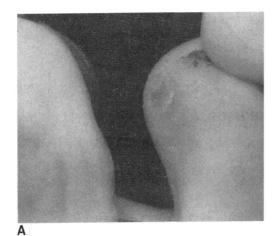

A

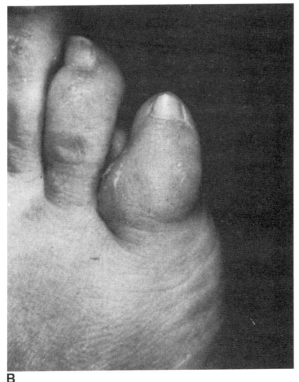

B

Figure 9-31 Clinical appearance of soft corns on the distal fifth toe **(A)**, and the base of fifth toe between fourth and fifth digits **(B)**. (From Coughlin MJ, Mann RA, editors: *Surgery of the foot and ankle*, ed 7, vol 2, St Louis, 1999, Mosby.)

toms. Corticosteroid injection into the joint can provide long-term relief for some patients. If conservative meas-

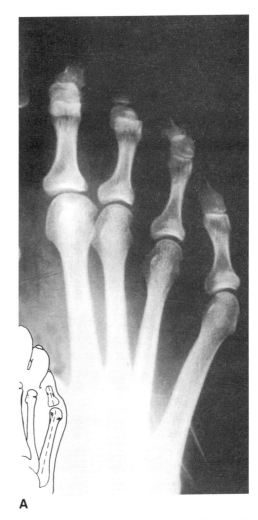

A

Figure 9-32 **A,** X-ray film and diagram of a bunionette deformity.

Continued

ures fail to provide relief, referral to an orthopedic surgeon is appropriate.

Pump Bump

Chronic rubbing of shoes, inversion of the heel, or an unstable calcaneus can lead to an inflammation of the bursa between the skin and Achilles' tendon. The posterior lateral aspect of the calcaneus becomes prominent (i.e., Haglund's deformity), and an exostosis may develop (Figure 9-34). The backs of certain types of shoes irritate the area.

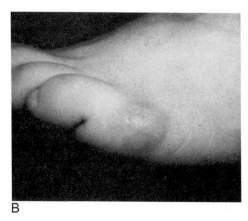

B

Figure 9-32, cont'd   B, Clinical appearance of the early development of a hard corn over a bunionette deformity. (From Coughlin MJ, Mann RA, editors: *Surgery of the foot and ankle,* ed 7, vol 1, St Louis, 1999, Mosby.)

The area of irritation may become a painful, erythematous bump, or it may remain a fairly small, indurated area at the posterior-superior edge of the calcaneus. If left untreated, the bursa may become permanently fibrotic.

The patient typically complains of posterior heel pain with certain types of shoes. He or she may have placed tape or some other type of padding over the bump to decrease pain. The bump on the back of the heel may be a concern for the patient.

Wearing shoes with open heels, a lower heel counter (i.e., back), or using heel pads to raise the heel can help reduce symptoms. NSAIDs may help decrease inflammation and pain. Referral to an orthotist or physical therapist may be appropriate for the fabrication of orthotics to stabilize the heel. Because of its proximity to the Achilles' tendon, corticosteroid injection should be avoided. In severe cases, the posterior lateral aspect of the calcaneus can be surgically excised.

Pes Planus (Acquired)

The contour of the foot's longitudinal arch is usually well established before reaching adulthood. A sudden onset of a new flatfoot deformity (i.e., acquired pes planus) frequently indicates a problem of the PTT. Associated additional injury to the spring ligament or the sinus tarsi is not uncommon with acute PTT injury.[3]

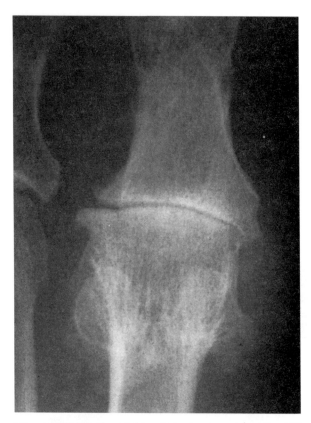

Figure 9-33   Hallux Rigidus. Note the narrowing of the MTP joint space and the formation of osteophytes at the joint line. (From Mercier LR: *Practical orthopedics,* ed 5, St Louis, 2000, Mosby.)

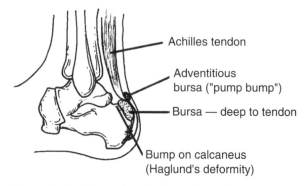

Achilles tendon

Adventitious bursa ("pump bump")

Bursa — deep to tendon

Bump on calcaneus (Haglund's deformity)

Figure 9-34   "Pump bump" shows the relationship of a Haglund's deformity and the development of the adventitious bursa known as the pump bump. (From Coughlin MJ, Mann RA, editors: *Surgery of the foot and ankle,* ed 7, vol 2, St Louis, 1999, Mosby.)

Inversion of the foot and maintenance of the longitudinal arch of the foot are two principal functions of the PTT. An acute injury to the PTT is often overlooked, or symptoms are attributed to a medial ankle sprain.

Disruption or dysfunction of the tendon causes a flattening of the medial longitudinal arch, valgus position of the heel, and painful or impossible of the foot. Over time, these changes can lead to a fixed deformity of the foot.

Diagnosis can be difficult, since there is something of a continuum of tendon dysfunction.[19] Subtle, progressive PTT dysfunction can be seen with diabetes, hypertension, and obesity.[40] Initially pain and discomfort occur along the tendon. Walking or standing can cause aching or complaints of fatigue along the plantar-medial foot and ankle. With an acute rupture or over time, pain may be more prominent laterally. As the arch flattens, the foot tends to pronate, and wearing shoes becomes difficult.

Examination of both feet reveals a flattened arch and pronation of the affected foot (Figure 9-35). When viewed from behind, the standing patient will have the "too many toes" sign. Inversion of the foot is painful and/or weak. One of the best tests to evaluate PTT function is the single-limb heel-rise test. To perform this test, the patient is asked to stand on tiptoe on the affected foot while the other foot is raised off the floor. If the PTT is weak or disrupted, the patient will be unable to perform this test.[27,40]

An acute injury resulting in symptoms of PTT dysfunction should be quickly referred to an orthopedic surgeon. Progressive loss of function or mild dysfunction can be treated with applications of ice, use of NSAIDs, rest, and cast immobilization or a removable cast boot for 6 to 8 weeks. Weight bearing is permitted while the foot is immobilized.

Surgical repair of the tendon can be performed if conservative measures fail. In the case of acute rupture, prompt referral to an orthopedic surgeon can reduce the incidence of complications and permanent instability or deformity.

Plantar Fasciitis

Plantar fasciitis has been variously termed a part of heel pain syndrome or the end result of other foot disorders.

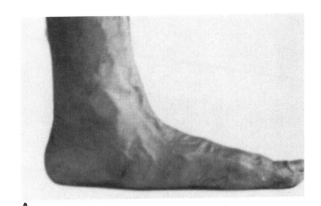

A

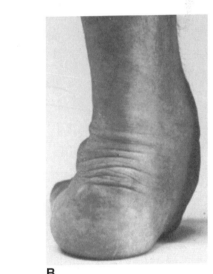

B

Figure 9-35 Typical findings of posterior tibial tendon dysfunction. Note the flat arch **(A)** and valgus position of the heel **(B)**. (From Coughlin MJ, Mann RA, editors: *Surgery of the foot and ankle*, ed 7, vol 1, St Louis, 1999, Mosby.)

Regardless of whether it is called painful heel syndrome, medial arch sprain, stone bruise, or calcaneal periostitis, inflammation of the plantar fascia is a common cause of hindfoot pain.

The plantar fascia is a thickened fibrous band of tissue in the subcutaneous layer of the foot (Figure 9-36). Beginning at the medial tuberosity of the calcaneus, the plantar fascia divides into five bands at the midfoot. The

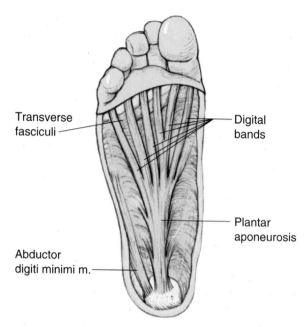

Transverse fasciculi

Digital bands

Abductor digiti minimi m.

Plantar aponeurosis

Figure 9-36 The plantar fascia of the foot. (From Mathers LH, editor: C.L.A.S.S.: *Clinical anatomy principles*, St Louis, 1996, Mosby.)

bands attach to the proximal phalanges just distal to the MTP joints. The plantar fascia helps support the tarsal bones, the arch of the foot, and the ligaments by acting as a truss or a windlass.[34] (A windlass is a system of ropes and pulleys used to lift heavy weights.) One of the plantar fascia's major functions is to act as a shock absorber when increased loads are placed on the foot.[49]

Stress overload results in a chronic degenerative-reparative process that causes pain. This process frequently occurs at or near the calcaneal insertion of the fascia. With continued overuse, destructive collagen changes occur and scar tissue is formed in the plantar fascia. Although the process is most often unilateral, it can be bilateral.

History. Patients tend to complain of a gradual onset of a sharp or sometimes burning pain on the sole of the foot. Usually there is no history of trauma, but a history of increased weight-bearing activities is not uncommon. Pain is characteristically worse first thing in the morning or when standing after a period of sitting. Symptoms improve once the patient begins walking or

---

Box 9-1	*Factors Contributing to Plantar Fasciitis*

Abnormal Biomechanics:

Pes cavus or planovalgus
Excessive pronation
Foot sprain
Posterior tibialis tendon dysfunction

Secondary Inflammation from Bony Disorders (Accessory navicular, Tarsal coalition, Fracture)

Systemic Problems:

Obesity
Infection
Gout, sarcoidosis, inflammatory arthritis

Training Errors:

Overuse
Sudden change in activity
Incorrect footwear
Hard surfaces (questionable)

---

exercising. The initial stiffness and pain are a reflection of the extent of stiffness and contracture in the fascia.

Physical examination and diagnosis. Examination and history frequently provide the diagnosis. Point tenderness over the plantar aspect of the medial calcaneal tuberosity is the cardinal sign of plantar fasciitis. Passive dorsiflexion of the ankle or toes can often reproduce symptoms.[33,49]

A multitude of factors contribute to the development of plantar fasciitis (Box 9-1), but both pes planus and pes cavus, which cause excessive strain on the plantar fascia, are commonly implicated. The presence of a heel spur is not uncommon in patients with plantar fasciitis, but symptoms frequently occur without radiographic evidence of any exostosis. X-ray studies are usually unnecessary for diagnosing plantar fasciitis. Tarsal tunnel syndrome can mimic symptoms of plantar fasciitis, but pain is usually worse at night or toward the end of the day.

Treatment. Treatment is directed toward relieving pain, identifying and removing predisposing factors when possible, and preventing the recurrence of symptoms. A rehabilitation program is an integral part of treatment. Many patients have complete resolution of symptoms with conservative therapy. They should be made aware, however, that it may take 6 months or more for symptoms to resolve.[17,49]

A formal physical therapy (PT) program with ice massage, iontophoresis, and electro-muscle stimulation may be helpful. A great deal of symptom relief can be obtained through home-based measures. Reducing or modifying activity to decrease repetitive stress on the foot is important. To maintain physical conditioning, the patient should be encouraged to substitute swimming, bicycling, or a stair-climbing machine for running or jogging.

Stretching the plantar fascia is one of the most successful ways to treat symptoms. The patient places a tennis ball or soft-drink bottle on the ground and then rolls the arch of the affected foot back and forth over the ball or bottle to provide low-stress massage to the plantar fascia. Hyperextending the toes while dorsiflexing the foot serves to stretch the fascia. This can be accomplished by asking the patient to place a rubber exercise band or a bicycle tire inner tube around the ball of the foot and then pull on the band to passively dorsiflex the foot.

Heel cord (i.e., Achilles' tendon) stretching is also useful in reducing symptoms. The patient stands on the edge of a bottom stair, facing upstairs. While grasping the handrail for support, the patient lowers his or her heel below the edge of the step and holds that position for a count of 5 to 10 seconds. Another method involves asking the patient to stand approximately 16 to 18 inches away from a wall, facing it. Maintaining the sole flat against the floor, the patient then leans forward toward the wall, stretching the calf and Achilles' tendon; this stretch is held for 5 to 10 seconds.

Night splints, which are commercially available, have been successful in reducing symptoms, even in recalcitrant cases.[17,33] The splints, worn while sleeping, maintain the foot in 5 degrees of dorsiflexion to keep the plantar fascia under constant, mild tension.

Other devices that may be useful include heel cups to thicken an atrophic fat pad, rubber heel cushions (e.g.,

Tuli cups), and orthotics to correct biomechanical deformities. The utility of strapping or taping the foot remains controversial.[17,33]

Medications include NSAIDs and steroid injection. As a rule NSAIDs offer only temporary relief of symptoms. If used, a course of 2 to 3 weeks should be prescribed to allow an adequate trial. Corticosteroid injections can be extremely helpful, but they should not be considered a first-line therapy because of associated risks, including rupture of the plantar fascia.

The majority of patients respond to conservative therapy within 6 to 10 months. In difficult cases, a last step before surgery is application of a short leg walking cast. Unfortunately, casting is often awkward for the patient, who may find wearing a cast for 6 weeks unacceptable. An orthopedic surgeon should make the decision for either casting or surgery.

JOINT PROBLEMS

Arthritis

Both RA and OA affect the foot. In either type of arthritis, other joints are usually involved before those in the feet. RA tends to affect the small joints of the hands first and may have other systemic manifestations before the feet become involved; however, the foot remains one of the most common sites for RA to occur. Usually, OA first affects larger weight-bearing joints.

In the foot, RA most often affects the metatarsals and phalanges.[1] Subluxation of the MTP joints is a significant problem with RA and surgical intervention is often necessary.[19] Synovitis of the MTP joints, rheumatoid nodules on the extensor tendons, plantar keratoses, and claw toe deformity of the lesser toes are common. Hallux valgus is another common manifestation of rheumatoid disease. Another frequent deformity is pes planovalgus, a flat foot with valgus deviation and abduction of the forefoot; this deformity is the result of an unstable subtalar joint. Any of these deformities, when present without another likely cause, should be evaluated as possible manifestations of RA (Figure 9-37).

RA should be managed in collaboration with a rheumatologist. Progressive pain and deformity in spite of disease-modifying antirheumatic drugs, orthotics,

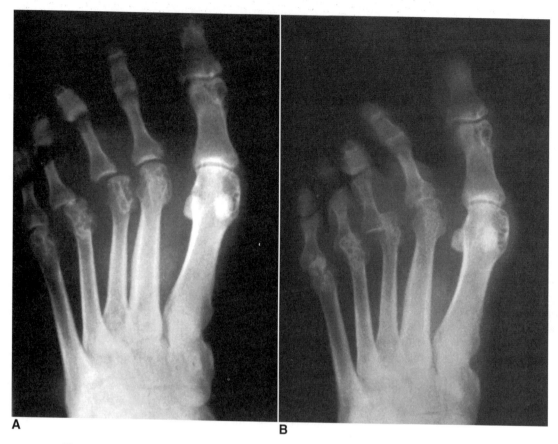

Figure 9-37 Radiographic appearance of rheumatoid arthritis progression over a 2-year period **(A, B)**. Note the increased subluxation of the metatarsophalangeal joints and cystic changes of the distal metatarsals. (From Mann RA, Coughlin MJ, editors: *Surgery of the foot and ankle*, ed 6, vol 1, St Louis, 1993, Mosby.)

assistive devices, and activity modification may require referral to an orthopedic surgeon for surgical stabilization of the foot.

OA is a degenerative condition that primarily affects weight-bearing joints. It is characterized by a loss of articular cartilage and bony hypertrophy of the joints. When the foot is involved the MTP joint of the great toe is often affected. Progressive development of osteophytes, or spurs, at the MTP joint can cause symptoms ranging from stiffness and decreased ROM (hallux limitus) to an inflexible joint (hallux rigidus). Other joints of the foot can also be involved, resulting in stiffness, pain,

and difficulty in walking. Stiffness, which is usually worse in the morning, tends to improve with activity.

Like OA of other sites, OA of the foot is managed with nonnarcotic analgesics, NSAIDs, and occasionally narcotic analgesics. Activity modification and assistive devices are also helpful. Referral to an orthopedic surgeon may be indicated if pain and joint deformity prevent normal ambulation.

Treatment of either arthritide should follow the guidelines of their pathogenesis and clinical course. Occupational therapy, PT, exercise, and diet modification are all essential components of treatment.

Rheumatoid disease more often necessitates a referral to a rheumatologist or orthopedic surgeon.

Gout

Gout is a term used to describe a collection of various disorders caused by the deposition of monosodium urate crystals in body tissue. Gout can be classified as either primary or secondary. Primary gout, which affects men ten times as often as women, is caused by an inborn error of purine metabolism that results in the overproduction or underexcretion of uric acid.

Secondary gout is associated with hyperuricemia, which is caused by other diseases or drugs that interfere with uric acid secretion. Secondary gout arises from a multitude of causes including endocrine disorders, lead poisoning, high-dose salicylates (more than 3 g per day), myeloproliferative disorders, and chronic renal disease.

The basic pathologic classification of gout is generally in one of two categories: overproduction or underexcretion of uric acid. A 24-hour urine collection is used to differentiate overproduction from underexcretion of uric acid.

Four phases are generally recognized in the development of gout. The first phase is asymptomatic hyperuricemia, which, as the name implies, is not associated with any clinical symptoms. There is evidence that the higher the level of an individual's serum uric acid, the greater the likelihood that acute gout will develop.[6] Typically the presenting symptom of acute gouty arthritis, the second phase, is a sudden, exquisitely painful monoarthropathy. Although any synovial joint can be affected, the most common site for this painful manifestation is the MTP joint of the great toe. This condition is called podagra. The third phase, the intercritical period, is the time between acute attacks. Most individuals develop a second episode of gout within 6 months to 2 years of the first attack. Untreated gout tends to result in more frequent, more severe attacks of longer duration. There are, however, some patients who never have a second attack. Finally, chronic tophaceous gout can develop.[5] Chronic gout results in bony destruction that is easily recognizable on x-ray films by its "punched out" appearance.[29] Tophi tend to appear anywhere between 2 years to more than 4 decades after the first onset of gout.[20] Tophi are sodium urate crystals that are deposited in the soft tissues and occur in up to 50% of patients with gout. The most common locations for tophi are the synovium, the prepatellar and olecranon bursae, the Achilles' tendon, and the helix of the ear.

The predominant risk factor for the development of gout is the presence of hyperuricemia. However, hyperuricemia alone is not diagnostic of gout; gout can occur in patients with normal levels of serum uric acid. Other risk factors for developing gout include obesity, excessive alcohol consumption, lead exposure (patients who consume "moonshine" whiskey have an even greater risk because moonshine tends to have a high lead content), and hypertension. Although the treatment of asymptomatic hyperuricemia is controversial, a blood uric acid level over 7 mg/dl may warrant treatment if the patient has other risk factors. Most clinicians recommend not treating asymptomatic hyperuricemia.

Up to 90% of persons with gout are underexcreters of uric acid. Normally the kidneys turn over approximately 700 mg/dl of uric acid per day. Of that amount, approximately 10% is excreted. Normal serum uric acid ranges from 2 to 7 mg/dl in men; the normal range for women is 2 to 6 mg/dl. Any factor that interferes with the glomerular and renal tubular resorption of uric acid can result in elevated serum uric acid levels.

Overproduction of uric acid is much less common than underexcretion and is often the result of another disease, frequently one associated with excessive rates of cell turnover. Hemolytic anemias, myeloproliferative and lymphoproliferative diseases, and psoriasis are examples of processes causing secondary gout attributable to overproduction of uric acid. Some inherited diseases and genetic abnormalities can cause primary gout as a result of overexcretion of uric acid.

The most important differential diagnosis to be made in a patient with gout is the exclusion of a septic joint. Orthopedic referral for joint aspiration may be appropriate if the practitioner is uncomfortable with the procedure or if materials with which to aspirate the joint are not available.

Definitive diagnosis is made by synovial fluid aspiration and examination. Fluid is sent for white blood cell count and differential, crystal analysis, and Gram's stain with culture. Examination of joint fluid using a polarized microscope will determine the presence of crystals. The presence of birefringent crystals in the synovial fluid does not exclude the possibility of infection, since gout and infection can coexist in a joint. As a result, care should be taken not to overlook a septic joint, especially in the presence of other constitutional symptoms of infection.

Once a diagnosis of gout has been made, the disease is managed primarily through pharmacologic and dietary measures. Treatment of acute gout usually begins with the use of NSAIDs (e.g., indomethacin, naproxen, and ibuprofen). Once NSAIDs are instituted, symptom relief is usually dramatic and significant improvement occurs within 24 hours. Allopurinol (a xanthine oxidase inhibitor) is used for long-term treatment. Long-term pharmacologic management of gout relies on NSAIDs, colchicine, uricosuric agents (e.g., probenecid and sulfinpyrazone), and xanthine oxidase inhibitors such as allopurinol.[12,20]

Dietary management includes avoiding foods high in purines and losing weight, if necessary. Consultation with a nutritionist is helpful in planning a realistic menu for the patient.

INFECTIONS

Diabetic Foot Infection

Among other problems, diabetes can result in peripheral neuropathy, abnormal functioning of polymorphonucleocytes, and increased severity of atherosclerotic vascular disease. This combination of factors increases the risk for developing unrecognized cellulitis, abscesses, ulcers, and even osteomyelitis.

Peripheral sensory neuropathy can be identified by an inability to perceive pressure from a 10-g monofilament or the vibration of a standard tuning fork placed over the affected area. Because of neuropathy, a diabetic patient may not experience the pain normally associated with a wound or infection. As a result an infected, deep ulceration or draining wound with cellulitis may occur before the patient seeks treatment.

For simplicity, diabetic foot infections can be divided into those that are nonlimb-threatening and those that are limb- or life-threatening.[16] Clinical differentiation of these two categories can sometimes be difficult because

the systemic signs of tachycardia, fever, and localized pain may be absent in the diabetic patient. Wounds having surrounding cellulitis greater in diameter than 2 cm, osteomyelitis, or a deep abscess are considered limb-threatening.[14]

Clinical examination of the wound is important in determining its severity. In the presence of neuropathy, using a blunt, sterile probe to assess the wound can be done in the office with little or no anesthesia. If any bone is palpable before débridement of the wound, there is an increased risk of osteomyelitis.[14,18] If osteomyelitis is suggested, either an immediate referral to an orthopedic surgeon for bone biopsy and consultation with or a referral to an infectious disease specialist should be made. The most common sites for osteomyelitis of the foot are the phalanges and metatarsals.

If no bone is palpable, the wound should be débrided and material sent for Gram's stain and aerobic and anaerobic cultures. If this analysis cannot be completed in the office setting, the patient should be admitted to a hospital. If the wound is not deep, draining, or malodorous, and if débridement consists solely of unroofing crusts, cultures can be taken in the office. In the case of cellulitis alone, the skin should be carefully inspected for evidence of breakdown, cracking, or puncture.

Even though superficial cultures do not correlate well with cultures from deep tissue, in most cases antibiotics that cover the superficial organisms will be adequate for initial therapy.[18] Empiric antibiotic therapy should begin as soon as wound cultures have been sent. Ideally the antibiotic selected should be effective against *Staphylococcus aureus*, streptococci, Enterobacteriaceae, and anaerobes. In the absence of pus, extensive cellulitis, unexplained hyperglycemia, flulike symptoms, or other evidence of a deep infection or systemic illness, oral antibiotics can be used as initial therapy.[18] Antibiotics should be adjusted once culture results are known. Under such circumstances, the patient requires close monitoring. If there is no improvement within 24 to 48 hours, the patient should be admitted to the hospital. Treatment of localized cellulitis in a diabetic patient may require intravenous antibiotics.

Diagnostic imaging studies can be helpful in evaluating the extent of infection. Plain x-ray films can show bony destruction and the presence of air within the soft tissues; both are evidence of a more serious infection. Because of its great sensitivity, triple-phase bone scan has long been the imaging standard for the diagnosing of osteomyelitis.[11] Bone scanning, however, remains non-specific. MRI has been shown to reveal bone changes associated with infection earlier than either bone scans or plain x-ray studies.

Treatment of a foot infection in a patient with diabetes requires a multifaceted approach. From an orthopedic standpoint, measures to be taken include the use of crutches or a walker to keep the affected limb on a completely nonweight-bearing status, padding around the wound to protect it, and simple, sterile dressings. Whirlpool, heat, and soaks are not recommended because of the potential for burns or tissue maceration attributable to a loss of normal sensation.[16] For mild infections, extra-depth shoes allow the use of padded, molded orthotics that can reduce pressure areas. Another way to avoid developing pressure areas on the feet is to encourage the patient to change footwear every 3 to 4 hours.

Consultation with or referral to an infectious disease specialist is appropriate for any deep wound or one that requires more than the simple unroofing of crusts. Referral to a general or orthopedic surgeon for débridement and culture of the wound is also appropriate in such cases. The presence of pus, lymphangitis, extensive cellulitis, or gangrene is a surgical emergency, and the patient should be immediately referred to a surgeon or emergency department.

Reflex Sympathetic Dystrophy/Complex Regional Pain Syndrome

Occasionally a patient will come to the primary care office with a swollen, painful, mottled, hyperesthetic foot. The history usually entails some trauma, ranging from a fracture to a relatively minor trauma, such as an ankle sprain or dropping something on the foot. The patient's complaints may also include changes in temperature and sweating patterns. Pain and vasomotor complaints often seem to be out of proportion to the mechanism of injury. As a result, the practitioner may ignore the patient and his or her complaints. Unfortunately, if left untreated this sympathetic nervous system dysfunction, commonly known as reflex sympa-

thetic dystrophy (RSD) can lead to a significant functional impairment. RSD is part of a group of disorders of the sympathetic branch of the autonomic nervous system. Other terms used to describe this disorder include Sudeck's atrophy (now rarely used), minor causalgia, spontaneous neuralgia, and posttraumatic neuralgia. More recently, RSD was classified as a complex regional pain syndrome (CRPS).[41]

The exact pathophysiology of CRPS is unknown; however, for some reason the pain of a noxious event is maintained by the sympathetic nervous system. There is no correlation between type or severity of injury and development of symptoms.[22,31] Although there is no reliable method of predicting when CRPS will follow an injury, slow healing or an unusual amount of pain after the injury may be an early indication of the syndrome.[26]

Symptoms usually begin within 6 weeks of injury. Cold intolerance is one of the earliest and most common complaints. An associated red to bluish-purplish skin color is not unusual. Either pitting or nonpitting edema can occur. Pain follows a nondermatomal distribution and can be caused by nonnoxious stimuli. Pain in a nonanatomic distribution is typical of sympathetically maintained pain.

On examination, excessive hair growth, smooth (sometimes shiny) skin, brittle nails, and even osteoporosis can be found to have developed. The affected foot is diffusely tender. Skin sensitivity with complaints of burning pain with a light touch is not uncommon. Normal activities such as walking or driving a vehicle can be difficult because of pain, swelling, and dysesthesia.

Diagnosis is often based on physical examination and a history of trauma followed by typical sympathetic nervous system changes. Bone scanning has often been used to identify CRPS by areas of diffusely increased uptake. A more definitive diagnosis can be made by referring the patient to a pain center or a qualified anesthesiologist for administration of a sympathetic blockade. The blockade may be intravenous, spinal, or epidural.[18]

Care must be taken not to miss RA or septic arthritis, cellulitis, systemic lupus erythematosus, or a peripheral neuropathy. Usually RA is bilateral and affects more than one area of the body. Unlike septic arthritis, CRPS does not usually involve constitutional symptoms such as fever, malaise, or leukocytosis. Peripheral neuropathies, including neuromas, tend to involve a specific dermatomal or nerve distribution.

Treatment is based on PT and sympathetic nerve blockade. Therapy includes active and active-assisted ROM and muscle-strengthening exercises, moist heat, and massage. A transcutaneous electrical nerve stimulation unit may be useful in controlling pain. The use of ice packs and passive ROM exercises should be avoided, since they tend to aggravate symptoms. The patient should be made aware that resolution of symptoms might take several weeks. Sympathetic stellate ganglion nerve blockade requires repeated injections by a qualified practitioner.

A number of medications are used to treat symptoms. Normal therapeutic doses of adrenergic agents (such as propranolol), calcium channel blockers, and tricyclic antidepressants (e.g., amytriptylline) are frequently used. Oral corticosteroids have also helped in some cases. Psychological counseling of the patient may be necessary during the course of treatment. Pamidronate, a bisphosphonate that is administered intravenously, has shown some promise in treating lower extremity CRPS. Overall, no definitive treatment yet exists for CRPS.[22]

INDICATIONS FOR REFERRAL

See the Red Flags box for referral information.

Red Flags *for Foot Disorders*

Patients with these findings may need to be referred for more extensive workup.

Signs and Symptoms	Response
Planar orientation of nail beds and comparison with contralateral foot show rotational deformity of fractured phalanx	Possible rotated fracture of the phalanx. Refer to orthopedic surgeon.
Radiograph of fractured toe reveals displacement	Displaced fracture of phalanx. Refer to orthopedic surgeon.
Swelling extending to dorsum and sometimes to sole of foot; point tenderness at site of metatarsal injury; pain may be described as deep aching or burning; pain becomes sharp when site is palpated or bears weight	Possible metatarsal fracture. Refer to orthopedic surgeon for further treatment.
Palpable deformity of fractured metatarsal	Possible displaced metatarsal fracture. Refer to orthopedic surgeon.
More than one metatarsal fracture	Refer to orthopedic surgeon.
Swelling over lateral dorsum of foot with or without discoloration; bruising may be apparent over inferior lateral border of foot; edema and ecchymosis may extend from ankle to lateral toes	Possible displaced fifth metatarsal fracture. Refer to orthopedic surgeon for evaluation.
Pain with weight bearing, difficulty walking, and excessive midfoot swelling after trauma to TMT area; clinical stress test for TMT instability is positive	Possible TMT fracture. Refer to orthopedic surgeon for surgical repair.
Heel pain increases with weight bearing; walking may be impossible because of pain; heel may appear widened or shortened in comparison with other foot; arch of foot may be flattened; fracture blisters may be present	Possible calcaneus fracture. Refer to orthopedic surgeon for surgical treatment.
X-ray film of possible sprained ankle reveals fractured talus	Immediately refer to orthopedic surgeon for open reduction and internal fixation.
X-ray films reveal small fractures of second cuneiform, cuboid, or navicular bones	Possible Lisfranc's fracture. Immediately refer to orthopedic surgeon.
Pain or swelling of toe; digit may be angular or deviated in some way; digit may be discolored and asymmetric	Possible dislocated toe. Refer to orthopedic surgeon for closed reduction, if practitioner is inexperienced in reducing dislocations.

Continued

Signs and Symptoms	Response
Symptoms of pain, burning, and numbness increase with weight bearing; symptoms may radiate to calf; diffuse medial foot or ankle pain; positive Tinel's sign	Possible tarsal tunnel syndrome. Refer to orthopedic surgeon for definitive treatment.
Failure of conservative treatment of metatarsalgia	Refer to orthopedic surgeon for further treatment.
Failure of conservative treatment of bunion or bunionette	Refer to orthopedic surgeon for possible surgical intervention.
Flexion deformity of PIP joint of toe resulting in distal phalanx "pointing down"; usually occurs in second toe; deformity is rigid and cannot manually be reduced	Possible fixed hammer toe; refer to orthopedic surgeon for surgical reduction.
Failure of conservative measures to treat hallux rigidus	Refer to orthopedic surgeon for further treatment.
Acute injury resulting in flattened arch and pronation of affected foot; inversion of foot is painful and weak; positive "too many toes" sign when patient is viewed from behind; positive single-limb, heel-rise test	Possible acute rupture of posterior tibial tendon. Immediately refer to orthopedic surgeon for surgical repair of tendon.
Any or all of these deformities: synovitis of MTP joints, rheumatoid nodules on the extensor tendons, plantar keratoses, claw toe deformity of the lesser toes, hallux valgus, and pes planovalgus	Possible RA. If no other possible cause, refer to rheumatologist or orthopedic surgeon.
Infected, deep ulceration or draining wound, possibly with cellulites	If bone is palpable before débridement of wound, possible osteomyelitis; refer to orthopedic surgeon. If no bone is palpable, admit patient to hospital for wound cultures if procedure cannot be performed in the office setting. If no improvement within 24 hours, admit patient to hospital for treatment. If it requires more than one simple unroofing of crusts, refer to infectious disease specialist. May refer to orthopedic or general surgeon for débridement and culturing of the wound.
Presence of pus, lymphangitis, extensive cellulitis, or gangrene	Medical emergency; refer to a surgeon or emergency department.

MTP, Metatarsophalangeal; *PIP,* proximal interphalangeal; *RA,* rheumatoid arthritis; *TMT,* tarsometatarsal.

REFERENCES

1. Abdo RV, Iorio LJ: Rheumatoid arthritis of the foot and ankle, *J Am Acad Orthop Surg* 2:326, 1994.

2. Archdeacon M, Wilber R: Fractures of the talar neck, *Orthop Clin North Am* 33:247, 2002.

3. Balen PF, Helms CA: Association of posterior tibial tendon injury with spring ligament injury, sinus tarsi abnormality, and plantar fasciitis on MR imaging, *Am J Roentgenol* 176:1137, 2001.

4. Barei DP et al: Fractures of the calcaneus, *Orthop Clin North Am* 33:263, 2002.

5. Buckley TJ: Radiologic features of gout, *Am Fam Physician* 54:1232, 1996.

6. Campion EW et al: Asymptomatic hyperuricemia. Risks and consequences in the normative aging study, *Am J Med* 82:421, 1987.

7. Chambers HG, Sutherland DH: A practical guide to gait analysis, *J Am Acad Orthop Surg* 10:222, 2002.

8. Coughlin MJ: Hallux valgus, *J Bone Joint Surg Am* 78A:932, 1996.

9. Coughlin MJ: The high cost of fashionable footwear, *J Musculoskelet Med* 11(12):40, 1994.

10. Dameron TB: Fractures of the fifth metatarsal: selecting the best treatment option, *J Am Acad Orthop Surg* 3:110, 1995.

11. Donohoe KJ: Selected topics in orthopedic nuclear medicine, *Orthop Clin North Am* 29:85, 1998.

12. Fam AG: 'Problem' gout: clinical challenges, effective solutions, *J Musculoskelet Med* 14(10):63, 1997.

13. Freeman DB: Corns and calluses resulting from hyperkeratosis, *Am Fam Physician* 65:2277, 2002.

14. Frykberg RG: Diabetic foot ulcers: pathogenesis and management, *Am Fam Physician* 66:1655, 2002.

15. Geppert MJ, Buckley PD: Pinpointing the cause of lower extremity injuries in the athlete, *J Musculoskelet Med* 15(1):8, 1998.

16. Gibbons GW, Habershaw GM: Diabetic foot infections, *Infect Dis Clin North Am* 9:131, 1995.

17. Gill LH: Plantar fasciitis: diagnosis and conservative management, *J Am Acad Orthop Surg* 5:109, 1997.

18. Grayson ML: Diabetic foot infections: antimicrobial therapy, *Infect Dis Clin North Am* 9:143, 1995.

19. Hillstrom HJ et al: Evaluation and management of the foot and ankle. In Robbins L et al, editors: *Clinical Care in the Rheumatic diseases*, ed 2, Atlanta, 2001, American College of Rheumatology.

20. Harris MD et al: Gout and hyperuricemia, *Am Fam Phys* 59:925, 1999.

21. Hochman MG et al: MR imaging of the symptomatic ankle and foot, *Orthop Clin North Am* 28:659, 1997.

22. Hogan CJ, Hurwitz SR: Treatment of complex regional pain syndrome of the lower extremity, *J Am Acad Orthop Surg* 10:281, 2002.

23. Judd DB, Kim DH: Foot fractures frequently misdiagnosed as ankle sprains, *Am Fam Phys* 66:785, 2002.

24. Lassus J et al: Bone stress injuries of the lower extremity: a review, *Acta Orthop Scand* 73:359, 2002.

25. Macintyre J, Joy E: Foot and ankle injuries in dancers, *Clin Sports Med* 19:351, 2000.

26. Merskey H, Bogduk N, editors: *Classification of chronic pain: descriptions of chronic pain syndromes and definitions of pain terms*, ed 2, Seattle, 1994, International Association for the Study of Pain.

27. Myerson MA: Acquired flatfoot deformity, *J Bone Joint Surg Am* 78A:780, 1996.

28. Novotny DA et al: Recurrent tarsal tunnel syndrome and the radial forearm free arm flap, *Foot Ankle Int* 17:641, 1996.

29. Ohta-Fukushima M et al: Characteristics of stress fractures in young athletes under 20 years, *J Sports Med Phys Fitness* 42:198, 2002.

30. Peterson WJ et al: The arterial supply of the lesser metatarsal heads: a vascular injection study in human cadavers, *Foot Ankle Int* 23:491, 2002.

31. Pittman DM, Belgrade MJ: Complex regional pain syndrome, *Am Fam Physician* 56:2265, 1997.

32. Prokuski LJ, Saltzman CL: Challenging fractures of the foot and ankle, *Radiol Clin North Am* 35:655, 1997.

33. Quashnick MS: The diagnosis and management of plantar fasciitis, *Nurse Pract* 21(4):50, 1996.

34. Ridola C, Palma A: Functional anatomy and imaging of the foot, *Ital J Embryol* 106:85, 2001.

35. Quill GE: Fractures of the proximal fifth metatarsal, *Orthop Clin North Am* 26:353, 1995.

36. Rosenberg GA, Sferra JJ: Treatment strategies for acute fractures and nonunions of the proximal fifth metatarsal, *J Am Acad Orthop Surg* 8:332, 2000.

37. Rudicel SA: Evaluating and managing forefoot problems in women, *J Musculoskel Med* 16:562, 1999.

38. Sanders RW et al: Symposium: the treatment of displaced intraarticular fractures of the calcaneus, *Contemp Orthop* 32:187, 1996.

39. Schenck RC, Heckman JD: Fractures and dislocations of the forefoot, *J Am Acad Orthop Surg* 3(2):70, 1995.

40. Smith AM, Teasdall R: Managing tendon disorders of the foot and ankle, *J Musculoskel Med* 19:196, 2002.

41. Stanton-Hicks SM et al: Reflex sympathetic dystrophy: changing concepts and taxonomy, *Pain* 63:127, 1995.

42. Teng AL et al: Functional outcome following anatomic restoration of tarsal-metatarsal fracture dislocation, *Foot Ankle Int* 23:922, 2002.

43. Reference deleted in proofs.

44. Trepman E, Yodlowski M: Occupational disorders of the foot and ankle, *Orthop Clin North Am* 27:815, 1996.

45. Trevino SG, Kodros S: Controversies in tarsometatarsal injuries, *Orthop Clin North Am* 26:229, 1995.

46. Reference deleted in proofs.

47. Verma RB, Sherman O: Athletic stress fractures: Part I: history, epidemiology, risk factors, radiography, diagnosis and treatment, *Am J Orthop* 30:798, 2000.

48. Verma RB, Sharma O: Athletic stress fractures: Part II. The lower body. Part III. The upper body—with a section on the female athlete, *Am J Orthop* 30:848, 2001.

49. Young CC et al: Treatment of plantar fasciitis, *Am Fam Phys* 63:467, 2001.

50. Yu WD, Shapiro MS: Fractures of the fifth metatarsal: careful identification for optimal treatment, *Phys Sportsmed* 26(2):47, 1998.

Chapter 10

Injections for Musculoskeletal Disorders

The judicious use of corticosteroid and anesthetic injections can be helpful in treating disorders such as bursitis, tenosynovitis, and arthritis, as well as in aiding in the diagnosis of certain musculoskeletal conditions. However, corticosteroid injections are not free of risks. Contraindications to injection are shown in Table 10-1.

In addition, if there is any question regarding either the need for or the technique of injection, the practitioner in the primary care setting should refer the patient to a specialist.

Improperly administered injections can cause additional problems, ranging from nuisances to serious consequences. For example, injecting a corticosteroid while withdrawing the needle can cause subcutaneous fat necrosis, skin atrophy, and hypopigmentation. Repeated corticosteroid injections can weaken tendons.[2] Nerve damage can result if fluid is injected into the nerve itself. Infections, ranging from cellulitis to septic joints to necrotizing fasciitis, have been reported.[1,7]

The patient should be warned in advance that injections could be painful for several days after the initial injection. This postinjection flare is thought to be caused by precipitation of corticosteroid crystals within the tissue or synovium.[12,19] As a result, the solution is more of an irritant for the first several days; it requires time to work through its antiinflammatory mechanism. After the injection, the patient should be advised that the injected area needs a period of 1 to 3 days of relative rest. This is especially true of weight-bearing joints.[18]

MATERIALS AND METHODS

The use of injections in orthopedics involves an understanding not only of the indications, medications, and methods to be used, but also of the materials with which the medicines are delivered. For instance, a knee injection may require a 10-ml syringe with a large needle (e.g., a 22-gauge) to allow easy delivery of the medication. In fact, this is less painful to the patient than using a 25-gauge needle.

Often the volume of fluid is in question. Some practitioners are far more generous with the amount of local anesthetic than the amount of corticosteroid, whereas others prefer a 1:1 ratio. In larger joints, 1- to 2-ml of steroid should be adequate.[13] In smaller joints or with tenosynovitis, 1 ml of corticosteroid is typically used.[17] The amount of local anesthetic is somewhat variable.

The use of local anesthetics is often a matter of personal choice. For example, bupivacaine (Marcaine) 0.5% provides longer-lasting local anesthesia than lidocaine (Xylocaine). Some providers prefer lidocaine because of its shorter duration of action, particularly if the injection is for a diagnostic rather than a therapeutic purpose.

Selecting a corticosteroid is frequently based on the medication's antiinflammatory potency and cost. There is no consensus on the appropriate corticosteroid dosage for various injections.[14] With a relative potency of 1, hydrocortisone preparations can be considered fairly mild. Prednisolone tebutate, methylprednisolone acetate, and triamcinolone acetate fall into the 4 to 5, or

TABLE 10-1   Contraindications to Joint Injections

Absolute Contraindications	Relative Contraindications
Septic joint	Anticoagulant therapy
Bacteremia	Lack of response after two to four injections
Severe coagulopathy	Joint prosthesis
Overlying cellulitis	Lack of response to previous injections
Unstable joint	Clotting disorders
More than three injections per year in weight-bearing joint	Severe immunocompromise
Inaccessible joint	Poorly controlled diabetes
Intraarticular fracture	Patient with a history of noncompliance to other treatment
Known hypersensitivity to material(s) being injected	Tumor at site of injection
Adjacent osteomyelitis	Immunosuppression (AIDS, chemotherapy)
Acute local tissue trauma	

moderate, range. Both betamethasone and dexamethasone acetate, which fall into the 20 to 30 range, are considered potent antiinflammatory agents.[12] Other considerations in choosing an agent include its half-life, which is considered an indication of the length of its therapeutic effect. Generally water-soluble corticosteroids have a shorter half-life than water-insoluble agents. Methylprednisolone acetate and triamcinolone acetate are slightly soluble. Dexamethasone acetate, prednisolone acetate, and triamcinolone acetonide are relatively insoluble.[4]

In general, a 22-gauge needle can be used for larger joints such as shoulders, hips, and knees. This size allows easier delivery of the medications. For shoulders and knees, 2 ml of a corticosteroid combined with 6 to 8 ml of local anesthetic can be used. For smaller areas a 25-gauge needle on a 3-ml syringe is useful. Table 10-2 summarizes some common needle sizes and dosages of a representative corticosteroid for various orthopedic injections.

UPPER EXTREMITY

The use of injections in the upper extremity can be helpful not only for their therapeutic effect, but also for differentiating confusing clinical findings. This phenomenon is particularly true around the shoulder. Injections into the subacromial space can be quite helpful not only

in treating patients but also in helping one delineate between acromioclavicular joint problems versus rotator cuff problems.[9,10]

In any upper extremity injection, pain can be a problem for several days after the injection. Nonsteroidal antiinflammatory drugs (NSAIDs) or narcotics can often prevent late-night phone calls from irate patients. Before injection, it is helpful to educate the patient about the expected pain and the prescribed appropriate medication.

Shoulder

Shoulder injections are commonly used for treatment of impingement syndrome, subacromial spurring, and AC arthritis, as well as aiding in the diagnosis of rotator cuff abnormalities.[3] They can also be helpful in alleviating pain in patients with pathologic shoulder conditions who are poor surgical candidates.

The subacromial injection is the most common one prescribed for the shoulder. Several techniques can be used for this injection.[5] One is the anterior approach (Figure 10-1), which is not recommended in this text; it is the most painful for the patient because most of the irritation is anterior in conditions such as bursitis. Access to the subacromial space is more difficult in the anterior approach, and this too can cause increased pain for the patient.

It is easier, more helpful, and less painful to enter the subacromial space posteriorly (Figure 10-2). The first

TABLE 10-2 Typical Sites, Needle Sizes, and Medication Dosages for Injections

Structure	Needle Gauge	Dose of 1% Lidocaine (ml)	Dose of Methylprednisolone Acetate (mg)
Radiohumeral joint	22	3-5	10-20
Lateral or medial epicondyle	22-25	4	10-20
Olecranon bursa	22	2-3	10-20
Finger and toe joints	22-25	0.5-1	4-10
Abductor tendon of thumb	25 (1.5 inch)	3-4	10-20 (de Quervain's disease)
Flexor tendon sheath	25 (1 inch)	0.25	4-10 (trigger finger)
Wrist	22-25	1-2	10-40
Carpal tunnel	25 (1.5 inch)	1	20-40
Ganglion of wrist	18-20	0.25-0.5	4
Subacromial bursa of shoulder	20 (1.5 inch)	5-7	20-40
Biceps tendon	22 (1.5 inch)	5-10	10-20
Acromioclavicular joint	22-25	2-4	4-10
Rotator cuff tendon	18-20 (1.5 inch)	5	20-40
Intraarticular space of shoulder	20 (1.5 inch)	5-7	20-40
Hip joint	20 (2.5-3 inch)	5	40-80
Trochanteric bursa	22	5-10	20-40
Anserine bursa	22-25	5	20-40
Prepatellar bursa	20	3	20-40
Intraarticular space of knee	20 (1.5 inch)	5	20-80
Calcaneal bursa	22 (1.5 inch)	5	20-40
Trigger point	25	3-5	10-20
Ankle	22	3-5	20-40

From Pfenninger JL, Fowler GC, editors: *Procedures for primary care physicians,* ed 2, St Louis, 2003, Mosby.

step in using the posterior approach is locating an appropriate insertion point. Placing the index finger on the coracoid process anteriorly and palpating the inferior lateral border of the posterior aspect of the acromion with the thumb locate this point. Approximately 2 to 3 cm below the acromion, there is usually a well-defined space that is palpated as a small indentation. Once this space is identified, the needle can be inserted underneath the acromion, aiming it upward and anteriorly toward the index finger, which is overlying the coracoid process.

Before injecting any solution, aspiration should be attempted to make certain the needle is not in a blood vessel. Once the needle is in place, the plunger should be pulled back to check for blood. If there is blood in the needle hub, withdraw the syringe a few millimeters and reposition it. If the bottom of the acromion is struck by

the needle, the practitioner should pull back slightly before injecting the solution. During the injection, minimal resistance indicates that the needle is in the subacromial space. Generally total injection volume is 5 to 10 ml of fluid.

The lateral injection can also be useful for bursitis or calcific tendinitis (Figure 10-3). As one would expect, this injection is given lateral to the acromion. After palpating the lateral edge of the acromion, the practitioner inserts the needle just under it and advances the needle into the subacromial space, where the injection can be administered.

The patient should be reassessed at least 10 to 15 minutes after a subacromial injection to ensure that the patient receives some relief, at least from the local anesthetic used in the injection. Waiting and reassessing the patient are helpful to make certain that the injection is

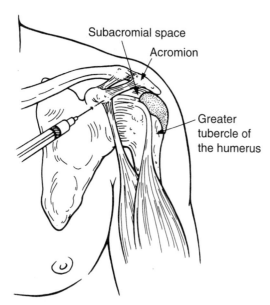

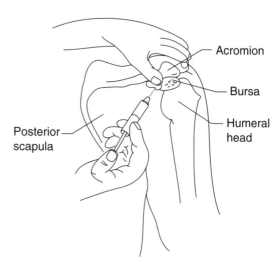

Figure 10-2   Posterior approach for subacromial injection.

Figure 10-1 Anterior Approach for Injecting the Subacromial Space. Note the proximity of the biceps tendons, as well as the relatively small subacromial space. (From Pfenninger JL, Fowler GC, editors: *Procedures for primary care physicians,* ed 2, St Louis, 2003, Mosby.)

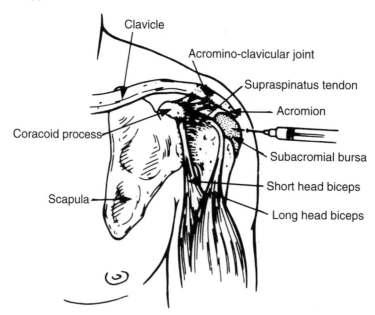

Figure 10-3   Lateral approach for subacromial injection. This approach may be more useful in cases of calcific tendinitis. (From Pfenninger JL, Fowler GC, editors: *Procedures for primary care physicians,* ed 2, St Louis, 2003, Mosby.)

administered in the appropriate area and that the medicine is where it is desired. If the patient has no relief, other possible diagnoses should be investigated, including a torn rotator cuff, biceps tendon rupture, osteonecrosis (ON), tumor, or unusual possibilities such as a lung abscess or another pathologic lung condition.

Elbow

Generally the use of injections around the elbow in the primary care setting should be limited to injection of the medial and lateral epicondyles. Lateral epicondylar inflammation and periostitis is classically known as tennis elbow. Medial epicondylitis is known as golfer's elbow.

Lateral injections are quite common and generally result in few complications. It cannot be emphasized enough that *the medial injection is quite dangerous because the ulnar nerve is very superficial at the medial epicondyle.* Inadvertent injection into the ulnar nerve can cause permanent damage. If the practitioner has any question about the technique required, the patient should be referred to a specialist.

With either lateral or medial epicondylitis, the injection should be given in the area of the patient's maximal tenderness. The practitioner should palpate to find the area of maximum tenderness and then mark the skin by making an **X** with a fingernail or make a small circle using a ballpoint pen with the pen point retracted. The needle is gently placed down to the level of the epicondyle itself; then the practitioner should gently pull back off the bone and inject the medication, using a "peppering" technique of multiple redirections of the needle. In this particular injection, a solution of 1 ml of 0.5% bupivacaine or 2% lidocaine and 1 ml of corticosteroid should be used.

With the medial injection, the practitioner must be very careful of nerve symptoms such as paresthesias in the ulnar nerve distribution when the needle is inserted. If the patient reports any pain or tingling in the arm or hand, the practitioner must immediately withdraw the needle without administering the injection. Some individuals can have a subluxing ulnar nerve, which can make this injection difficult by increasing the risk of intraneural injection.

Injection on the lateral side is somewhat simpler (Figure 10-4). Again, the practitioner should elicit and

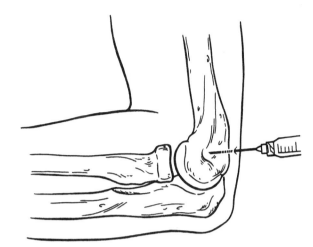

Figure 10-4   Injection technique for lateral epicondylitis or tennis elbow. The needle is introduced at a 90-degree angle to the lateral epicondyle. (From Pfenninger JL, Fowler GC, editors: *Procedures for primary care physicians,* ed 2, St Louis, 2003, Mosby.)

mark the patient's point of maximal tenderness. Using a total volume of approximately 2 ml of solution, the needle should be inserted down to the lateral epicondyle and then withdrawn slightly; the injection should then be given. The patient should have relief of symptoms within 10 to 15 minutes of injection. Reassessing the patient is helpful to assure the practitioner that the medication was injected in the correct area.

WRIST AND HAND

Wrist

Injection around the wrist in the primary care setting includes carpal tunnel syndrome (CTS) and de Quervain's disease. Injections into these areas must proceed cautiously. Nine flexor tendons and the median nerve lie within the carpal tunnel.[8] Carpal tunnel injection is not a first-line therapy. It is generally performed after splinting, NSAIDs, and activity modification have been tried. Corticosteroid injection improves symptoms in a majority of CTS patients, but relief is usually temporary.[8] De Quervain's disease responds very well to corticosteroid injection.[15] However, care must be taken when injecting because the very sensitive dorsal sensory

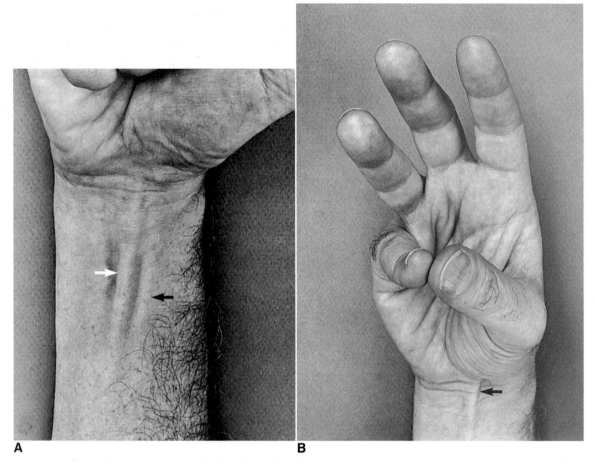

Figure 10-5   Location of Palmaris Longus Tendon. A, The palmaris longus tendon *(white arrow)* and flexor carpi ulnaris tendon *(black arrow)*. **B,** Opposition of the thumb and little finger makes the palmaris longus more prominent. (From Reider B: *The orthopaedic physical examination,* Philadelphia, 1999, WB Saunders, p.113)

branch of the radial nerve lies in close proximity to the first dorsal compartment.

To inject the carpal tunnel, first the palmaris longus tendon (Figure 10-5) is located. Needle entry is at the proximal wrist crease, just ulnar to the palmaris longus tendon. Entering at a 30-degree angle, the needle is directed toward the ring finger and advanced approximately 1 to 2 cm. If the needle moves when the patient makes a fist, the needle is in the tendon and should be withdrawn slightly before slowly injecting the solution.[18]

For de Quervain's disease, the technique of injection begins by asking the patient to hold his or her thumb in the extended position. The practitioner can then palpate down to the radial styloid. Moving the examining finger approximately one to two fingerbreadths proximal to the styloid, the needle is inserted at a 45-degree angle, aiming in a distal direction (Figure 10-6). The needle is placed into the first compartment and down to the bone. After gently pulling the needle away from the bone, the solution is injected. In this situation, 1 ml of

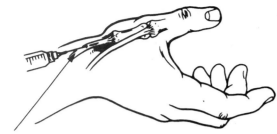

Abductor pollicis longus

Figure 10-6   Approach for injecting the first dorsal tendon sheath compartment in de Quervain's disease. The needle is directed distally at a 45-degree angle. (From Pfenninger JL, Fowler GC, editors: *Procedures for primary care physicians*, ed 2, St Louis, 2003, Mosby.)

corticosteroid along with 1 ml of local anesthetic should be injected.

As the injection is administered, the practitioner should feel the tendon sheath of the first dorsal compartment fill with the injection fluid. Often the practitioner will feel a pop; this sensation is the synovium filling with the injection material. After administering injections such as this, it is appropriate to ask the patient to wait a few minutes to allow the anesthetic time to work and to confirm that the injection was given in the appropriate area. Once again, if the diagnosis or technique is in question, the patient should be referred to a specialist.

Hand

Intraarticular injection of the digits should be referred to a rheumatologist, hand surgeon, or orthopedic surgeon who is experienced in small joint injections. In the hand, injections should be limited to trigger-finger abnormalities. Stenosing flexor tenosynovitis, or trigger finger, occurs in the area of the A1 pulley, which is in the area of the palmar crease in the hand. If trigger finger is present, a patient usually has pain and swelling in the area of the A1 pulley.

Trigger finger injection is more successful if performed within the first 4 months of symptom onset. Various approaches can be used to inject the area in and around the A1 pulley.[16,18] Regardless of approach, care must be taken to inject the center of the A1 pulley because the neurovascular bundles lie on the radial and ulnar aspects of the fingers. Permanent nerve or arterial damage to the digit can result if steroid is injected into the neurovascular bundle.

A simple technique for this injection is using a total volume of approximately 2 ml of corticosteroid and local anesthetic solution. Using a 25-gauge needle, the needle is inserted directly on the palmar aspect at a 30- to 60-degree angle into the area of the A1 pulley, passing through the tendon, down to the metacarpal bone (Figure 10-7). It may be helpful to have the patient wiggle the affected finger. If slight grating at the tip of the needle can be felt with movement, it has been accurately placed in the tendon sheath.[16] After the metacarpal is approached, the needle is withdrawn slightly, and then the material is injected. The practitioner can place a finger over the volar aspect of the proximal phalanx to allow palpation of the digit as it fills with solution.

LOWER EXTREMITIES

Corticosteroid injection of the lower extremities has been shown to be beneficial in treating bursitis, meralgia paresthetica, arthritic conditions of the hip, sacroiliac and knee joints, popliteal cysts, synovitis, and tendinitis.[6,11,17] Intraarticular injections into the sacroiliac and hip joints are technically difficult[3] and should be performed by a specialist.

In the primary care setting, injection around the hip and knee is helpful, especially in the case of bursitis. Lower extremity injections for tendon problems, especially Achilles' tendinopathy, are not recommended in the primary care setting because of the high risk of rupture.

Hip

Greater trochanteric bursitis, one of the more common problems seen in primary care, usually responds favorably to injection. With the patient lying on the unaffected side, the greater trochanter is located on the lateral aspect of the hip and is typically an easy landmark to locate. The area of greatest tenderness should be palpated and marked. Injecting this area is relatively simple. In a large area such as this, a 10-ml syringe with a 22-gauge needle of appropriate length is used to inject 2 ml of steroid combined with 5 to 6 ml of anesthetic. The needle is inserted down to bone (Figure 10-8).

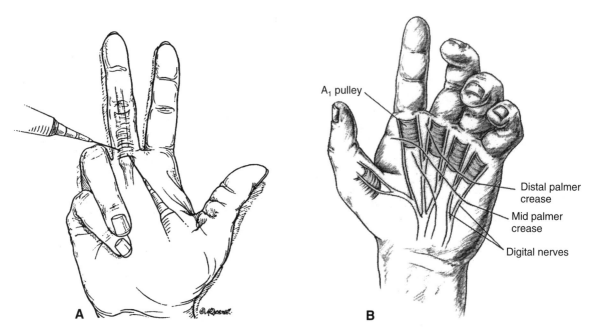

A

B

Figure 10-7   Trigger Finger Injection. A, Location of injection point over A1 pulley of the finger. **B,** Diagram showing location of A1 pulleys. Pulleys are located about one third the distance from the distal palmar crease and two thirds the distance from the base of the digits. (A from Idler RS: Helping the patient who has wrist or hand tenosynovitis. Part 2, Managing trigger finger, de Quervain's disease, *J Musculoskel Med* 14(2):62-75. Artist: Teri McDermott. **B** from Fitzgerald RH, Kaufer H, Malkani AL: Orthopaedics, St Louis, 2002, Mosby.)

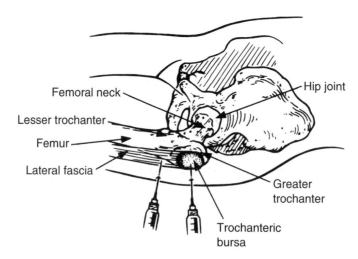

Figure 10-8   Location of Injection Site(s) for Trochanteric Bursitis. The trochanteric bursa is large and may occasionally require more than one injection. (From Pfenninger JL, Fowler GC, editors: *Procedures for primary care physicians,* ed 2, St Louis, 2003, Mosby.)

Care should be taken to palpate the bony prominence of the trochanter and not to stray posteriorly with the needle, because the sciatic nerve can reside in the posterior area. Once on the bone, the needle is pulled back slightly, and the solution gently injected. No resistance should be felt during the injection, after which the patient should wait 10 to 15 minutes to ascertain efficacy of analgesia. Usually there should be rapid improvement in pain once the local anesthetic has had time to take effect. Occasionally a second, more distal injection may be necessary if the patient continues to have pain 10 to 15 minutes after injection.

Knee

There are multiple injection techniques for the knee joint. The most frequently used techniques are with the knee extended, but it is increasingly common to have the patient seated with the knee flexed. Having the knee flexed tends to slightly open the joint space. With either position, the medial or lateral approach can be used (Figure 10-9). Needle insertion may also be either superior or inferior to the patella.

Using the inferior patellar approach, the practitioner palpates the proximal patellar tendon. At this point, the undersurface of the patella can be palpated, and the needle can be easily inserted beneath the patella into the knee joint. Needle entry should be either slightly medial or lateral to the patellar tendon, with the needle angled about 45 degrees in a slightly posterolateral or posteromedial direction, respectively.[7] The superior patellar approach uses the superior pole of the patella for a landmark. Needle entry is approximately 1 to 1.5 cm above and lateral to the pole.[19]

When inserting the needle, there should be minimal to no resistance until the joint is entered. As the needle pierces the synovium, a slight pop can often be felt. While injecting the solution, there should be no resistance; if injecting is difficult, the needle may be in a ligament or lying against bone. Some practitioners prefer the lateral approach, since there are fewer superficial nerves to cause problems and pain. Injection into the knee should consist of 2 ml of steroid along with 5 ml or more of a local anesthetic.

Bursitis

Inflammation of the pes anserine bursa, located on the anteromedial aspect of the tibia approximately 2.5 cm below the medial tibial joint line, is a frequent cause of knee pain and swelling. The prepatellar and infrapatellar bursae are also commonly afflicted by inflammation (Figure 10-10). Unlike a joint effusion, bursitis does not significantly limit knee flexion and extension. Clinically, swelling with bursitis can be marked.

As with other areas of bursitis, injection can offer sustained relief, but great caution must be used to rule out

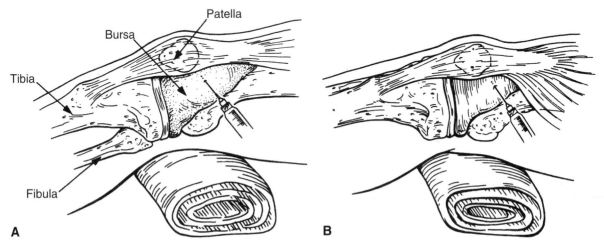

Figure 10-9   Lateral **(A)** and medial **(B)** approaches for injecting the knee joint. (From Pfenninger JL, Fowler GC, editors: *Procedures for primary care physicians,* ed 2, St Louis, 2003, Mosby.)

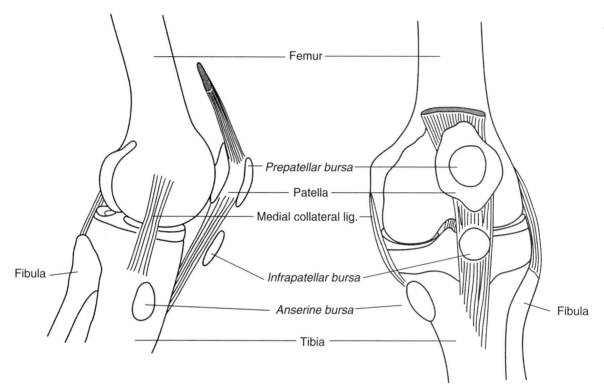

Figure 10-10   Schematic representation of commonly inflamed peripatellar bursae. (From Noble J, editor: *Textbook of primary care medicine,* ed 3, St Louis, 2001, Mosby.)

an infected bursa or intraarticular problem before injection. Once history and clinical examination confirm the diagnosis, it is appropriate to inject a combination of 1 ml of corticosteroid and 1 ml of local anesthetic into the bursa. This is done by gently inserting the needle in the fluctuant area of maximal tenderness until there is contact with bone. After withdrawing the needle 2 to 3 mm, the solution is injected.

Heel

Another area that is commonly injected is the symptomatic plantar heel spur or plantar fasciitis. This can be a very difficult and painful injection. Generally a 25-gauge, 1½-inch needle and 3-ml syringe are used. If the practitioner has any question about the technique or safety of injection, referral to a specialist is indicated.

One can usually pinpoint the worst area of tenderness on the bottom of the foot at the plantar fascial insertion into the distal calcaneus. Once identified, the area of maximal tenderness is marked. The injection is given from the medial side, and the needle is inserted onto the calcaneus (Figure 10-11). Once on the bone, the needle is gently pulled back, and the medication is injected. The solution should infuse without any resistance.

It is critical that the practitioner take care not to damage any of the deep nerves in the foot. The use of an extra cubic centimeter of local anesthetic may be useful, especially if the patient is allowed to sit for an extra 15 minutes. This time allows for alleviation of some pain before the patient begins to walk on the heel.

POSTINJECTION INSTRUCTIONS

As previously indicated, it is important that the practitioner instruct the patients that the problem can be

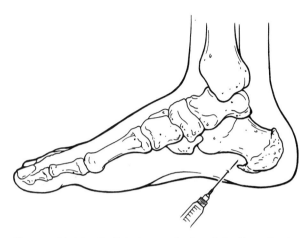

Figure 10-11 Medial Approach for Injecting Plantar Fasciitis. This approach reduces the likelihood of causing plantar fat pad atrophy. (From Pfenninger JL, Fowler GC, editors: *Procedures for primary care physicians*, ed 2, St Louis, 2003, Mosby.)

worse for several days after injection. NSAIDs, along with mild narcotics, can be prescribed to make this period less troublesome. Immediately after injection, the patient should be asked to rest the affected area for a few days to reduce steroid clearance from the area and reduce pain.[4] Once the rest period is over, physical therapy rehabilitation can increase range of motion and improve flexibility and strength. Patients should be aware that postinjection flushing could occur with higher doses of steroid.[19] The patient should be reassessed 6 weeks after injection to determine if improvement is noted.

CONCLUSION

The injection of cortisone-type material for the treatment of musculoskeletal problems is often quite helpful in an orthopedic or primary care setting. However, judicious use of injections is recommended, and, if any question regarding the need for injection or the technique of injection remains, it is strongly recommended that the patient be referred to an appropriate specialist. This chapter is not intended to be all-encompassing

with regard to injections; rather, it describes some of the most often used injections for common musculoskeletal problems encountered in the primary care setting.

REFERENCES

1. Birkinshaw R, O'Donnell J, Sammy I: Necrotising fasciitis as a complication of steroid injection, *J Accid Emerg Med* 14(1):52, 1997.
2. Cardone DA, Tallia AF: Joint and soft tissue injection, *Am Fam Physician* 66: 283, 2002.
3. Ebraheim NA et al: Sacroiliac joint injection: a cadaveric study, *Am J Orthopedics* 26:338, 1997.
4. Fadale PD, Wiggins ME: Corticosteroid injections: their use and abuse, *J Am Acad Orthop Surg* 2:133, 1994.
5. Fongemie AE, Buss DD, Rolnick SJ: Management of shoulder impingement syndrome and rotator cuff tears, *Am Fam Physician* 57:667, 1998.
6. Handy JR: Popliteal cysts in adults: a review, *Semin Arthritis Rheum* 31:108, 2001.
7. Hofmeister E, Englehardt S: Necrotizing fasciitis as a complication of injection into greater trochanteric bursa, *J Am Acad Orthop Surg* 30:426, 2001.
8. Katz JN, Simmons BP: Carpal tunnel syndrome, *N Engl J Med* 346:1807, 2002.
9. Larson HM, O'Connor FG, Nirschl RP: Shoulder pain: the role of diagnostic injections, *Am Fam Physician* 53:1637, 1996.
10. Noerdlinger MA, Fadale PD: The role of injectable corticosteroids in orthopedics, *Orthopedics* 24:400, 2001.
11. Plant MJ et al: Radiographic patterns and response to corticosteroid hip injection, *Ann Rheum Dis* 56:476, 1997.
12. Rifat SF, Moeller JL: Basics of joint injection, *Postgrad Med* 109(1):157, 2001.
13. Rifat SF, Moeller JL: Site-specific techniques of joint injection, *Postgrad Med* 109(3):123, 2001.
14. Rozental TD, Sculco TP: Intra-articular corticosteroids: an updated overview, *Am J Orthopedics* 29:18, 2000.
15. Sakai N: Selective corticosteroid injection into the extensor pollicis brevis tenosynovium for de Quervain's disease, *Orthopedics* 25:68, 2002.
16. Saldana MJ: Trigger digits: diagnosis and treatment, *J Am Acad Orthop Surg* 9:246, 2001.

17. Shbeeb MI et al: Evaluation of glucocorticosteroid injection for the treatment of trochanteric bursitis, *J Rheumatol* 23:2104, 1996.

18. Tallia AF, Cardone DA: Diagnostic and therapeutic injection of the wrist and hand, *Am Fam Physician* 67:745, 2003.

19. Zuber TJ: Knee joint aspiration and injection, *Am Fam Physician* 66:1497, 2002.

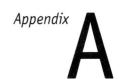

Keys to Common Diagnoses

CERVICAL SPINE

Diagnosis	Signs/Symptoms
Cervical strain	Muscular tenderness posttrauma, overuse. No-focal neurologic findings.
Degenerative disk disease	Decreased disk space on x-ray, radicular symptoms may occur, decreased ROM, pain may occur.
Fracture	Compression forces common, also distraction-extension, compressive-flexion.
Herniated nucleus pulposus (herniated disk)	Decreased sensation, decreased or absent reflexes, muscle weakness of upper extremity.
Infection	Diskitis, osteomyelitis, TB usually associated with systemic symptoms (fever, chills), localized pain.
Ligamentous instability	Forced flexion/hyperextension injury, age, rheumatoid disease, infection.
Locked facets	Acute injury, usually after trauma, but may occur spontaneously. Inability to turn head.
Osteoarthritis	Morning stiffness, osteophytes causing disk space narrowing on x-ray. C5-6 most common.
Rheumatoid disease	Systemic involvement, progressive inflammation, destruction of articular surfaces, may affect C1-2 stability.
Spinal stenosis	Radiographic finding. Often associated with radiculopathy or myelopathy.
Spondylosis	C5-6, C6-7 most common. Degenerative changes in disk, narrow cervical canal or neural foramen.
Torticollis	Spasm of neck muscles causing tilting and rotation of the head.
Tumor	Increasing, expanding pain. May have radicular symptoms. CT, MRI, bone scan, x-ray to diagnose.

SHOULDER

Diagnosis	Signs/Symptoms
Acromioclavicular separation	Tenderness or pain over AC joint, varying degree of deformity.
Adhesive capsulitis (frozen shoulder)	Decreased abduction, forward flexion, often painless. Restricted passive motion.
Bicipital tendonitis	Tenderness over bicipital groove, pain and weakness with resisted elbow flexion, forearm supination.
Cervical degenerative disk disease	C5—abduction and external rotation diminished; C6, C7, and C8—adduction and internal rotation diminished.
Cervical nerve root irritation	No restricted range of motion or local tenderness. Pain, numbness, and tingling referred from cervical spine.
Dislocation	Anterior—external rotation and/or hypertension. Posterior—shoulder variably flexed, adducted, internally rotated.
Fracture	Acute pain, swelling, decreased ROM, ecchymosis over shoulder, arm, anterior chest wall not uncommon.
Glenohumeral injury or instability	Clicking, popping, pain, especially anterior joint; decreased ROM; muscle and joint guarding.
Gout (rare)	Negatively birefringent crystals in synovial fluid aspirate, culture negative.
Impingement syndrome	Painful arc, decreased forward flexion, abduction.
Infection	Pain, warmth, erythema, edema, decreased ROM. Systemic symptoms (fever, chills, nausea usually present).
Instability	Traumatic or atraumatic; positive sulcus sign, apprehension, relocation tests.
Long thoracic nerve palsy	Weakness, posterior protrusion of scapula (scapular winging) with raising ipsilateral arm; early in process may have significant pain.
Osteoarthritis	Morning stiffness, pain. May have other joint symptoms. Osteophytes, joint space narrowing on x-ray.
Osteochondritis dissecans	Painful catching in joint; x-ray, MRI to show osseous changes.
Pancoast tumor (lung)	Pain, numbness, weakness of arm, medial hand. Horner's syndrome usually present.
Post-traumatic arthritis	Pain, decreased ROM, osteophytes on x-ray. History of injury (recent or remote).
Reflex sympathetic dystrophy	Pain, swelling, sensory changes.
Rheumatoid disease	Systemic disease, single or multiple joints affected; rheumatoid serology usually positive.
Rotator cuff tear	Inability and weakness of external rotation, abduction, pain in varying degrees; decreased internal rotation with subscapularis.
Rotator cuff tendinitis	Pain, weakness with abduction, external rotation; painful arc.
SLAP lesion	Arthroscopic diagnosis; pain, "locking," or "snapping" with overhead activities.
Spinal accessory nerve paralysis	Unilateral shoulder droop; weakness of trapezius muscle.

SHOULDER—cont'd

Diagnosis	Signs/Symptoms
Subluxation	Anterior more common, often voluntary; generalized ligamentous laxity.
Suprascapular nerve entrapment	Pain but primarily weakness with external rotation of shoulder.
Tendon rupture	Rotator cuff, biceps most common. Pain and weakness with contraction of affected muscle.
Thoracic outlet syndrome	Pain, paresthesia, weakness, easy fatiguing of extremity, cold intolerance. Positive provocative tests.
Tumor	Uncommon, but when present, constant, expanding pain, possible lesion on x-ray examination; MRI helpful especially for soft tissue lesions with bony extension.

ARM AND ELBOW

Diagnosis	Signs/Symptoms
Bursitis	Fluid-filled sac at point of elbow. May be inflammatory, hemorrhagic, or septic.
Collateral ligament injury	History of trauma; increased laxity of ligament.
Cubital tunnel syndrome	Local pain, paresthesias of hand and fingers; positive Tinel's over cubital tunnel.
Dislocation	Obvious joint deformity post-trauma with swelling, pain and ↓ ROM.
Fracture	Localized pain, swelling; ecchymosis after few days. Positive posterior fat pad sign on lateral x-ray (elbow fracture).
Golfer's elbow (medial epicondylitis)	Medial epicondyle pain, aggravated by resisted flexion of elbow and wrist.
Gout	Acute pain, erythema, swelling warmth localized to joint; ↓ ROM.
Infection	Acute pain, hot joint, erythema, swelling. Systemic manifestations often present: fever, chills.
Tennis elbow (lateral epicondylitis)	Point tenderness over lateral epicondyle, aggravated by resisted extension of elbow and wrist.

WRIST AND HAND

Diagnosis	Signs/Symptoms
Anterior interosseous syndrome	Elbow or forearm pain, weakness of thumb and index finger flexion; can't make the "okay" sign.
Avascular necrosis (AVN)	Lunate most common (Kienböck's disease); pain with palpation, movement. Ulna minus a frequent associated finding.
Carpal dislocation, instability	Acute or chronic pain. Pain worse with specific movements. Diagnosis best left to orthopedic hand surgeon.
Carpal tunnel syndrome, other entrapment neuropathy	Nighttime "wake and shake" of hand; positive Phalen's, Tinel's; positive EMG/NCS testing. Late involvement—muscle atrophy.
Cervical disk disease	C5-6; weak wrist extension; C6, C7, C8, T1 nerve roots.
Cervical nerve root irritation	C6, C7: thumb, index long finger sensory symptoms; neck pain.
Collateral ligament injury	Joint swelling, pain greater with bilateral compression than AP compression. Variable joint laxity.
Compartment syndrome	Pain, pallor paresthesia, paralysis, no pulse (latter two are late findings); pain with passive stretch. Often after a crush injury. Pain, pallor, paresthesia, paralysis, no pulse.
de Quervain's disease	Positive Finkelstein's test; swelling and tenderness over first dorsal compartment at the wrist.
Dislocation	Trauma with obvious deformity; pain and decreased ROM, swelling usually associated with fracture. Obvious deformity of joint, inability to move joint. X-ray to fully evaluate position of dislocated bones, possible fracture.
Distal radioulnar joint injury	Ulnar-sided pain—includes TFCC. CT, MRI, arthrogram to diagnose subluxing tendon(s), triangular fibrocartilage tear.
Dupuytren's contracture	Progressive flexion contracture of fingers (ring finger common), men more than women. May begin as palmar nodule.
Extensor tendon injury	Inability to extend finger(s); DIP injury results in mallet finger deformity.
Felon	Abscess of fingertip pulp; deep infection that may have multiple compartments; refer to surgeon.
Flexor tendon injury	Inability to flex finger(s); surgical emergency in acute injury—should be repaired within seven days.
Fracture	Pain, swelling, possible deformity, decreased movement after trauma; point tenderness.
Gamekeeper's thumb	Pain, varying degrees of ulnar collateral ligament laxity at MCP joint. May have associated avulsion fracture.
Ganglion cyst	Firm/smooth, fluctuant, round tumor of tendon or tendon sheath. Size varies with activity.
Guyon's tunnel syndrome	Numbness and tingling of little and ring fingers, positive Tinel's over ulnar nerve at wrist. EMG/NCS to diagnose.
Infection	Pain, swelling, erythema, limited ROM. Surgical emergency if tendon sheaths involved. Erythema, pain, warmth, decreased motion. May be localized or spreading. Any involvement of tendon sheaths, deep tissues, or due to bites should be referred to hand surgeon.

WRIST AND HAND—cont'd

Diagnosis	Signs/Symptoms
Kienböck's disease	Avascular necrosis of lunate with progressive collapse of bone; initial x-ray may be negative. MRI for earlier diagnosis.
Muscle strain	Overuse or overstretching. Diffuse pain aggravated by movement. Neurovascular intact.
Osteoarthritis	Morning stiffness, pain relieved by rest; degenerative changes on x-ray; ↓ ROM. DIP joints. Morning stiffness, "gelling." Pain relieved by rest; may have some weakness, swelling (bony hypertrophy).
Paronychia	Infection of eponychial fold; usually involves only one side of nail bed.
Pronator syndrome	Diffuse aching of forearm, paresthesias of median nerve, weak thumb flexion, sensory loss on thenar eminence.
Radial tunnel syndrome	Radial nerve entrapment from lateral epicondyle to supinator muscle.
Raynaud's disease, phenomenon	Disease is idiopathic, phenomenon is secondary to other processes (connective tissue disorders, hypothyroidism), intermittent blanching or cyanosis of digits after exposure to cold, emotional stress.
Rheumatoid disease	Systemic disease, rheumatoid nodules, positive rheumatoid serology. Often DIP joint abnormalities—boutonnière, swan neck, mallet, ulnar drift of digits at MCP joint synovitis, other small joint involvement (may be seronegative).
Sprain	Swelling, pain aggravated by movement post-injury. Diffuse tenderness; no point tenderness or neurologic deficit. Pain, stiffness, tenderness over ligament; varying degrees of joint instability.
Tendonitis/tenosynovitis	Pain with movement. Tendon may be thickened, palpable crepitus. Either extensor or flexor tendons affected. Overuse or overstretching injury; pain with stretching, movement of associated muscle, often wrist extensors or flexors.
Triangular fibrocartilage complex (TFCC) tear	Usually acute injury involving hyperextension of wrist; can also occur with forced flexion. Pain over distal radioulnar and ulnocarpal area.
Trigger finger	Flexor tendon becomes trapped in A-I pulley (MCP joint at palm of hand); reactive nodule often present. Finger "locks" in flexion; ring and middle fingers most often affected.

LUMBAR SPINE

Diagnosis	Signs/Symptoms
Abdominal aortic aneurysm	Deep, aching, poorly localized pain. May have LE neuro symptoms.
Ankylosing spondylitis	Loss of lordotic curve, decreased motion; HLA-B27; associated ↓ ROM of hips and chest; diaphragmatic breathing.
Arthritic conditions	Other weight-bearing joints (hips, knees) often affected, morning stiffness, osteophytes and joint space narrowing on x-ray.

Keys to Common Diagnoses

Continued

LUMBAR SPINE—cont'd

Diagnosis	Signs/Symptoms
Fracture	Localized pain over bony area. X-ray, CT to diagnose. Usually acute.
GI disease	Careful history and physical examination. No back findings on examination.
Gynecologic disorders	Referred pain. May have seeding of infection to lumbar area; GYN exam needed.
Herniated disk	Severe pain, usually radiates into lower extremity, often weakness, diminished reflexes. Bladder dysfunction or incontinence represents a cauda equina syndrome—surgical emergency.
Infection	Recent history of GI, GU infection, untreated TB, STD, brucellosis.
Osteomalacia	Demineralization of vertebrae on x-ray. Decreased serum calcium and phosphorus. May have liver disease (advanced).
Osteoporosis	History, risk factors; bone densitometry; atraumatic compression fracture, anterior wedging of vertebral bodies.
Pancreatic disease	Also abdominal pain, glucose, lipase abnormalities; CT or ERCP (Endoscopic Retrograde Cholangiopancreatography) to diagnose.
Peptic ulcer	Back pain may be sign of perforation; bleeding, acute emergency.
Prostate problems	Spinal metastases from prostate cancer; referred pain from prostatitis or seeding of infection.
Renal disorders (calculi, infection, tumor)	CVA tenderness, urinary symptoms (hematuria, abnormal IVP).
Sacroiliac joint dysfunction	Pain lateral to spine; sclerotic bone on x-ray examination.
Scoliosis	Clinical or radiographic curvature of spine; vertebral wedging or rotation on x-ray.
Spinal cord injury	Cauda equina syndrome—surgical emergency.
Spinal stenosis	Insidious pain, decreasing range of motion; pain worse with walking or standing; worse with lumbar extension.
Spondylolisthesis	Displacement of one vertebra on another.
Tumor/metastases	Osteoporosis, spinal fracture or wedging out of proportion to age, abnormal calcium metabolism.

HIP AND THIGH

Diagnosis	Signs/Symptoms
Avascular necrosis	Dull ache or throbbing in groin, lateral hip, or buttock. Pain usually of gradual onset.
Bursitis	Localized tenderness over bursal area; worse with prolonged sitting, certain movements. Normal ROM.

HIP AND THIGH—cont'd

Diagnosis	Signs/Symptoms
Dislocation	Inability to move hip. May have obvious deformity of joint. High-energy trauma or post-TJA. Posterior: hip flexed, adducted, internally rotated. Anterior: hip abducted, externally rotated. Shortened limb.
Fracture (stress, osteoporotic, femoral, avulsion, acetabular)	Pain, especially with weight-bearing. Antalgic gait, decreased ROM, shortening of thigh.
Herniated nucleus pulposus	Diminished reflexes, sensory changes, back pain. Leg pain often worse than back pain. Focal motor weakness.
Inguinal hernia	Tenderness or pain to palpation, often palpable mass in groin.
Muscle contusion, hematoma	Bruising, swelling, pain and tenderness over injured area. May have defined area of fluctuance or induration.
Muscle strain, tear, rupture	Varies from soreness to actual palpable/visible defect; pain with stretch and weakness with contraction in active ROM.
Nerve entrapment	Lateral femoral cutaneous nerve; solely sensory with pain, dysesthesia over lateral thigh (meralgia paresthetica).
Osteoarthritis	Gradual, progressive pain; morning stiffness; decreased joint space, spurring on x-ray.
Osteoporosis	Risk factors noted. Antalgic gait, increasing pain with weight-bearing. Associated kyphosis, possible spine compression fractures.
Piriformis syndrome	Pain along sciatic distribution worsened with prolonged sitting, athletic activities. Pain with passive internal rotation of hip. MRI may show compression of nerve by piriformis muscle.
Sciatica	Often sudden onset; associated back pain common. Pain radiates below knee (into ankle or foot).
Sickle-cell disease	Arterial occlusion due to crisis; increased risk for avascular necrosis of femoral head.
Slipped capital femoral epiphysis (SCFE)	Occurs only with open epiphyses. Spontaneous or posttraumatic pain, limp. Groin or anterior thigh pain. Unilateral or bilateral. External rotation of leg with walking.
Stress fracture	Progressive pain with weight-bearing, antalgic gait. Bone scan or MRI to diagnose.
Tumor/metastases	Increasing pain that becomes constant, swelling, bony tenderness, antalgic gait, deformity, radiographic evidence of lesion, previous history of malignancy. Rule out pelvic mass.

KNEE AND LEG

Diagnosis	Signs/Symptoms
Achilles tendon rupture	Acute pain, palpable defect in tendon, inability to plantar flex foot or perform single-limb toe raises. Positive Thompson's test.
Baker's cyst	Popliteal fullness, tenderness that is increased with flexion. Rarely palpable. MRI or ultrasound to confirm.
Bursitis	Usually painless swelling unless pressure applied; full ROM; swelling usually localized.
Collateral ligament strain, tear	History of injury with tenderness, pain, and varying instability of affected ligament.
Compartment syndrome	Pain, pallor, paresthesias, lack of pulse, paralysis.
Crystal arthropathy	History, x-ray may show chondral calcifications, joint aspiration shows crystals.
Deep vein thrombosis	Deep, aching, often poorly localized pain, positive Doppler (ultrasound) or venogram. Calf pain with compression, increased pain with foot dorsiflexion but may have swelling alone.
Extensor mechanism dysfunction	Inability to extend knee against resistance; often with palpable defect over quadriceps or patellar tendon.
Fracture	Point tenderness, pain, swelling, decreased ROM. Weight-bearing may be difficult.
Gout	Acutely hot, red, extremely painful joint. Few systemic symptoms. Presence of negatively birefringent crystals on polarized light microscopy.
Iliotibial band syndrome (ITBS)	Pain along lateral femoral condyle, especially in runners. Positive Noble's, Ober's tests.
Infection	Acutely hot, red, painful joint. Fever, chills, malaise common. May have recent history of other infection, STD.
Intraarticular ligament strain, tear	Direct or indirect trauma; often with history of "pop." Subjective instability, swelling within hours. Effusion, increased laxity on exam (positive Lachman's, anterior or posterior drawer, or Godfrey's tests). MRI to diagnose.
Loose body in joint	Clicking, catching, locking, giving way. X-ray may show loose body in joint. May need MRI or arthroscopy.
Meniscus tear	Twisting injury, swelling within 24 hours. Locking, catching or giving way. Descending stairs worse than climbing. Positive McMurray's, Steinman's, or Apley's compression tests. MRI or arthoscopy to diagnose.
Muscle strain, tear	Localized pain, tenderness and swelling. Muscle weakness. Large tear may have hematoma, visible/palpable bulge.
Osgood-Schlatter's disease	Adolescent; prominent tibial tubercle, with pain and swelling. Fragmentation of tibial tubercle seen on lateral x-ray.
Osteoarthritis	Gradual onset of pain; morning stiffness lasting more than 30 minutes, bony hypertrophy. Osteophytes; joint space narrowing on x-ray; $\downarrow$ ROM; +/− joint effusion.
Osteochondritis dissecans	Pain, stiffness, and swelling may progress to locking, catching, giving way. X-ray shows lesion (most often medial femoral condyle). Wilson's test, x-ray to diagnose.

KNEE AND LEG—cont'd

Diagnosis	Signs/Symptoms
Patellar malalignment	Increased Q angle, relatively more lateral tibial tubercle. Patellar knee pain; often crepitus.
Peripheral vascular disease	Pain, ache, or cramp with exercise, initially relieved by rest; may progress to rest pain. Diminished peripheral pulses. Poor nail and hair growth on extremity; foot cool to touch.
Plantaris tendon rupture (very rare)	Acute pain medial to Achilles tendon, ecchymosis present 24 to 48 hours after rupture. No motor deficit.
Referred pain from hip, low back	L3-4:sensory deficits in anterior knee, medial leg, diminished patellar reflex. L4-5:sensory deficit in anterior lateral leg. No reflex changes.
Shin splints	Progressive tibial (usually distal) pain after exercise, initially relieved by rest. Local tenderness to palpation. Excessive foot pronation not unusual.
Stress fracture	Progressive pain unrelieved by rest. Pain with remote percussion of bone. Positive bone scan.
Tendonitis	Contraction of associated muscle(s). Tendon may be thicker than contralateral structure.
Tendon strain, rupture (quadriceps)	Palpable defect if acute;inability to actively extend knee against resistance. Tenderness at defect.
Tennis leg	Acute calf pain;tenderness or pain and swelling over medial gastrocnemius.
Tumor	Expanding pain, mass, restricted ROM. Constitutional symptoms (weight loss, fever, malaise) may be present. Visible abnormality on x-ray. Computed tomography, radioimmunoassay MRI to diagnose;vague pain may be only symptom.

ANKLE

Diagnosis	Signs/Symptoms
Bursitis (retrocalcaneal most common)	Pain anterior to Achilles tendon (just above its insertion onto calcaneus) aggravated by squeezing area anterior to tendon.
Chronic ligamentous laxity	Aching, swelling after prolonged activity, otherwise may have few symptoms. Tenderness over ligaments.
Fracture	Pain, swelling, difficulty or inability to bear weight. Decreased ROM. Obvious bony disruption on x-ray.
Loose body in joint	Catching, locking, instability. May have osteochondritis dissecans of talus.
Nerve entrapment	May be due to ankle fracture, dislocation, or traction injury. Tibial nerve:loss of ankle plantar flexion, toe flexion, weak ankle inversion.
Osteonecrosis	History of steroids, SLE, sickle-cell disease, nontraumatic ankle pain worse with weight-bearing;variable pain at rest. X-ray, MRI to evaluate.

Keys to Common Diagnoses

Continued

ANKLE—cont'd

Diagnosis	Signs/Symptoms
Peroneal tendon subluxation	Pain, "snapping" over posterior distal fibula. Pain worse with active eversion of dorsiflexed foot. May have palpable/visible movement of tendons.
Posterior impingement syndrome	Pain, with swelling of posterior ankle. Worse with plantar flexion. Dancers (ballet) more likely to develop. Pain with resisted plantar or dorsiflexion of great toe. Os trigonum present on lateral x-ray.
Referred pain	Disk herniation L5-SI: sensory deficit over lateral malleolus, weak eversion, decreased Achilles reflex.
Sprain (lateral, medial, syndesmosis)	Lateral: most common. Foot inverted, plantar flexed. Pain, swelling over lateral collateral ligaments. Varying ecchymosis, instability. Medial: foot neutral or dorsiflexed. Medial malleolar pain, swelling. Variable instability, ecchymosis. Syndesmosis: positive squeeze test.
Tendon rupture (Achilles, posterior tibial)	Achilles: palpable defect; positive Thompson's test. Inability to plantar flex foot, toe raise. Tibialis posterior: acute acquired flat foot: pain and swelling of medial malleolus.
Tumor	Increasing pain, restricted ROM; may have palpable mass. X-ray, CT, MRI shows lesion.

FOOT

Diagnosis	Signs/Symptoms
Calluses	Usually found on plantar surface of metatarsal heads; circumscribed, hypertrophied horny layer, usually with a smooth surface, may be silvery or brownish.
Claw toe	Flexion of PIP joint and hyperextension of DIP joint. Callus over dorsal PIP.
Compartment syndrome	Pain (out of proportion to injury), pallor, paresthesias, pulselessness, paralysis.
Complex regional pain syndrome (CRPS) or reflex sympathetic dystrophy (RSD)	Stiffness, swelling, pain out of proportion to injury, vasomotor changes following trauma (often minor).
Corns	Keratotic lesions commonly found over or between digits. Pain more common with corn than callus.
Dislocation	Obvious deformity (e.g., swelling, angulation) after acute trauma, inability to move joint.
Fracture	Swelling, discoloration, point tenderness at site of injury. Pain with weight-bearing or with moving affected structure.
Gout	Acute onset of exquisitely painful, hot, red joint. Known as podagra when it affects first MTP joint. Few systemic symptoms. Incidence increases with age, alcohol, certain foods. Negatively birefrigent crystals on polarized microscopy.
Hallux rigidus	Pain, stiffness, and restricted movement of first MTP joint, area tender to palpation, bony hypertrophy often palpable. Exostosis, joint space narrowing on x-ray.
Hallux valgus (bunion)	Tender, prominent first MTP joint with lateral deviation of great toe; often positive family history. Pain worsened by wearing shoes.

FOOT—cont'd

Diagnosis	Signs/Symptoms
Hammertoe	Flexion deformity of PIP, DIP joints that also results in hyperextension of the MTP joint; can be fixed or supple.
Infection	Increased risk in diabetics, immunocompromised patient. H/O trauma, burns, puncture wounds, insensate foot. Swelling, erythema, possibly draining wound. Variable degree of diffuse pain.
Lumbar disk disease	L4-5—sensory deficit, over dorsum of foot, weak extension of great toe. L5-SI—sensory deficit over lateral heel and foot, fourth and fifth web space, decreased or absent ankle reflex, decreased ankle flexion (see Figure 9-6).
Mallet toe	Flexion deformity of DIP joint alone.
Metatarsalgia	Pain beneath metatarsal heads, increased with weight-bearing. Lateral compression of metatarsal heads usually does *not* increase pain. May have plantar callus over metatarsal head.
Morton's neuroma	Interdigital nerve entrapment, most often between third and fourth toes. Pain worse with wearing shoes, manual compression between third and fourth MT heads or lateral compression of forefoot. Palpable nodule may be present.
Neuropathy (diabetic, alcoholic, vascular)	Diminished sensation, proprioception; paresthesias, abnormal reflexes. May have progressive joint instability, swelling.
Osteoarthritis	Pain relieved by rest, morning stiffness. Joint space narrowing, osteophytes on x-ray.
Plantar fasciitis, fibromatosis	Heel pain worse with first steps in morning or after prolonged sitting; tenderness over medial calcaneal tubercle. Palpable nodules may be present with fibromatosis. Heel spur on x-ray is often an incidental finding.
Reflex sympathetic dystrophy (RSD)	See complex regional pain syndrome (CRPS).
Rheumatoid disease	Multiple small joint involvement; systemic disease, positive or negative serology; periostitis but no osteophytes on x-ray.
Spondyloarthropathy (ankylosing spondylitis, psoriatic arthritis, Reiters syndrome)	Referred pain from L4, L5, SI nerve roots (see Figure 9-6).
Sprain	Mild to moderate diffuse tenderness and swelling, varying ecchymosis and instability, pain worse with weight-bearing.
Stress fracture	Second metatarsal most common, also (rarely) tarsal navicular. Progressive localized pain over bone; diffuse swelling of foot. Pain with remote percussion. Positive bone scan.
Tarsal tunnel syndrome, other nerve entrapment syndromes	Shooting, burning pain, and/or numbness and tingling from plantar foot into toes. Positive Tinel's over tarsal tunnel. EMG/NCS to confirm.
Tendonitis	Achilles—thickened, tender; crepitant tendon, posterior heel or ankle pain. Toe raises increase pain. Peroneal—lateral foot pain extending proximally into lateral calf, pain and/or weakness with resisted eversion of foot. Tibialis—posterior tender, swollen posterior medial malleolus, may have palpably thickened tendon. Pain worse with single-limb toe raise.

Index